ASPHYXIA AND FETAL BRAIN DAMAGE

ASPHYXIA AND FETAL BRAIN DAMAGE

Edited by

Dev Maulik, M.D., Ph.D.

WILEY-LISS

A JOHN WILEY & SONS, INC., PUBLICATION

New York • Chichester • Weinheim • Brisbane • Singapore • Toronto

This book is printed on acid-free paper. ♾

Published simultaneously in Canada.

Library of Congress Cataloging-in-Publication Data:

Asphyxia and fetal brain damage / edited by Dev Maulik.
p. cm.
Includes bibliographical references and index.
ISBN 0-471-18427-6 (cloth : alk. paper)
1. Fetal brain—Abnormalities. 2. Fetal brain—Diseases.
3. Asphyxia neonatorum—Complications. I. Maulik, Dev.
[DNLM: 1. Brain Injuries—in infancy & childhood. 2. Asphyxia Neonatorum. 3. Fetal Diseases. WS 340 A839 1998]
RG629.B73A85 1998
618.3′268—dc21
DNLM/DLC
for Library of Congress 97-52695

Printed in the United States of America.

10 9 8 7 6 5 4 3 2 1

To Shibani
and
Devika and Davesh
with my love

CONTENTS

PREFACE

Asphyxial injury to the fetal central nervous system is one of the most vital, and yet highly controversial, areas of concern in perinatal medicine. The spectrum of neurological compromise that may result from such an insult extends from behavioral and learning disabilities to severe cerebral palsy. The cause and effect relationship, however, is often uncertain and contentious as debate continues about defining the clinical and laboratory parameters of perinatal asphyxia. Most cases of perinatal neurological compromise do not demonstrate any defined antecedents, and most cases of clinically labeled perinatal asphyxia do not result in any demonstrable neurodevelopmental deficit. Although evidence has existed to the contrary, birth asphyxia has been blamed for most cases of perinatal neurological compromise. The issue is clouded by the fact that changes in obstetrical practice over the last two decades, including electronic fetal heart rate monitoring and increased cesarean deliveries, have failed to reduce the incidence of perinatal neurological compromise, and the prevalence of cerebral palsy has remained virtually static over the last two decades.

These controversies reflect deficiencies in our knowledge regarding many critical aspects of asphyxial injury to the developing brain. Recent investigations, however, have made significant contributions in elucidating and managing this complex problem. It is now recognized that prenatal insult is likely to be a greater offender than intrapartum events in the causation of fetal neuronal injury, and that asphyxial insult to the fetus is often chronic and repetitive. Current evidence also provides considerable insight into the molecular mechanisms of hypoxia-ischemia induced neuronal injury, which essentially starts with neuronal energy failure and culminates in either immediate or delayed neuronal death. As the former is an acute event, the possibility of any therapeutic intervention is obviously quite limited. In contrast, the latter may offer a beneficial window of opportunity for therapeutic strategies for neuronal protection or rescue. In the clinical arena, advances in perinatal neuroimaging have not only provided superb diagnostic tools but also advanced our understanding of the pathogenic mechanisms, their ontogeny, and the temporal evolution of neural lesions. The latter phenomenon has immense clinical and medicolegal implications, and has generated considerable interest and controversy. Significant progress has also been made in elucidating the physiopathological processes underlying fetal compensation and decompensation, and thus providing a rational foundation for the optimal utilization of fetal surveillance.

These advances are not only altering our fundamental perspectives on this issue, but may have far reaching practical consequences. The purpose of this book is to offer the current knowledge and insights of internationally recognized clinical and basic investigators involved in this area. I can express nothing but profound admiration for and gratitude to our distinguished contributors whose enthusiastic participation made this project a reality. I am also deeply grateful to our publishers, John Wiley & Sons and especially to Mr. Shawn Morton, the Senior Editor, for their generous support and competent assistance. Our endeavor will be amply rewarded if this text proves intellectually stimulating and useful to our prospective readers, especially those who are involved and interested in improving perinatal outcome.

Dev Maulik, M.D., Ph.D.

ACKNOWLEDGMENTS

I would like to express my gratitude to Kristin Cooke, Assistant Managing Editor at John Wiley & Sons, Inc., for facilitating the editorial and production work. I would also like to extend my sincere thanks to my editorial assistants, Maria Troia and Wendie Irving at Winthrop-University Hospital for their invaluable assistance in the preparation of this book.

CONTRIBUTORS

Myoung Ock Ahn, M.D., Ph.D., M.P.H., Department of Obstetrics and Gynecology, Cha Women's Hospital, Seoul, Korea

Domenico Arduini, M.D., Department of Obstetrics and Gynecology, University of Rome "Tor Vergata", Policlinico Nuovo "S. Eugenio", 00144 Rome, Italy

David Boas, Ph.D., Electro-Optics Technology Center, Tufts University School of Engineering and Computer Science, Medford, MA 02155

Yoshihide Chiba, M.D., Ph.D., Department of Clinical Physiology, Clinical Chemistry and Perinatology, National Cardiovascular Center, Suita, Osaka 565-8565, Japan

Lawrence D. DeVoe, M.D., Department of Obstetrics and Gynecology, Medical College of Georgia, Augusta, GA 30912

Tom Farrell, M.R.C.O.G., Department of Obstetrics and Gynaecology, Ninewells Hospital and Medical School, Dundee DD1 9SY, Scotland

Francesco Giacomello, M.D., Department of Obstetrics and Gynecology, University of Rome "Tor Vergata", Policlinico Nuovo "S. Eugenio", 00144 Rome, Italy

Flavio Giannini, M.D., Department of Obstetrics and Gynecology, University of Rome "Tor Vergata," Policlinico Nuovo "S. Eugenia," 00144 Rome, Italy

Christopher R. Harman, M.D., Department of Obstetrics, Gynecology and Reproductive Sciences, University of Maryland Medical Center, Baltimore, MD 21201

Alexander H. Hoon, Jr., M.D., M.P.H., Johns Hopkins University School of Medicine and Kennedy Kreiger Institute, Baltimore, MD 21205

Michael V. Johnston, M.D., Johns Hopkins University School of Medicine and Kennedy Kreiger Institute, Baltimore, MD 21205

Lisa M. Korst, M.D., Department of Obstetrics and Gynecology, Cedars-Sinai Medical Center, Los Angeles, CA 90048

James A. Low, M.D., Department of Obstetrics, Gynaecology and Paediatrics, Queen's University, Kingston, Ontario, Canada K7L 3N6

Frank A. Manning, M.D., Sloane Hospital for Women, Columbia-Presbyterian Medical Center, New York, NY 10032

Dev Maulik, M.D., Ph.D., F.A.C.O.G., F.R.C.O.G., Department of Obstetrics and Gynecology, Winthrop-University Hospital, Mineola, NY 11501

Savas M. Menticoglou, M.D., Department of Obstetrics, Gynecology and Reproductive Sciences, University of Manitoba, Winnipeg, Canada R3E 0L8

Gary J. Mires, M.D., M.R.C.O.G., Department of Obstetrics and Gynaecology, Ninewells Hospital and Medical School, Dundee DD1 9SY, Scotland

Ana Monteagudo, M.D., Department of Obstetrics and Gynecology, Division of Maternal-Fetal Medicine, New York University Medical Center, New York, NY 10016

Ian Morrison, M.B., Ch.B., St. Boniface General Hospital, University of Manitoba, Winnipeg, Canada R3E 0L8

Richard L. Naeye, M.D., Department of Pathology, Milton S. Hershey Medical Center, The Pennsylvania State University College of Medicine, Hershey, PA 17033

Philip Owen, M.D., M.R.C.O.G., Department of Obstetrics and Gynaecology, Stobhill Infirmary, Glasgow, G21 3UW Scotland

Naren B. Patel, P.R.C.O.G., Department of Obstetrics and Gynaecology, Ninewells Hospital and Medical School, Dundee, DD1 9SY Scotland

Jeffrey M. Perlman, M.B., Department of Pediatrics, University of Texas Southwestern Medical School, Dallas, TX 75235

Jeffrey P. Phelan, M.D., Department of Obstetrics and Gynecology, Pomona Valley Hospital Medical Center, Pasadena, CA 91767

Bryan S. Richardson, M.D., F.R.C.S.C., Departments of Obstetrics/Gynaecology and Physiology, The Lawson Research Institute, St. Joseph's Health Centre, The University of Western Ontario, London, Ontario, Canada N6A 4V2

Carolyn M. Salafia, M.D., Department of Pathology, Montefiore Medical Center, 1825 Eastchester Road, Bronx, NY 10461

Miljan R. Stankovic, M.D., Ph.D., Department of Obstetrics and Gynecology, Boston University School of Medicine, 80 East Concord Street, Boston, MA 02118

Robert H. Stigter, M.D., Department of Obstetrics and Gynecology, University Hospital, 3508 GA Utrecht, The Netherlands

Phillip G. Stubblefield, M.D., Department of Obstetrics and Gynecology, Boston University School of Medicine, Boston, MA 02118

Ilan E. Timor-Tritsch, M.D., Department of Obstetrics and Gynecology, Division of Maternal-Fetal Medicine, New York University Medical Center, New York, NY 10016

Herbert Valensise, M.D., Department of Obstetrics and Gynecology, University of Rome "Tor Vergata," Policlinico Nuovo "S. Eugenio," 00144 Rome, Italy

Robert C. Vannucci, M.D., Department of Pediatrics, The Pennsylvania State University College of Medicine, The Milton S. Hershey Medical Center, Hershey, PA 17033

Gerard H. A. Visser, Ph.D., Department of Obstetrics and Gynecology, University Hospital, 3508 GA Utrecht, The Netherlands

ASPHYXIA AND FETAL BRAIN DAMAGE

1

ANTECEDENTS OF LONG-TERM HANDICAP

Tom Farrell, M.R.C.O.G., Gary J. Mires, M.D., M.R.C.O.G., Philip Owen, M.D., M.R.C.O.G., and Naren B. Patel, P.R.C.O.G.

Department of Obstetrics and Gynaecology, Ninewells Hospital and Medical School, Dundee, Scotland (TF, GJM, NPB); and Department of Obstetrics and Gynaecology, Stobhill Infirmary, Glasgow, Scotland (PO)

INTRODUCTION

Cerebral palsy is a disorder of posture or movement which is persistent and is caused by a nonprogressive lesion of the brain, acquired at a time of rapid brain development. It is usually manifest in early infancy and involves one or more limbs and results in muscular spasticity or paresis (1). Its incidence is estimated at 1.5–2.5 per 1000 births (2), a figure which has remained unchanged despite changing obstetric practice (3,4). The prevalence of brain-damaged children, however, is increasing as a result of increasing survival in very premature infants (5). Cerebral palsy can result from events occurring either in prenatal, perinatal, or postnatal periods; however, the specific event is in most cases unknown (6–8). Intrapartum asphyxia accounts for around only 10% of cases of cerebral palsy (6,9) despite its occurrence being synonomous with a "difficult" or "negligent" birth by those parents involved. The interest in intrapartum causes of cerebral palsy centers around (a) the issue of any avoidable factors present and (b) improvements in the current methods of diagnosing fetal distress. Confusion arises when a medical definition of intrapartum asphyxia

Asphyxia and Fetal Brain Damage, Edited by Dev Maulik, M.D., Ph.D.
ISBN 0-471-18427-6

is attempted. The obstetrician views meconium staining, abnormal fetal heart rate patterns, and low fetal scalp and umbilical cord pH as evidence of a possible hypoxic insult, whereas the pediatrician views hypoxia as low Apgar scores, prolonged interval to first spontaneous breath, and abnormal neonatal neurological signs. All with exception of the latter are commonly seen but rarely associated with cerebral palsy (10–13). In many cases these observed parameters which are considered to represent fetal distress reflect the physiological response of the fetus to the stress of labor. When used as markers of fetal compromise, increased intervention without benefit will result (14). Therefore, in obstetric terms the challenge remains to develop a method of intrapartum fetal assessment which has sufficient sensitivity and specificity to allow intervention before the onset of permanent fetal damage.

This chapter will consider the association between methods of fetal and neonatal assessment and adverse neurological outcome and possible obstetric antecedents of cerebral palsy.

FETAL RESPONSE TO "HYPOXIA" AND "BIRTH ASPHYXIA"

The question as to whether birth asphyxia was responsible for a case of cerebral palsy is a difficult one to answer when based on the traditional markers of fetal distress as previously described. Extreme birth asphyxia is defined as suffocation with anoxia and rising carbon dioxide levels in the fetal blood. In reality, however, acute or chronic hypoxia and not anoxia is usually present. A normal fetus is well adapted to the periods of hypoxemia/hypoxia which are universally experienced during labor as a result of uterine activity. The exposure of the fetus to hypoxia results in a response which may be adaptive or compromising. The response will be modified by factors such as intrauterine growth retardation and the degree of hypoxia. Healthy adaptive responses include (a) the shunting of blood to the brain—especially the brain stem—at the expense of peripheral organs (15), (b) release of catecholamines from adrenal glands (16), and (c) utilization of liver glycogen reserves (17). If the period of hypoxia/ischemia persists, then decompensation occurs with peripheral vasodilatation, hypotension, and decreased cardiac output which results in reduced cerebral and myocardial blood flow (18). The result of the cerebral hypoxia is accumulation of lactic acid which has been found to disturb neuronal transmitters and disrupt energy production in monkeys. In these studies, anoxia for 10 minutes resulted in profound hypoxemia, hypercapnia, and severe acidosis associated with marked hypotension (19). Recent studies have suggested that hypoxia is the primary insult but that secondary damage can occur during the period of reoxygenation and reperfusion with the release of toxic free radicals (20).

If the hypoxia is severe or prolonged, it results in irreversible neuronal impairment (21). The area mostly affected is the watershed area of the parasagittal regions in the border zones supplied by the anterior, middle, and posterior cerebral arteries (22) which lie principally between occipital and parietal lobes. Neuronal necrosis can also occur in the basal ganglia and thalamus. This distribution of neuropathological findings parallels those of children with hypoxic-ischemic brain injury documented at the time of postmortem examination (23). This supports the concept of damage due to a period of hypoxia.

THE DIAGNOSIS OF INTRAPARTUM "ASPHYXIA" AND THE ASSOCIATION OF CURRENTLY USED METHODS WITH ADVERSE NEURODEVELOPMENTAL OUTCOME

The cardiotocograph (CTG) was introduced in an effort to reduce perinatal mortality and is considered by some to be responsible in reducing long-term handicap (24,25). Despite being poorly specific with a low positive predictive value (26), it continues to be the "gold standard" of intrapartum monitoring. Because of its poor specificity, intervention for suspected "fetal distress" has resulted in increased cesarean section rates without fetal benefit (27). However, the chance of a fetus being acidotic is greater with increasingly abnormal patterns (28), and reassurance can be obtained from a normal tracing (29). The addition of fetal scalp pH values improves the specificity of the CTG (30,31).

Abnormalities in the fetal heart rate pattern—particularly late decelerations—suggest uteroplacental insuffuciency leading to acidosis (32,33); however, most abnormal cardiotocographs result in nonacidotic infants (33). Although no specific fetal heart rate pattern predicts subsequent abnormal neurological development (34), Shields and Schifrin (35) found that 56% of cerebral palsy cases in their review had a chronically abnormal fetal heart rate pattern associated with a fixed baseline rate and reduced variability. These abnormalities were noted to persist throughout labor and were associated with other markers of fetal compromise such as meconium, reduced amniotic fluid, and growth retardation, suggesting chronic placental insufficiency with antenatal origins. Spencer et al. (36) demonstrated that for every case of neonatal encephalopathy associated with an abnormal cardiotocogram there will be 83 abnormal cardiotocograms in which there is no evidence of subsequent neonatal encephalopathy. Phelan and Myoung (37), who considered the admission CTG, suggested that a fixed baseline fetal heart rate represented underlying fetal neurological impairment, whereas a tracing which was initially reactive and subsequently became nonreactive represented an intrapartum event. In this way they were able to differentiate those infants who were damaged in the intrapartum period from those who already had suffered damage antenatally. Spencer et al. (36) suggested that a reduction in fetal heart rate variability associated with the absence accelerations suggests a disturbance secondary to hypoxia in the normal fetal behavioral cycle which may relate more closely to neonatal encephalopathy than traditional markers of intrapartum hypoxia such as late decelerations which do not relate to irreversible long-term central nervous system (CNS) injury (38).

Screening for potential fetal compromise using the labor admission CTG and umbilical Doppler has also been demonstrated to correlate poorly with short-term outcome measures (39) and is no better than clinically assigned risk.

Another marker for suspected intrapartum hypoxia is meconium staining of the liquor. However, 20% of fetuses will pass meconium during labor, particularly if they are postdates (40), and its passage is poorly correlated with adverse neurodevelopment (12,41). In a search for improved methods of intrapartum surveillance, Westgate et al. (42) demonstrated a 46% reduction in operative deliveries for fetal distress and showed a trend towards fewer low 5-minute Apgar scores and less metabolic acidosis when the fetal electrocardiogram (ECG) was used in combination with the CTG.

Therefore, the use of the fetal ECG in conjunction with the CTG appears to result in less intervention without apparent short-term fetal compromise. The ECG analysis in this study was based on changes in the ST segment, with elevation of the T/QRS ratio correlating with anaerobic metabolism of myocardial glycogen stores (43,44). A negative T wave has also been demonstrated to be associated with endocardial hypoxia (45). In addition to changes observed in the ST segment of the fetal ECG, Pardi et al. (46) and Murray (47) demonstrated that the normal negative relationship between the fetal heart rate and PR interval of the ECG becomes positive with fetal acidosis. This relationship (conduction index), if positive for greater than 20 min, is associated with an increased risk of fetal compromise (48,49). Current methods of assessing the intrapartum condition of the fetus therefore remain poorly predictive of those fetuses who may be genuinely compromised and may benefit from obstetric intervention aimed at reducing or limiting the effects of hypoxia. Newer techniques (e.g., fetal ECG, pulse oximetry, near-infrared spectroscopy, continuous tissue pH) may provide an adjunct to the currently available methods but require evaluation by properly controlled randomized controlled trials with adequate long-term neurodevelopmental follow-up. Others require improvements in technology and therefore remain research tools which provide opportunities to add to physiological and pathophysiological knowledge from previously inaccessible areas.

MODE OF DELIVERY AND ITS ASSOCIATION WITH ADVERSE NEURODEVELOPMENT

The association of the breech infant and cerebral palsy may be explained by an antenatal predisposition (see later) or associated with mode of delivery. The association between cerebral palsy and vaginal breech delivery is a controversial issue. Because of fears of litigation resulting from vaginal breech delivery, there has been an increase in cesarean section rates for breech presentation without a comparitive reduction in rates of cerebral palsy (50). Vaginal breech delivery has been shown by some not to affect the risk of cerebral palsy (6,51–53) and to increase the risk by others (54,55) in term and preterm infants. There is, however, a lack of evidence from randomized controlled trials to support elective cesarean section (CS) or vaginal breech delivery as the delivery route of choice for the breech presenting whether at term or preterm.

A recent audit of CSs in Scotland (56) demonstrated that 11% of CSs were elective for breech presentation, and it recommended that there is a need for (a) randomized controlled trials (RCTs) of external cephalic version and (b) elective CS versus vaginal breech for the fetus presenting at term.

For the preterm infant presenting as a breech in labor there is equal controversy. Breech presentation is more common in preterm infants and causes a higher risk for the infant. This has led to the concept that CS is a safer option. In 1980 Crowley and Hawkins (57) reviewed studies which had compared CS versus vaginal delivery in the preterm breech. They concluded that for infants weighing 1500–2500 g, neonatal survival is independent of mode of delivery, but between 1000–1500 g CS appears to confer an advantage. The problem with studies contributing to this conclusion is that they were not RCTs. Despite attempts to allow for confounding variables, they do not compare like with like. Infants delivered by CS were more likely to have delivery planned and therefore to have been preceded by a thorough assessment of fetal condition. They are also more likely to be of an advanced gestation and hence of greater birthweight. In comparison, infants delivered by the vaginal route are more likely to be considered too premature or sick to benefit from CS and are more likely to occur in mothers who present in advanced labor. They are also less likely to have had the benefit of antenatal steroids and to have delivered in the absence of a senior neonatologist. Attempts to undertake RCTs to answer the question of which method of delivery is more advantageous have been unsuccessful. To date there have been six attempted trials, all of which have been abandoned primarily because of inability to recruit patients. However, Grant (58) performed a meta-analysis of the 104 women recruited to five of these trials. The results suggest that there are fewer low Apgar scores and less intubation in these infants undergoing elective CS but these differences were not statistically significant. Thornton and Lilford (59) included the patients recruited to the sixth abandoned study (60) and demonstrated in the women recruited to all six studies a nonsignificant trend to reduced perinatal mortality but with increased maternal morbidity in women delivered by CS.

Traumatic vaginal delivery is now an uncommon cause of cerebral palsy in the developed world. Macrosomic babies at particular risk now have the lowest rates of cerebral palsy (61). Petridou et al. (62) found no association with a forceps delivery or birth trauma in the absence of a coexisting prenatal risk factor.

CONDITION AT BIRTH AND ITS ASSOCIATION WITH SUBSEQUENT NEURODEVELOPMENT

Birth asphyxia is a biochemical process best identified on the basis of fetal acid–base status reflected in umbilical arterial blood. It reflects the degree of anaerobic metabolism required during periods of increased oxygen demand or hypoxia during which lactic acid is produced. The prevalence of intrapartum metabolic acidosis ranges from 0.5% to 2% (63,64). Metabolic acidosis is a good measure of the severity of intrapartum asphyxia, but it does not determine the timing of the intrapartum asphyxial event (65). A difference between the umbilical arterial and venous buffer base of less than 6 mmol/liter suggests a long asphyxial insult (63) which may help to time the onset of the asphyxial insult to an antenatal event.

What level of acidosis reflects asphyxia has recently been questioned. Previously a pH of less than 7.2 was considered acidotic because this represented two standard deviations from the mean in population studies (66). However, it has been suggested that this level is too high because it is not associated with increased neonatal complications due to asphyxia and a pH of less than 7 should be used (67–69). Even a pH of this value is, however, poorly predictive of neurological deficit because a severely acidotic infant will usually have a normal outcome (32,68,70), unless associated with low Apgar scores (68,70). The presence of acidosis reflected by a fall in pH may be reflecting the physiological switch to anaerobic metabolism, which is a healthy response to hypoxia, and paradoxically it may be the fetuses who are unable to mount this response and therefore have "normal" umbilical gases in the face of hypoxia who may suffer long-term neurological sequelae (13). In addition, it could be anticipated that an insult occurring in the antenatal period would not result in abnormal blood gases at delivery. Umbilical blood gas values may therefore aid in excluding intrapartum asphyxia and not confirming its presence (68).

The Apgar score was developed to quickly identify the newborn infant in need of resuscitation (71). Hypoxia in utero from whatever cause may be responsible for low Apgars as may other factors such CNS abnormalities, prematurity, cardiorespiratory problems, and maternal medication. The Apgar score has been found to be associated with adverse neurological sequelae (34,72–74) especially if the Apgar score is depressed for more than 10 min (34,72,73), which would suggest a greater degree of asphyxia. A persistently depressed Apgar score has been associated with death in more than half of the cases, or neurological deficit in 25% of the surviving infants suggesting an "all or nothing" effect (73).

Not suprisingly, studies looking at neurological outcome in infants with low Apgar scores at 1 and 5 minutes with metabolic acidosis at delivery demonstrated a similiar association (35,37). This group may have represented the asphyxiated infant previously noted in other studies to have prolonged depressed Apgar scores. However, despite the association, a low Apgar and metabolic acidosis failed to predict which infants would develop cerebral palsy (37).

Sarnat and Sarnat (75) first used the principal of hypoxic-ischemic encephalopathy (HIE) to assess the degree of asphyxia in a group of neonates. HIE is characterized by abnormalities of tone, feeding, level of consciousness, and, in the more severe cases, seizures and coma developing within the first few days of life. The severity of the condition is graded as mild (no seizures), moderate (seizures), and severe (coma) (76).

A stepwise degree of asphyxial damage seems to be present, initially with the development of acidosis and depressed Apgar scores, which are poor predictors of cerebral palsy (32,37,68,70,72,74), followed by the development of HIE on reaching a certain threshold. There is a more substantial association between the latter and neonatal death and cerebral palsy (32,36,75,77). Yudkin et al. (32) demonstrated no cases of cerebral palsy in any infant in the absence of HIE despite the presence of other poor parameters. This suggests that a threshold of asphyxia exists before the development of cerebral palsy and does not support the theory that "a small amount of asphyxia results in a small amount of damage" (65).

Not all degrees of HIE, however, carry the same risk. Mild HIE carries good long-term prognosis, whereas severe HIE results in infant death or severe handicap in all cases (25,75,77). It is the moderate form which provides the difficulty in assigning a prognosis, with 20–30% developing a major handicap (77).

Encephalopathy is not the whole answer to the problem of determining whether intrapartum asphyxia has occurred (25,78). It had been postulated that perhaps an antenatal cerebral insult before the onset of labor which escaped standard monitoring or a structural abnormality of the fetal brain results in impairment in the ability of the fetus to cope with the normal stresses of labor, making intrapartum asphyxia more likely.

THE PARTICULAR PROBLEMS OF THE PRETERM INFANT

As a consequence of advances in neonatal intensive care, more preterm infants are surviving, with a significant proportion of these survivors having adverse neurodevelopmental sequelae often in the form of major handicap. Pharoah et al. (4), reviewing a register of infants with cerebral palsy in the Mersey region between 1967 and 1984, demonstrated no significant increase in the prevalence of cerebral palsy in normal-birthweight infants (>2500 g) but showed a significant increase in infants of low birthweight (<2500 g). They concluded that these changes in prevalence could be a consequence of improved survival of prenatally impaired infants because of improvements in medical care or a reflection of failure to maintain optimal conditions at or around the time of birth. The advent of cerebral ultrasound has provided a means of studying the evolution of periventricular hemorrhage (PVH) and hypoxic ischemic lesions (periventricular leukomalacia: PVCL) (79). These abnormalities are associated with adverse neurodevelopmental outcome in this group of infants, with both major PVH and PVCL being associated with cerebral palsy (80–84).

Associations have been made between the development of PVH and low-gestation, low-birthweight hypercarbia at birth and respiratory distress syndrome (85–87).

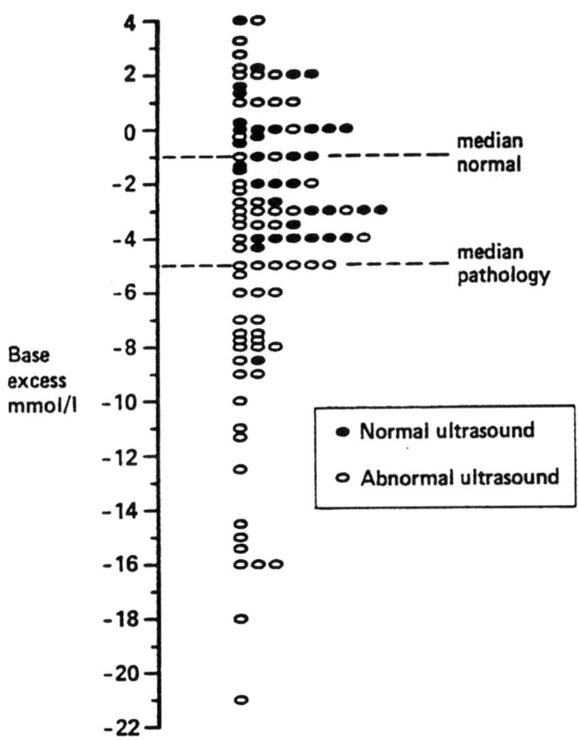

Figure 1. Comparison of base deficit in infants with birthweight < 1500 g with normal and abnormal ultrasound scans. Reproduced with permission from Reference 89.

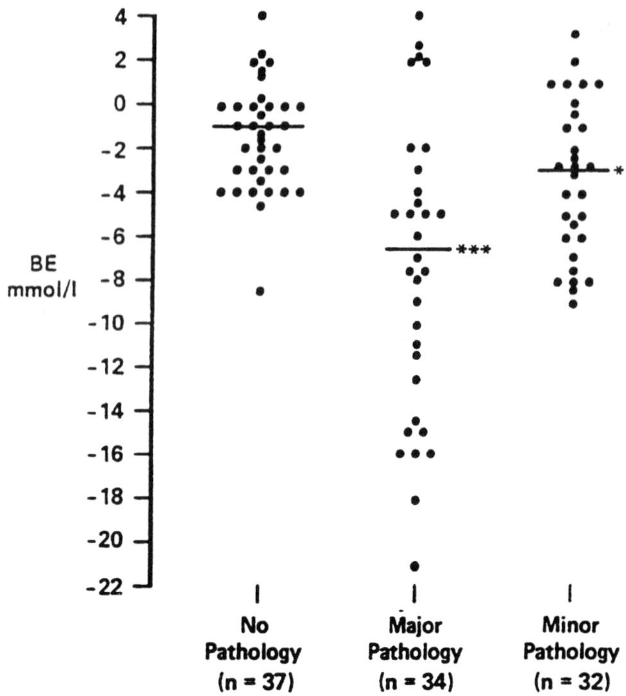

Figure 2. Base deficit within 1 hour of birth in infants with normal ultrasound scans, major cerebral pathology, and minor cerebral pathology. *** $P < 0.001$ compared with normals; * $P < 0.02$ compared with normals. Reproduced with permission from reference 89.

Ischemic white matter lesions (PVCL) have been associated with growth retardation and oligohydramnios (84), antepartum hemorrhage (87), and respiratory distress syndrome (88).

In a study from Dundee, 103 infants with a birthweight of less than 1500 g and delivering before 32 weeks' gestation had a capillary blood sample taken within an hour of birth and serial cranial ultrasound scans performed during the first weeks of life. The subsequent development of intracranial pathology was found to be significantly associated with gestation at delivery, birthweight, and base deficit within 1 hour of birth. The strongest association was in infants with major pathology (grade III/IV PVH and PVCL) where a base deficit of > 5 mmol/liter had a positive predictive value of 97% and a sensitivity of 51% for the development of pathology (Figures 1 and 2) (89). In a further study on a group of 217 infants delivering before 37 weeks' gestation, multiple regression analysis of a number of antenatal, peripartum, and neonatal factors identified gestation at delivery, umbilical arterial base deficit, and 5-minute Apgar scores as being significantly and independently associated with the development of cerebral pathology. In those infants delivering before 32 weeks who subsequently developed major cerebral pathology, as well as in a similar multiple re-

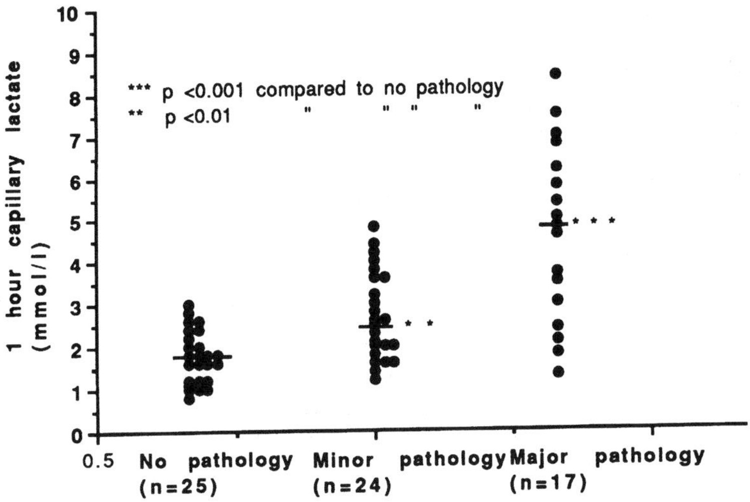

Figure 3. One-hour capillary lactate and cerebral pathology in infants delivering at less than 32 weeks' gestation.

gression analysis of antenatal, peripartum, and neonatal factors, Mires (90) identified 1-hour capillary lactate, umbilical arterial base deficit, and umbilical arterial lactate as being significantly and independently associated with the development of this pathology (Figures 3 and 4).

These findings provide support for the hypothesis that condition at birth in preterm infants is an important predisposing factor for the development of cerebral pathologies which have been associated with adverse neurodevelopmental outcome. Major cerebral pathology has also been demonstrated to be more likely in those infants in whom the metabolic acidosis persists beyond delivery.

Improved surveillance of the very preterm infant during labor and at birth, with the aim of reducing the incidence of metabolic acidosis at birth, may therefore help to reduce subsequent intracranial pathology and thereby perinatal and long-term morbidity.

In a randomized controlled trial of electronic fetal monitoring (EFM) in the preterm infant, Luthy et al. (91) demonstrated no significant differences in the prevalence of low 5-min Apgar scores, intrapartum acidosis, intracranial hemorrhage, or frequency of cesarean section between the fetuses undergoing EFM and those having periodic ascultation of the fetal heart. Subsequent follow-up of these children at 18 months failed to demonstrate improved neurologic development in the infants who had EFM. In fact there was a 2.9-fold increase in cerebral palsy in the EFM group, possibly as a result of a longer diagnosis of fetal heart rate abnormalities to delivery interval in this group. The risk of cerebral palsy was demonstrated to increase with the duration of the fetal heart rate abnormalities (92).

The controversial issue of delivery of the preterm breech was discussed earlier in this chapter.

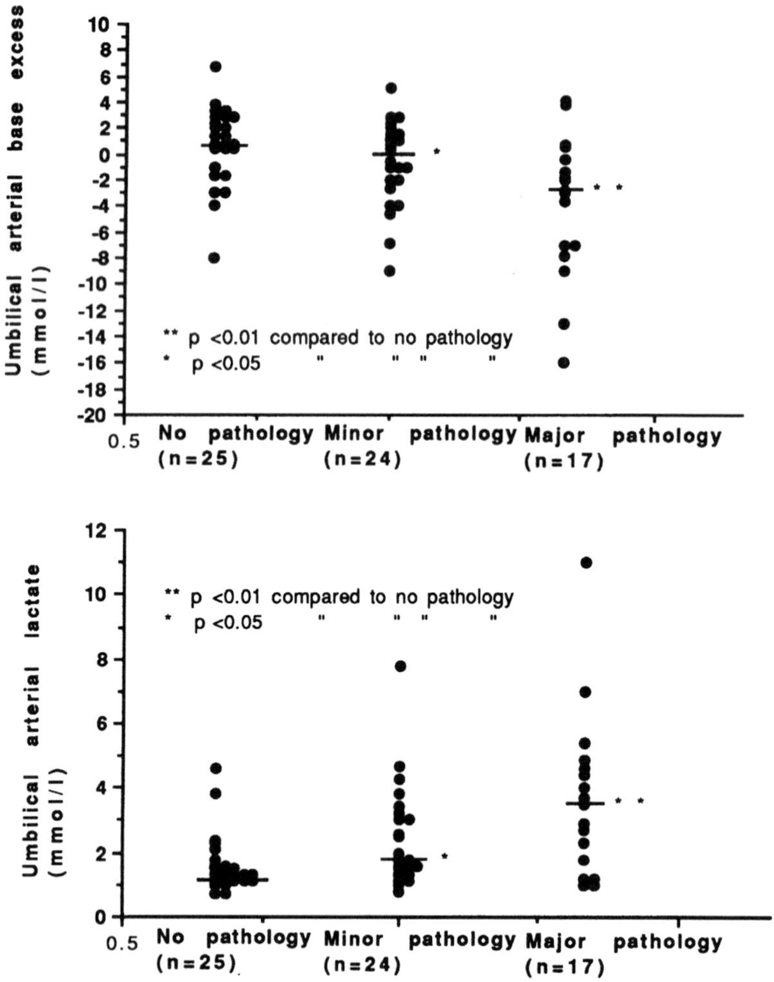

Figure 4. Umbilical arterial base excess and lactate and cerebral pathology in infants delivering at less than 32 weeks' gestation.

ANTENATAL CONSIDERATIONS AND NEURODEVELOPMENTAL OUTCOME

Small for Gestational Age

The answer to whether a small for gestational age (SGA) infant is at increased risk of poor neurodevelopmental outcome is not entirely clear despite a number of long-term follow-up studies. A number of population-based studies are available from which some conclusions regarding birthweight and cerebral palsy can be drawn.

Ellenberg and Nelson (93) compared the gestational ages and birthweights of children with cerebral palsy, children free of cerebral palsy but with seizure disorders, and children free from these conditions amongst a prospectively studied cohort of 54,000 singleton births. This is an important study since previous reports either included twins in their sample or were of very small numbers (94,95). Ellenberg and Nelson (93) described an increase in risk of cerebral palsy with shorter gestational age and lower birthweight. When birthweight was adjusted for gestational age, very few infants fell below the tenth percentile for gestational age, although, as a group, infants with cerebral palsy also born prematurely had lower percentile birthweight distributions than those born at term. As regards seizure disorders, neither low birthweight, prematurity, or being SGA were significantly associated with afebrile seizures in this population. While birthweight among cerebral palsy children as a group is reduced compared to the nonaffected population, very few fall within the current categorization of being SGA.

Cases from the Cerebral Palsy Register of Western Australia form the index population of the investigation by Blair and Stanley (96) into birthweight, gestational age, and risk of spastic cerebral palsy. Three controls were selected for each case of cerebral palsy and were matched for birthweight, sex, and year of birth, but not for gestational age. They described a strong relationship between decreasing birthweight and risk of cerebral palsy amongst infants born at less than 34 weeks' gestation with the strongest relationship seen between 34 and 37 weeks; no such relationship existed for infants born at more than 37 weeks. Nearly 50% of cerebral palsy cases born between 34 and 37 weeks' gestation may be attributable to having a birthweight less than the tenth percentile for the population. This is important data suggesting a strong association between low birthweight and risk of cerebral palsy in infants delivered at certain gestational ages. It is unable, however, to determine whether cerebral palsy is a consequence of growth failure, is a feature of some genetically small infants, or is itself responsible for the apparently poor growth observed in cerebral palsy children.

The neonatal anthropometric features of the same population of cerebral palsy children were subsequently reported in an effort to distinguish the nature of the growth abnormality or insult associated with and possibly responsible for the disability (97). The morphological variables included birthweight, length, and head circumference for gestational age together with "thinness" reflected by the Ponderal index. Compared to controls, there was a 44% excess of morphological abnormalities seen amongst the cerebral palsy cases. These were separately analyzed according to gestational age at delivery. Short infants (<10th percentile) contributed a greater proportion of cerebral palsy children than did thin infants who were not short, with the highest proportion being short but not thin, although the highest risk of cerebral palsy was experienced by infants who were both thin and short. All the thin and short infants were delivered at term. If, as seems likely, one accepts that different types of growth retardation, reflected by different anthropometric features at birth, are a consequence of insults to the fetus at differing times in gestation (98,99), then an insult in the first half of pregnancy seems more likely to result in a child with cerebral palsy than a later insult. This may be because of the susceptibility of the developing brain in early pregnancy or that a combination or sequence of events is necessary which must begin in early pregnancy and be exacerbated by a persistently adverse intrauterine environment. The precise nature of these insults is far from clear and represents an ongoing challenge to those determined to unravel the relationship between antenatal life, fetal growth, and cerebral palsy.

Multiple Pregnancy

Cerebral palsy is more common in multiple pregnancy, with risks of 0.2%, 1.3%, and 7.6% for singleton, twin, and triplet pregnancies respectively being reported by Stanley and Petterson (100) for the period 1960–1989 in Western Australia. Much of the excess risk in multiple pregnancies can be accounted for by differences in birthweight distribution, with infants from multiple pregnancies being much more likely to be of low birthweight than singletons. However, when adjustments are made for gestational age at delivery and birthweight, there is no difference in neurological morbidity between singleton and multiple births (100).

Another factor contributing to the increased cerebral palsy rates in multiple pregnancy is the higher rates of preterm delivery in this group. Both Stanley and Petterson (100) and Grether et al. (101), however, demonstrated a higher risk of cerebral palsy in multiple births where the birthweight was greater than 2500 g, suggesting that as twin pregnancies approach term the risk of disability exceeds that in twins of lower birthweight.

Laplaza et al. (102), in a hospital-based study of cerebral palsy in twins, found that 10 of the 80 cerebral palsied twins had survived the fetal death of their co-twin; five of these deaths occurred before 20 weeks' gestation, highlighting this as a cause of neurological morbidity.

Breech Presentation

The question of the influence of route of delivery and subsequent neurological outcome has already been discussed in relation to the term and preterm infant presenting as a breech. However, an alternative hypothesis to support the increased risk of adverse neurological outcome in the term breech infant is that a preexisting prenatal neurological deficit may be the cause of the infant presenting as a breech. It is suggested that a neurological deficit in the fetus affects the normal control of the limbs, leading to extension of the fetal legs and prevention of normal fetal attitude. This neurological deficit may explain the increased rates of neurological handicap in these infants (51,103).

Other Maternal/Fetal Considerations

Pregnancy-induced hypertension has been linked to minor neurological problems (104) but no increased risk of cerebral palsy. Murphy et al. (105) found that preeclampsia lowered the risk of cerebral palsy in preterm babies.

Antepartum hemorrhage may imply placental separation and a subsequent degree of hypoxia, and therefore it is a possible etiological factor for cerebral palsy (54). However, in these cases, preterm delivery may be a confounding variable (106). In a case control study by Taylor and Howie (107) the association between prenatal complications and neurodevelopmental disability was stronger than retarded growth alone.

The relative risk of handicap increased from 1.4 in infants who were small for gestational age in the absence of antenatal complications to 6.6 in infants who were small for gestational age and had associated complications. The complications included severe hypertension, unclassified antepartum hemorrhage, and preterm uterine activity.

Congenital infections such as toxoplasmosis, rubella, and cytomegalovirus are reported to cause long-term neurological handicap. Cytomegalovirus, usually an asymptomatic neonatal infection which often goes unrecognized at birth, can be a cause of cerebral palsy (108) secondary to the intracranial calcifications which result from the virus. Congenital toxoplasmosis infection also results in intracranial calcification, and in the absence of effective treatment in the neonatal period it can lead to major neurological handicap such as cerebral palsy in 75% of cases (109). Congenital rubella if associated with other major systemic features can also result in cerebral palsy.

CONCLUSION

Despite changing obstetric and neonatal practice, the incidence of cerebral palsy has remained constant but the prevalence is increasing probably as a consequence of increased survival in preterm infants. Avoidance and early detection of intrapartum asphyxia, the cause of approximately 10% of cases of cerebral palsy, remains the aim of every obstetric unit. This is, however, difficult with current methods of fetal and neonatal assessment which are poorly associated with long-term neurological outcome. The challenge remains to improve these techniques. Current research interest is focused on the attempts to understand the underlying cellular and molecular events associated with brain damage in the fetus and newborn particularly when associated with hypoxia-ischemia. This may lead to the introduction of potential pharmacological tools to prevent or treat brain injury in the newborn.

The majority of cases of cerebral palsy are likely to be the result of an antenatal insult of unknown origin and may be multifactorial. Certain groups are at more risk than others, such as the preterm infant, the small-for-gestational-age infant, and infants delivered from multiple pregnancy, and there is a need for continued research in these areas, particularly long-term follow-up studies of infants born to these complicated pregnancies.

REFERENCES

1. Rosen M, Hobel C. Prenatal and perinatal factors associated with brain disorders. *Obstet Gynaecol* 1986;68:416.
2. Pharoah P. Epidemiology of cerebral palsy: a review. *J R Soc Med* 1981;74:516.
3. Stanley FJ. The changing face of cerebral palsy. *Dev Med Child Neurol* 1987;29:263.
4. Pharoah PD, Cooke T, Cooke RWI, et al. Birthweight specific trends in cerebral palsy. *Arch Dis Child* 1990;65:602.
5. Fawer CL, Diebold P, Calame A. Periventricular leucomalacia and neurodevelopmental outcome in preterm infants. *Arch Dis Child* 1987;62:30.

6. Nelson KB, Ellenberg JH. Antecedents of cerebral palsy: multivariate analysis of risks. *N Engl J Med* 1986;315:81.
7. Freeman J, Nelson K. Intrapartum asphyxia and cerebral palsy. *Paediatrics* 1988;82:240.
8. Kitchen WH, Doyle LW, Ford GW, et al. Cerebral palsy in very low birthweight infants surviving to 2 years with modern perinatal intensive care. *Am J Perinatol* 1987;4:29.
9. Stanley FJ, Watson L. The cerebral palsy in Western Australia: trends 1968 to 1981. *Am J Obstet Gynaecol* 1988;158:89.
10. Sykes GS, Malloy PM, Johnston F, et al. Do Apgar scores indicate asphyxia? *Lancet* 1982;ii:494.
11. Low JA, Galbraith RS, Muir DW. Intrapartum fetal hypoxia: a study of long term morbidity. *Am J Obstet Gynecol* 1983;145:129.
12. Dijxhorn MJ, Visser G, Fiddler JJ. Apgar score, meconium and acidaemia at birth in relation to neonatal and neurological morbidity in term infants. *Br J Obstet Gynaecol* 1986;93:217.
13. Dennis J, Johson A, Mutch L, et al. Acid–base status at birth and neurodevelopmental outcome at four and one-half years. *Am J Obstet Gynecol* 1989;161:213.
14. MacDonald D, Grant A, et al. Dublin randomised control trial of intrapartum fetal heart rate monitoring. *Am J Obstet Gynecol* 1985;152;524.
15. Peeters LL, Sheldon RD, Jones MD, et al. Blood flow to fetal organs as a function of arterial oxygen content. *Am J Obstet Gynaecol* 1979;135: 637.
16. Nylund L, Lagercrantz H, Lunell NO. Catchecholamines in fetal blood during birth in man. *J Dev Physiol* 1979;1:427.
17. Irested L, Lagercrantz H, Belfrage P. Causes and consequences of maternal and fetal sympathoadrenal activation during parturition. *Acta Obstet Gynaecol Scand* 1984; 118:111.
18. Richardson BS, Rurak G, Patrick JE et al. Cerebral oxidative metabolism during sustained hypoaemia in fetal sheep. *J Dev Physiol* 1989;11:37.
19. Ranck JB, Windle WF. Brain damage in the monkey *Macaca mulatta* by asphyxia neonatorum. *Exp Neurol* 1959;1:130.
20. Longo LD, Packianathan S. Hypoxic-ischaemia and the developing brain: hypotheses regarding the pathophysiology of fetal neonatal brain damage. A review. *Br J Obstet Gynaecol* 1997;104:652.
21. Roth SC, Edwards AD, Cady EB, et al. Relation between cerebral oxidative metabolism following birth asphyxia and neurodevelopmental outcome and brain growth at 1 year. *Dev Med Child Neurol* 1992;34:285.
22. Brierly J, Brown AW, Excel BJ, Meldrum BS. Brain damage in the rhesus monkey from profound arterial hypotension. 1. Its nature, distribution and general physiological correlates. *Brain Res* 1969;13:68.
23. Wigglesworth, J. Brain development and its modification by adverse influences. In Stanley F and Alberman E (Eds). *Epidemiology of the cerebral palsies*. Oxford: Blackwell Scientific, 1984:18.
24. Ingemarsson E, Ingemarsson I, Svenningsen N. Impact of routine fetal monitoring during labour on fetal outcome with long term follow up. *Am J Obstet Gynaecol* 1981; 141:29.

25. Hull J, Dodds K. Falling incidence of hypoxic ischaemic encephalopathy in term infants. *Br J Obstet Gynaecol* 1992;99:386.
26. Machachlan NA, Spencer JAD, Harding K. Fetal acidaemia, the cardiotocogram and the T/QRS ratio of the fetal ECG in labour. *Br J Obstet Gynaecol* 1992;99:26.
27. Haverkamp AD, Thompson HE, McFee JG, et al. The evaluation of continuous fetal heart rate monitoring in high risk pregnancies. *Am J Obstet Gynaecol* 1976;125:310.
28. Beard, RW, Filschie GM, Knight CA, Roberts GM. The significance of the changes in the continuous fetal heart rate in the first stage of labour. *J Obstet Gynaecol Br Commonw* 1971;78:865.
29. Zuspan FP, Quilligan EJ, Iams JD, et al. Predictors of intrapartum fetal distress. The role of electronic fetal monitoring. *Am J Obstet Gynecol* 1979;35:287.
30. Westgren M, Ingemarsson E, Ingemarsson I, Solum T. Intrapartum electronic fetal monitoring in low risk pregnancy. *Obstet Gynaecol* 1980;56:301.
31. Young D, Gray J, Luther E, et al. Fetal scalp blood pH sampling. Its value in an active obstetric unit. *Am J Gynecol* 1980;136:276.
32. Yudkin PL, Johnson A, Clover LM, et al. Clustering of perinatal markers of birth asphyxia and outcome at age 5 years. *Br J Obstet Gynaecol* 1994;101:774.
33. Gilstrap LC, Hanth SC, Toussant S. Second stage fetal heart rate abnormalities and neonatal acidosis. *Obstet Gynaecol* 1984;63:209.
34. Rosen GM, Dickinson JC. The paradox of electronic fetal monitoring: more data may not enable us to predict or prevent infant neurologic morbidity. *Am J Obstet Gynecol* 1993;168:745.
35. Shields JR, Schifrin BS. Perinatal antecedents of cerebral palsy. *Obstet Gynaecol* 1988;71:899.
36. Spencer JAD, Badowi N, Burton P, et al. The intrapartum CTG prior to neonatal encephalopathy at term: a case control study. *Br Obstet Gynaecol* 1997;104:25.
37. Phelan JP, Myoung OA. Perinatal observations in 48 neurologically impaired term infants. *Am J Obstet Gynecol* 1994;171:424.
38. Painter MJ, Scott M, Hirsch RPO, et al. Fetal heart rate patterns during labour: neurologic and cognitive development at 6 and 9 years of age. *Am J Obstet Gynaecol* 1988;159:854.
39. Farrell T, Mires GJ, Howie P. A prospective evaluation of the value of intrapartum biophysical and Doppler parameters in identifying the compromised fetus. *J Obstet Gynaecol* 1997;17:452.
40. Steer PJ, Eigbe F, Lissauer TJ, Beard RW. Interrelationships among abnormal cardiotocograms in labour, meconium staining of the amniotic fluid, arterial cord blood pH and Apgar scores. *Obstet Gynaecol* 1989;74:715.
41. Nelson KB, Ellenberg JH. Obstetric complications and risk factors for cerebral palsy and seizure disorders. *JAMA* 1984;251:1843.
42. Westgate J, Harris M, Curnow J, et al. Plymouth randomised trial of the CTG versus St waveform plus CTG for intrapartum monitoring in 2400 cases. *Am J Obstet Gynecol* 1993;169:1151.
43. Rosen KG, Isaksson O. Alterations in fetal heart rate and ECG correlated to glycogen creatinine phosphate and ATP levels during graded hypoxia. *Biol Neonate* 1976;30:17.

44. Green KR, Dawes GS, Lilja H, et al. Changes in the ST waveform of the fetal ECG with hypoxaemia. *Am J Obstet Gynecol* 1982;144:950.
45. Widmark C, Jansson T, Lindercrantz K, et al. ECG waveform, short term heart rate variability and placental catchecholamine concentrations in response to hypoxia in intrauterine growth restricted guinea pigs. *J Dev Physiol* 1991;15:161.
46. Pardi G, Tucci E, Uderzo A, Zawini D. Fetal ECG changes in relation to fetal heart rate patterns during labour. *Am J Obstet Gynecol* 1974;118:243.
47. Murray HG. The fetal ECG: current clinical developments in Nottingham. *J Perinat Med* 1986;14:399–400.
48. Murray HG. Evaluation of the fetal ECG. MD thesis, University of Nottingham, 1992.
49. Mohajer MP, Sahota DS, Reed NW, et al. Cumulative changes in the fetal ECG and biochemical indices of fetal hypoxia. *Eur J Obstet Gynecol Reprod Biol* 1994;55:63.
50. Scheller J, Nelson K. Does Caesarean delivery prevent cerebral palsy or other neurologic problems of childhood? *Obstet Gynaecol* 1994;83:624.
51. Svenningsen N, Westgren M, Ingemarsson I. Modern strategy for the term breech delivery—a study with a 4 years follow up of the infants. *J Perinat Med* 1985;13:117.
52. Croughan-Minihane M, Petitti D, Gordis L, Golditch I. Morbidity among breech infants according to method of delivery. *Obstet Gynaecol* 1990;75:821.
53. Koike T, Minakaim H, Sasaki M, et al. The problem of relating fetal outcome with breech presentation to mode of delivery. *Arch Gynaecol Obstet* 1996;258:119.
54. Mayer P, Wingate M. Obstetric factors in cerebral palsy. *Obstet Gynaecol* 1978;51:399.
55. Kato E, Yamada H, Matsumoto Y, et al. Relation between perinatal factors and outcome of very low birthweight infants. *J Perinat Med* 1996;24:677.
56. Audit of Caesarean section in Scotland 1994. Report for the clinical audit and resources group of the Scottish Office. Department of Health, 1997.
57. Crowley P, Hawkins DF. Premature breech delivery: the Caesarean section debate. *J Obstet Gynaecol* 1980;1:2.
58. Grant A. Elective versus selective Caesarean section of the small baby. Pregnancy and childbirth module of the Cochrane Database of Systematic Reviews, 1995.
59. Thornton JG, Lilford RJ. Preterm breech babies and randomised trials of rare conditions. Commentary. *Br J Obstet Gynaecol* 1996;103:611.
60. Penn Z, Steer PJ, Grant A. A multicentre randomised controlled trial comparing elective and selective caesarean section for the delivery of the preterm breech. *Br J Obstet Gynaecol* 1996;103:684.
61. Cummins S, Nelson K, Grether J, Velie E. Cerebral palsy in 4 Northern California counties, births 1983 through 1985. *J Paediatr* 1993;123:230.
62. Petridou E, Koussouir M, Toupadaki N, et al. Risk factors for cerebral palsy: a case control study in Greece. *Scand J Soc Med* 1996;24:14.
63. Low JA, Panagiotopoulos C, Derrick EJ. Newborn complications after intrapartum asphyxia with metabolic acidosis in the term fetus. *Am J Obstet Gynecol* 1994;170:1081.
64. Low JA. *Intrapartum fetal asphyxia. A critical appraisal of fetal surveillance.* Amsterdam: Elsevier, 1994:411.
65. Low JA, Galbraith RS, Muir DW, et al. Motor and cognitive deficits after intrapartum asphyxia in the mature fetus. *Am J Obstet Gynecol* 1988;158:356.

66. ACOG Technical Bulletin N.127. Assessment of fetal and newborn acid–base status. ACOG, 1989.

67. Gilstrap LC, Levene KJ, Burris J, et al. Diagnosis of birth asphyxia on the basis of fetal pH, Apgar score and newborn cerebral dysfunction. *Am J Obstet Gynecol* 1989;161:825.

68. Winkler H, Houth J, Tucher J, et al. Neonatal complications at term as related to the degree of umbilical artery acidaemia. *Am J Obstet Gynecol* 1991;164:637.

69. Goldaber KG, Gilstrap LC, Levene KJ, et al. Pathologic fetal acidaemia. *Obstet Gynaecol* 1991;78:1103.

70. Socol ML, Garcia PM, Riter S. Depressed Apgar scores, acid–base status and neurologic outcome. *Am J Obstet Gynecol* 1994;170:991.

71. Apgar V. A proposal for a new method of evaluation of the newborn infant. *Curr Res Anaesth Analg* 1953;32:260.

72. Nelson K, Ellenberg J. Neonatal signs as predictors of cerebral palsy. *Paediatrics* 1979;64:225.

73. Nelson K, Ellenberg J. Apgar scores are predictors of chronic neurologic disability. *Paediatrics* 1981;68:36.

74. Levene M, Sands C, Grindulis H, Moore J. Comparison of two methods of predicting outcome of perinatal asphyxia. *Lancet* 1986;1:67.

75. Sarnat HB, Sarnat MS. Neonatal encephalopathy following fetal distress. *Arch Neurol* 1976;33:696.

76. Levene M, Kornberg J, Williams TH. The incidence and severity of post asphyxial encephalopathy in full term infants. *Early Hum Dev* 1985;11:21.

77. Robertson C, Finer N. Term infants with hypoxic ischaemic encephalopathy: outcome at 3.5 years. *Dev Med Child Neurol* 1985;27:473.

78. Menticoglou S, Manning F, Harman C, et al. Severe fetal brain injury without evident intrapartum asphyxia or trauma. *Obstet Gynaecol* 1989;74:457.

79. Levene MI, Williams JL, Fawer CL. *Ultrasound of the infant brain*. Oxford: Blackwell Scientific Publications, 1985.

80. Luthy DA, Shy KK, Strickland D, et al. Status of infants at birth and risk of adverse neonatal events and long term sequelae; a study of low birthweight infants. *Am J Obstet Gynecol* 1987;157:676.

81. Graham M, Levene MI, Trounce JQ, et al. Prediction of cerebral palsy in very low birthweight infants: prospective ultrasound study. *Lancet* 1987;ii:593.

82. Cooke RWI. Early and late cranial ultrasonographic appearances and outcome in very low birthweight infants. *Arch Dis Child* 1987;62:931.

83. Levene MI. Cerebral ultrasound and neurological impairment: telling the future. *Arch Dis Child* 1990;65:469.

84. Gaffney G, Sqvier MV, Johson A, et al. Clinical association of prenatal ischaemic white matter injury. *Arch Dis Child* 1994;70:F101.

85. Cooke RW. Factors associated with periventricular haemorrhage in the very low birthweight infants. *Arch Dis Child* 1981;56:425.

86. Levene MI, Fawer CL, Lamont RF. Risk factors for the development of intraventricular haemorrhage in the preterm neonate. *Arch Dis Child* 1982;57:410.

87. Weindling AM, Wilkinson AR, Cooke J, et al. Perinatal events which precede periventricular haemorrhage and leukomalacia in the newborn. *Br J Obstet Gynaecol* 1985;92:1218.

88. Larroche JL. *Developmental pathologies of the neonate.* Amsterdam: Excerpta Medica, 1977.

89. Mires GJ, Agustsson P, Forsyth JS, et al. Cerebral pathology in the very low birthweight infant: predictive value of peripartum metabolic acidosis. *Eur J Obstet Gynecol Reprod Biol* 1991;42:181.

90. Mires GJ. A study of cerebral pathology in the preterm infant and associated peripartum antecedents. MD thesis, University of Dundee, 1994.

91. Luthy DA, Shy KK, Van Bell G, et al. A randomised controlled trial of electronic fetal heart rate monitoring in preterm labour. *Obstet Gynaecol* 1987;69:687.

92. Shy KK, Luthy DA, Bennett FC, et al. Effects of electronic fetal heart rate monitoring compared to periodic ascultation on the neurologic development of premature infants. *N Engl J Med* 1990;322:588.

93. Ellenberg JH, Nelson KB. Birthweight and gestational age in children with cerebral palsy or seizures disorders. *Am J Dis Child* 1979;133:1044.

94. Hagberg G, Hagberg B, Olow I. The changing panorama of cerebral palsy in Sweden 1965–1970. III. The importance of foetal deprivation supply. *Acta Paediatr Scand* 1976;65:403.

95. Sabel KG, Olegard R, Victorin L. Remaining sequelae with modern perinatal care. *Paediatrics* 1976;57:652.

96. Blair E, Stanley F. Intrauterine growth and spastic cerebral palsy. I. Association with birthweight for gestational age. *Am J Obstet Gynecol* 1990;162:229.

97. Blair E, Stanley F. Intrauterine growth and spastic cerebral palsy. II. The association with morphology at birth. *Early Hum Dev* 1992;28:91.

98. Villar J, Belizan JM. The timing factor in the pathophysiology of the intrauterine growth retardation syndrome. *Obstet Gynaecol* 1982;37:499.

99. Fay RA, Ellwood DA. Categories of intrauterine growth retardation. *Fetal Mat Med Rev* 1993;5:203.

100. Stanley F, Petterson B. Cerebral palsy in multiple birth: the changing epidemiological patterns. In Ward RH, Whittle M (eds). *Multiple pregnancy.* London: RCOG Press, 1995:309.

101. Grether JW, Nelson WB, Cummins SK. Twinning and cerebral palsy: experience in four northern Californian Countries, births 1983 through 1985. *Paediatrics* 1993;92:854–858.

102. Laplaza FJ, Root L, Tassanawipas A, et al. Cerebral palsy in twins. *Dev Med Child* 1992;34:1053.

103. Cox C, Kendall AC, Hommers C. Changing prognosis of breech presenting low birthweight infants. *Br J Obstet Gynaecol* 1982;89:881.

104. Spinillo A, Iasci A, Capuzzo E, et al. Two year infant neurodevelopmental outcome after expectant management and indicated preterm delivery in hypertensive pregnancy. *Acta Obstet Gynaecol Scand* 1994;73:625.

105. Murphy DJ, Sellers S, MacKenzie IZ, et al. A case control study of antenatal and intrapartum risk factors for cerebral palsy in very preterm singleton babies. *Lancet* 1995;346:1449.

106. Palmer L, Blair E, Petterson B, et al. Antenatal antecedents of moderate and severe cerebral palsy. *Paediatr Perinat Epidemiol* 1995;9:171.

107. Taylor DJ, Howie P. Fetal growth achievement and neurodevelopmental disability. *Br J Obstet Gynaecol* 1989;96:789.

108. Pass RF, Stagno S, Myers GJ. Outcome of symptomatic congenital cytomegaolovirus infection: results of long term longitudinal follow up. *Paediatrics* 1980;66:758.

109. Eichenwald H. A study of congenital toxoplasmosis. In Sam JC (ed). *Human toxoplasmosis*. Copenhagen: Munskgaard, 1960:41.

2

FETAL ASPHYXIA AND OUTCOME

James A. Low, M.D.

Department of Obstetrics, Gynaecology, and Paediatrics, Queen's University, Kingston, Ontario, Canada

Fetal asphyxia has been a concern since the first report of an association between perinatal events, asphyxia neonatorum, and the mental and physical condition of the child (1). Subsequently, fetal exposure to asphyxia during the antepartum period was proposed (2). In spite of continuing clinical experience, the contribution of fetal asphyxia to brain damage remained obscure.

It was recognized that an animal model was required to permit the systematic examination of the effect of asphyxia and ischemia on the fetus. Dr. Baillie, Director of the National Institute of Neurological Disease, speaking to a symposium marking the beginning of studies of the fetus in the monkey colony in Puerto Rico, stated "Medical research in regard to cerebral palsy and other neurological disorders has been relatively neglected. The focus should be on those adverse biological factors which operate in the perinatal period. The proper point of departure is through controlled animal observations" (3).

Since that time a number of research models have examined the effect of asphyxial exposure in the fetal monkey and fetal lamb. Asphyxia has been induced by maternal hypoxemia, reduced uteroplacental blood flow, and umbilical cord occlusion, while cerebral ischemia has been caused by carotid artery occlusion. Two relevant

Asphyxia and Fetal Brain Damage, Edited by Dev Maulik, M.D., Ph.D.
ISBN 0-471-18427-6

questions examined include (1) the fetal response to asphyxial exposure and (2) the occurrence of cerebral dysfunction and brain damage after an asphyxial exposure.

FETAL RESPONSE TO ASPHYXIA

The concept of fetal cardiovascular compensation has been established by laboratory studies in the fetal lamb. The effect of fetal asphyxia due to maternal hypoxemia (4–7), reduced uteroplacental blood flow (8–11), and cord occlusion (12,13) on fetal cardiovascular function has been examined. There has been a remarkable consistency of the fetal cardiovascular response in these different models (Table 1).

The initial response of the fetus to an asphyxial exposure is an increase of arterial pressure due to increased systemic vascular resistance mediated by the autonomic nervous system (14). This response may be initiated through arterial chemoreceptors (15) and possibly by circulating endogenous opiates (16).

There is a redistribution of cardiac output with decreased blood flow to the lungs, kidney, gastrointestinal system, and body, along with a centralization of the circulation with increased blood flow to the brain, heart, and adrenals. Fetal hypoxia due to partial cord occlusion is associated with decreased placental blood flow. The fetus compensates by increasing the blood flow through the ductus venosus with reduced blood flow through the liver.

This cardiovascular response is important to the integrity of the central nervous system during the compensatory phase of an asphyxial exposure. Cerebral oxygen requirements are reduced with an increase of high-voltage electrocortical activity (17). Cerebral oxygen metabolism is maintained because of a combination of increased cerebral blood flow and oxygen extraction. Similarly, myocardial oxygen requirements continue to be met because of increased myocardial blood flow and decreased myocardial work.

Table 1. Initial fetal response to asphyxial exposure

Reference	Year	Model[a]	Duration (minutes)	Mean Arterial Pressure	Blood Flow				
					Brain	Heart	Adrenal	Kidney	Carcass
Cohn et al. (4)	1974	1	4–44	↑	↑	↑	↑	↓	↓
Peeters et al. (5)	1979	1	60	↑	↑	↑	↑	↓	↓
Richardson et al. (6)	1989	1	420	↑	↑				
Field et al. (8)	1990	2	90	↑	↑	↑	↑	↓	↓
Reid et al. (9)	1991	2	20	↑	↑	↑	↑	↓	↓
Jensen et al. (10)	1991	2	35	↑	↑	↑	↑	ϕ	↓
Ball et al. (11)	1994	2	90	ϕ	ϕ	↑	↑	↓	↓
Itskovitz et al. (12)	1987	3	5	↑	↑	↑	↑	ϕ	ϕ
Ball et al. (13)	1994	3	90	↑	↑	ϕ	↑	↓	↓

[a]Model 1, maternal hypoxemia; model 2, reduced uteroplacental blood flow; model 3, umbilical cord occlusion; ϕ, change not statistically significant.

If the asphyxial exposure persists, a threshold of decompensation will occur. When fetal oxygen saturation falls below 30%, a progressive metabolic acidosis will develop. The threshold of cerebral dysfunction characterized by suppression of electrocortical activity and seizures in the fetal lamb occurs when the metabolic acidosis is severe (i.e., base deficit greater than 16 mmol/liter). Decompensation with a severe metabolic acidosis is associated with a fall of arterial pressure due to either a decrease of cardiac output or a failure to maintain peripheral vascular resistance. The combination of asphyxia and ischemia due to hypotension results in a decrease of cerebral oxygen consumption and, if sustained, brain damage.

FETAL BRAIN DAMAGE

Cerebral Ischemia

The effect of cerebral ischemia has been examined with a carotid artery occlusion model in chronically instrumented fetal lambs (Table 2). After 10–20 minutes of ischemia, the electroencephalogram was briefly depressed and then progressively recovered. Mild selective neuronal necrosis was seen on postmortem examination. After 30–40 minutes of ischemia, electroencephalographic activity remained depressed for 8 hours, followed by a transition to low-frequency epileptiform activity that reached maximum intensity at 10 hours. This sequence was associated with laminar necrosis of the parasagittal cortex, with necrosis in the hippocampus, basal ganglia, and thalamus (18).

The electrophysiologic and histologic consequences of isolated brief episodes of reversible cerebral ischemia at 1- and 5-hour intervals have been examined. The effect of frequent episodes of brief cerebral ischemia alters the pattern of brain injury, with basal ganglia damage a major feature. The pattern of the ischemia may be an important factor regarding the resultant neuropathology (19).

GLOBAL ASPHYXIA

A series of experiments in the monkey and lamb examined the effect of global asphyxia on the fetal brain (Table 3). Global asphyxia in the fetal monkey for more than 10 min resulted in profound hypoxemia with a severe metabolic acidosis and

Table 2. Brain damage after cerebral ischemia

				Neuropathology	
Reference	Year	Model[a]	Duration (minutes)	Cerebrum	Basal Ganglia Thalamus
Williams et al. (18)	1992	1	10	+	
		1	40	+++	+
Mallard et al. (19)	1993	1	10 × 3	++	+++

[a]Model 1: Lamb—carotid artery occlusion.

Table 3. Brain damage after global asphyxia

Reference	Year	Model[a]	Duration (minutes)	Fetal Response		Neuropathology		
				Acidosis	Hypotension	Cerebrum	Basal Ganglia Thalamus	Brain Stem
Ranck and Windle (20)	1959	1	8–30	+	+	+	++	+++
Mallard et al. (21)	1992	2	10	+	+	++	+	
Mallard et al. (22)	1995	2	Recurrent	+			++	
deHaan et al. (23)	1996	2	Recurrent	+	+	++	+	

[a]Model 1, monkey—placental separation; model 2, lamb—cord occlusion.

hypotension. The resultant neuropathology included neuronal necrosis principally in the brain stem, basal ganglia, and thalamus. On the basis of these studies it was concluded that global asphyxia for less than 8 min may not cause brain damage, while global asphyxia for more than 10 min invariably resulted in neuropathology (20).

This threshold for brain damage due to global asphyxia was confirmed by 10 min of cord occlusion in chronically instrumented fetal sheep (21). Cord occlusion resulted in acidosis (pH 6.9, lactate 6 mmol/liter) and hypotension. Postmortem examination demonstrated neuronal necrosis in the hippocampus and, to a lesser degree, in the basal ganglia and thalamus. There was a correlation between hypotension and the magnitude of neuronal necrosis.

Short but repeated episodes of global asphyxia are associated with different patterns of neuronal loss. Five minutes of cord occlusion repeated four times at 30-minute intervals affected principally the basal ganglia and specifically the striatal projection neurons (22). Cord occlusion for 1 min of every 2.5 min or for 2 min of every 5 min over several hours resulted in severe acidosis and hypotension. The predominant neuropathology was selective neuronal necrosis throughout the fetal brain (23).

The preterm fetus may be more resistant to global asphyxia. At mid-gestation before myelination has begun, 10 min (24) and 20 min (25) of cord occlusion caused no brain damage.

PARTIAL ASPHYXIA

The effects of sustained partial asphyxia have been examined in the fetal monkey and lamb (Table 4). Fetal monkeys were exposed to partial asphyxia for 1–3 hours. They were subsequently killed and their brains examined. Some monkeys had evidence of neuropathology, while others did not. Those monkeys with neuropathology had a severe acidosis with concurrent hypotension. The neuropathology ranged from a generalized to focal neuronal necrosis that principally involved the parasagittal regions and the junctional zones between the occipital and parietal lobes. Neuronal necrosis also occurred in the basal ganglia and thalamus (26).

Mid-gestational fetal lambs were exposed to 2 hours of maternal hypoxemia and fetal hypovolemia (27). Subsequent postmortem examination demonstrated that some lambs had evidence of brain damage while others did not. The fetuses with brain damage had a moderate acidosis and concurrent hypotension. There was a correlation between the severity of the hypotension and the extent of the neuropathology in the white matter, cerebral cortex, and basal ganglia.

Fourteen late-gestation fetal lambs were exposed to partial asphyxia (arterial oxygen content < 1.5 mmol/liter for 60 min) due to reduced uterine blood flow (28). Eight fetuses had evidence of brain damage. These fetuses had a severe acidosis (pH < 7.0) and concurrent hypotension. The predominant neuronal necrosis was in the parasagittal cortex and, to a lesser extent, in the basal ganglia. There was a correlation between the severity of the hypotension and the extent of the neuropathology.

Acidosis (pH 7.0) without hypotension due to partial asphyxia was induced by reduced uterine blood flow in seven fetal lambs (29). Histologic examination 3 days

Table 4. Brain damage after partial fetal asphyxia

Reference	Year	Model[a]	Duration (minutes)	Fetal Response		Neuropathology	
				Acidosis	Hypotension	Cerebrum	Basal Ganglia Thalamus
Myers (26)	1972	1	60–80	+	+	+++	++
Ting et al. (27)	1982	2	120	+	+	++	++
Gunn et al. (28)	1992	3	60	+	+	++	++
deHaan et al. (29)	1993	3	60	+	ϕ	+	
Ikeda et al. (30)	1996	4	60	+	+	++	+

[a]Model 1, monkey, reduced uteroplacental blood flow; model 2, lamb—maternal hypoxemia–fetal hypovolemia; model 3, lamb—reduced uteroplacental blood flow; model 4, lamb—partial cord occlusion.

after this exposure showed neuronal necrosis in a few fetuses principally in the cerebellum and, to a lesser extent, in the cerebral cortex.

Partial asphyxia was induced in eight near-term fetal lambs due to partial cord occlusion for approximately 60 min (30). This resulted in severe asphyxia (pH < 6.9, BD > 20 mmol/liter) with concurrent hypotension. The fetuses were sacrificed 3 days after exposure and the brain examined. There was a wide range of neuropathology in the cerebral cortex and basal ganglia. Again, the extent of the neuropathology was correlated with the severity of the hypotension.

These laboratory studies have confirmed that cerebral ischemia or global asphyxia of 10-min duration is consistently associated with brain damage. Sustained partial asphyxia of 1- to 3-hour duration may or may not be associated with brain damage. The key is the severity of the acidosis and the magnitude of the hypotension. Recent studies of repeated short episodes of cerebral ischemia or global asphyxial exposure suggest that the nature of the asphyxial exposure may be a factor contributing to the variability of the neuropathology observed in the different animals.

FETAL PATHOPHYSIOLOGY AFTER AN ASPHYXIAL EXPOSURE

The important feature of global asphyxia or cerebrovascular occlusion was the short duration of the sequence of events with limited compensation prior to the threshold of brain damage. These mechanisms may occur but are an infrequent cause of brain damage in a surviving newborn. On the other hand with partial asphyxia, the fetal brain is protected for variable periods (hours) before the threshold of metabolic acidosis and hypotension leading to brain damage has been reached. The variability of outcome after a fetal asphyxial exposure can be attributed to the concept emerging from these laboratory studies.

$$\text{Fetal exposure} + \text{Fetal response} = \text{Outcome}$$

This concept is expressed in greater detail in Figure 1. The fetus may be exposed to asphyxia with a developing metabolic acidosis. However, if the fetal compensatory cardiovascular response is maintained with increased blood flow to the brain, heart, and adrenals, then oxygen supply to these organ systems will be sustained and cerebral and other organ system dysfunction or damage will not occur. On the other hand, if the asphyxia persists with progression of the metabolic acidosis, then fetal decompensation with hypotension, decreased blood flow, and decreased oxygen supply to the brain will develop. The resulting tissue oxygen debt and anaerobic metabolism will initiate the cascade of biochemical events leading to brain cell dysfunction and death.

It is likely that this pathophysiological sequence of events in response to asphyxia operates in the human fetus. However, contrary to the animal studies in the laboratory, certain data are not available for the human fetus in the clinical setting. A fetal blood gas and acid–base assessment with a significant metabolic acidosis confirms that an asphyxial exposure has occurred and provides an indication of the severity at the time of sampling. However, the duration of the exposure or whether the exposure

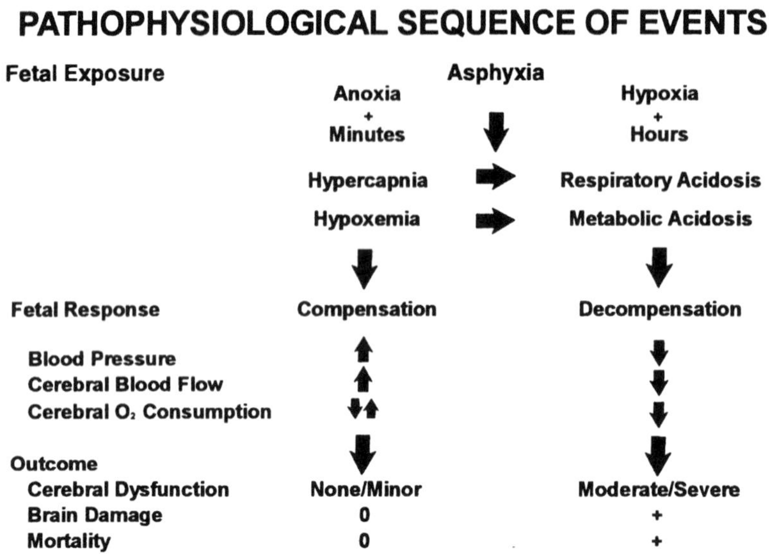

Figure 1. Fetal pathophysiology after an asphyxial exposure.

was continuous or intermittent is rarely known. Assessment of the fetal cardiovascular response as expressed by cardiac output, systemic blood pressure, and brain and other organ system blood flow is, in general, not available. Thus in the clinical setting, there is little information of fetal compensation or decompensation in response to the asphyxial exposure.

DEFINITION AND CLASSIFICATION OF FETAL ASPHYXIA

A task force set up by the World Federation of Neurology Group defined asphyxia as a condition of impaired gas exchange leading, if it persists, to progressive hypoxemia and hypercapnia (31). This is a good definition of asphyxia. However, in the fetus during labor, this may occur in a transient fashion which, although of physiological interest, has no pathological significance. Significant asphyxia leading to tissue oxygen debt with accumulation of fixed acids results in a metabolic acidosis. Thus for relevent fetal asphyxia during labor the following addition to this definition is proposed:

Fetal asphyxia is a condition of impaired blood gas exchange leading to progressive hypoxemia and hypercapnia with a significant metabolic acidosis.

The important question is the threshold of metabolic acidosis beyond which fetal morbidity or mortality may occur. There is a growing body of evidence from laboratory and clinical studies that the threshold for a significant metabolic acidosis is a

Table 5. Classification of intrapartum fetal asphyxia

Asphyxia	Metabolic Acidosis at Delivery[a]	Encephalopathy			Cardiovascular, Respiratory, and Renal Complications	
		Minor	Moderate	Severe	Minor	Moderate/Severe
Mild	+	+/–			+/–	
Moderate	+		+			+/–
Severe	+			+		+

[a]Umbilical artery base deficit ≥ 12 mmol/liter.

base deficit between 12 and 16 mmol/liter. Routine blood gas and acid–base assessment of umbilical artery blood at delivery has demonstrated an umbilical artery base deficit greater than 12 mmol/liter in 2% and greater than 16 mmol/liter in 0.5% of the total population. Thus during labor and delivery, 2% of fetuses have been exposed to asphyxia, which may affect their outcome.

A classification of the severity of a fetal asphyxial exposure is required to predict the long-term outcome in the child. Severity can be classified by determining the short-term outcome as expressed by newborn encephalopathy and other newborn organ system complications. This alternative is required because the duration of the asphyxia itself cannot be determined and the clinical measures of cardiovascular compensation and decompensation are not available. A classification of mild, moderate, and severe intrapartum fetal asphyxia is presented in Table 5. This is important for the 2% of newborns who experienced an asphyxial exposure. The majority of these events will be mild with little short- or long-term significance (32).

This classification is based on the evidence that at this time early onset newborn encephalopathy is the best single predictor of long-term outcome. Pelowski and Finer (33), in a review of five studies of term newborns, reported a good outcome for newborns with minor encephalopathy, whereas the risk of death or severe handicap in moderate encephalopathy was 5.6% and 20% and in severe newborn encephalopathy was 60% and 72%, respectively. Our experience of the frequency of handicaps in term newborns with moderate encephalopathy was 27% and with severe encephalopathy was 50% (34). Cardiovascular, respiratory, and renal complications provide a further indication of the severity of the asphyxial exposure.

CLINICAL STUDIES OF FETAL ASPHYXIA

The need has been for prospective clinical studies of biochemically determined fetal asphyxia to establish that, as in the animal studies, the human fetus can compensate with no morbidity or mortality until a particular threshold when decompensation occurs with morbidity or mortality. Current clinical studies have examined the association between fetal asphyxial exposure and outcome expressed by cerebral and other organ system dysfunction and brain damage.

NEWBORN MORBIDITY AFTER FETAL ASPHYXIA

Recent reports have examined the association between acidemia at delivery and newborn complications (35–38). All studies reported the occurrence of newborn complications when the acidosis was severe (i.e., an umbilical artery pH less than 7.0). These studies did not discriminate between a metabolic and respiratory acidosis and lacked a control group for the interpretation of outcome.

To determine the significance of respiratory acidosis, 51 term fetuses with no metabolic acidosis but a respiratory acidosis (umbilical artery $pCO_2 > 75$ mmHg) were compared to a control group with no respiratory or metabolic acidosis. There was no difference in the frequency or severity of newborn complications between the respiratory acidosis and control groups (39).

The significance of metabolic acidosis was determined in 59 term fetuses with metabolic acidosis (umbilical artery base deficit greater than 16 mmol/liter) matched with 59 term fetuses with normal blood gas measures at delivery. This study indicated that intrapartum fetal asphyxia with a severe metabolic acidosis was associated with a striking increase in the frequency and severity of complications in all systems. One factor discriminating the newborns with complications was the duration of the metabolic acidosis (expressed by the umbilical artery–vein base deficit difference) (39). Interpretation of the significance of fetal asphyxia in the preterm newborn is difficult. However, a matched case control study demonstrated that intrapartum fetal asphyxia with a severe metabolic acidosis in preterm newborns between 32 and 36 weeks' gestational age was associated with a striking increase in the frequency and severity of complications in all systems (40).

The threshold of metabolic acidosis in the term newborn associated with moderate and severe newborn complications was examined in a matched case control study comparing three groups defined by umbilical artery base deficit (UABD) at birth. The group criteria were UABD 4–8 mmol/liter, UABD 8–12 mmol/liter, and UABD 12–16 mmol/liter. These groups were compared to the term newborn with an UABD > 16 mmol/liter (Table 6). The frequency of moderate or severe newborn complications increases with increasing severity of the metabolic acidosis at delivery. The threshold of fetal metabolic acidosis at delivery when moderate and severe newborn complications and particularly central nervous system complications may occur was an umbilical artery base deficit of 12 mmol/liter (41).

Table 6. Threshold of metabolic acidosis in the term newborn

Newborn Complications Moderate/Severe	UABD 4–8 mmol/liter $n = 58$	UABD 8–12 mmol/liter $n = 58$	UABD 12–16 mmol/liter $n = 58$	UABD > 16 mmol/liter $n = 58$
CNS	2	0	5	24
Respiratory	0	3	9	8
Cardiovascular	0	1	1	18
Renal	0	1	2	8

There is a threshold of asphyxial exposure beyond which cerebral dysfunction and other organ system complications may occur. This dysfunction may be reversible and the clinical manifestations transient. However, in some cases, particularly those with moderate and severe newborn encephalopathy, brain damage may have occurred and account for subsequent motor and cognitive deficits.

BRAIN DAMAGE AFTER FETAL ASPHYXIA

The determination of the cause of brain damage in surviving newborns is complicated by the relatively low incidence of severe handicaps and the need for carefully controlled long-term follow-up to identify less severe handicap. Several studies have reported that metabolic acidosis in umbilical artery blood has been a poor predictor of subsequent neurological dysfunction (42–45). This is not suprising recognizing that asphyxia is only one of a number of mechanisms which may account for brain damage while the outcome after a fetal asphyxial exposure will be variable due to the complex pathophysiology.

Two studies indicate that asphyxial exposure of a duration or degree sufficient to cause major deficits may occur in surviving children. The occurrence of motor and cognitive deficits at 1 year of age has been examined in mature newborn infants after intrapartum fetal asphyxia (46). The outcome of 90 term infants with a metabolic acidosis at delivery (umbilical base deficit greater than 12 mmol/liter) was compared with that of 125 term infants with normal blood gas measures at delivery. Many children in the asphyxia group (72%) had normal motor and cognitive development at 1 year of age. However, the incidence of both major and minor deficits in the asphyxial group (28%) was significantly greater than that in the control group (15%).

The significance of intrapartum fetal asphyxia in the preterm fetus has also been examined in a matched case control study (47). Mortality with neuropathology on postmortem examination in the asphyxia group was significantly greater than that in the control group. Similarly, the incidence of major motor and cognitive deficits at 1 year of age in the surviving children of the asphyxia group (27%) was significantly greater than that in the control group (13%).

These studies highlight two points. There is a large number of newborns after an asphyxial exposure who do not exhibit evidence of brain damage. This implies that fetal compensation has protected the brain during the asphyxial exposure. On the other hand there was a small number with evidence of brain damage, with a correlation between the severity of the metabolic acidosis and the occurrence of motor and cognitive deficits.

In order to examine this question further, the outcome of term newborns after mild fetal asphyxia (i.e., metabolic acidosis UABD > 12 mmol/liter with no or mild newborn complications) was examined in a matched case control study. The incidence of motor and cognitive deficits at 1 year was of the same order in the asphyxia and control groups. Because of the possibility of less severe brain damage accounting for minor disabilities, the follow-up was continued to 8 years of age with assessment of motor and cognitive function and memory. Again, no significant difference was observed between the asphyxia and control groups (48).

These findings support the contention that the fetus has compensated and protected the brain in mild asphyxial exposures, and they are in keeping with previous reports that minor newborn encephalopathy is not associated with short-term major or long-term minor disability (49).

NEUROPATHOLOGY AFTER FETAL ASPHYXIA

The occurrence of brain damage has been confirmed in the human fetus by neuropathology following a perinatal death. Recent studies have examined the neuropathological findings in fetal and early neonatal deaths (50–53). The occurrence of neuropathology characteristic of asphyxia in these studies has emphasized the importance of antepartum asphyxia. It must be assumed that the fetus in these pregnancies has experienced a sublethal asphyxial exposure of a degree sufficient to cause brain damage. Although the neuropathology is characteristic of asphyxia, in the majority of cases the occurrence of the asphyxial exposure has not been confirmed biochemically. However, in recent years there have been a number of cases of confirmed asphyxial exposure with characteristic neuropathology on subsequent postmortem examination (54,55).

DISCUSSION

Laboratory research has provided the foundation of our understanding of fetal asphyxia. Fetal cardiovascular compensation in response to an asphyxial exposure protects vital organs, particularly the brain and heart. However, a sustained asphyxial exposure with a significant metabolic acidosis results in fetal decompensation with hypotension, decreased cerebral blood flow and cerebral tissue oxygen debt. In these circumstances brain damage may occur.

Global asphyxia results in brain damage after 10 min, followed by death shortly thereafter. Partial asphyxia is more complex. A wide range of duration and degree of asphyxia may occur either continuously or intermittently. The outcome is varied, ranging from no morbidity to short-term or long-term morbidity or mortality.

Clinical studies indicate that the common mechanism in the intrapartum period is partial asphyxia. The normal newborn outcome in the majority suggests that the asphyxial exposure has been mild and the fetal compensation has protected the fetus. On the other hand, there are some in whom the exposure has been more severe with evidence of cerebral and other organ system dysfunction; a few of these individuals will have brain damage expressed by (a) subsequent motor and cognitive deficits or (b) a fetal or neonatal death with neuropathology on postmortem examination.

A classification of asphyxia is important to predict outcome. The classification proposed includes a metabolic acidosis to confirm that an exposure has occurred; and the subsequent occurrence of newborn encephalopathy and other organ system complications reflects the severity of the exposure. Newborns after mild asphyxia will have normal motor and cognitive development. Newborns with moderate or severe asphyxia may or may not have evidence of brain damage with motor and cognitive handicaps in the surviving children.

The magnitude of the problem in the intrapartum period is now clear. Asphyxial exposure with a significant metabolic acidosis occurs in approximately 20 per 1000 births. Moderate and severe asphyxial exposure occurs in approximately 3 per 1000 births, of whom approximately 1 may have evidence of brain damage.

The responsibility of the caregiver is the early recognition of fetal asphyxia exposure and the prevention of morbidity and mortality. Since intrapartum asphyxia is usually partial and often intermittent, fetal compensation may be satisfactory for some time (i.e., hours). This is the window of opportunity during which the occurrence of asphyxial exposure can be confirmed and, when appropriate, intervention initiated before the threshold of decompensation has been reached.

REFERENCES

1. Little WJ. On the influence of abnormal parturition, difficult labour, premature birth and asphyxia neonatorum on the mental and physical condition of the child, especially in relation to deformities. *Trans London Obstet Soc* 1862;3:293–325.
2. Freud S. *Die infantile cerebral Lahmung.* Wien: A Holder. Translated by Russia IA as *Infantile cerebral paralysis.* Coral Gables, FL: University of Miami Press, 1968.
3. Windle WF (ed). *Neurological and psychological deficits of asphyxia neonatorum: with consideration of the use of primates for experimental investigations.* By twenty-eight contributors. Symposium in Neurology. Springfield, IL: Charles C Thomas, 1956.
4. Cohn HE, Sacks EJ, Heymann MA, Rudolph Am. Cardiovascular response to hypoxemia and acidemia in fetal lambs. *Am J Obstet Gynecol* 1974;120:817–824.
5. Peeters LL, Sheldon RD, Jones MD, Makowski EL, Meschia G. Blood flow to fetal organs as a function of arterial oxygen content. *Am J Obstet Gynecol* 1979;135:637–646.
6. Richardson BS, Rurak D, Patrick JE, Homan J, Carmichael L. Cerebral oxidative metabolism during sustained hypoxemia. *J Dev Physiol* 1989;11:37–43.
7. Richardson BS, Carmichael L, Homan J, Patrick JE. Cerebral oxidative metabolism in fetal sheep with prolonged and graded hypoxemia. *J Dev Physiol* 1993;10:77–83.
8. Field DR, Parer JT, Auslander RA, Cheek DB, Baker W, Johnson J. Cerebral oxygen consumption during asphyxia in fetal sheep. *J Dev Physiol* 1990;14:131–137.
9. Reid DL, Parer JT, Williams K, Darr D, Phermaton TM, Rankin JHH. Effects of severe reduction in maternal placental blood flow in blood flow distribution in the sheep fetus. *J Dev Physiol* 1991;15:183–188.
10. Jensen A, Roman C, Rudolph AM. Effects of reducing uterine blood flow on fetal blood flow distribution and oxygen delivery. *J Dev Physiol* 1991;15:309–323.
11. Ball RH, Espinoza MI, Parer JT. Regional blood flow in asphyxiated fetuses with seizures. *Am J Obstet Gynecol* 1994;170:156–161.
12. Itskovitz J, LaGamma EF, Rudolph AM. Effect of cord compression of fetal blood flow distribution and O_2 delivery. *Am J Physiol* 1987;252:H100–H109.
13. Ball RH, Parer JT, Caldwell LE, Johnson J. Regional blood flow and metabolism in ovine fetuses during severe cord occlusion. *Am J Obstet Gynecol* 1994;171:1549–1555.

14. Jensen A, Lang U. Fetal circulatory responses to arrest of uterine blood flow in sheep: effects of chemical sympathectomy. *J Dev Physiol* 1992;17:75–86.

15. Bartelds B, vanBel F, Teetel DF, Rudolph AM. Carotid not aortic chemoreceptors mediate the fetal cardiovascular response to acute hypoxemia in lambs. *Pediatr Res* 1993; 34:51–55.

16. LaGamma EF, Itskovitz J, Rudolph AM. Effect of naloxone on fetal circulatory responses to hypoxemia. *Am J Obstet Gynecol* 1982;143:933–940.

17. Richardson, BS, Patrick JE, Abduljabber H. Cerebral oxidative metabolism in fetal sheep: relationship to electrocortical state. *Am J Obstet Gynecol* 1985;153:426–431.

18. Williams CE, Gunn AJ, Mallard EC, Gluckman PD. Outcome after ischemia in the developing sheep brain: an electroencephalographic and histological study. *Ann Neurol* 1992;31:114–121.

19. Mallard EC, Williams CE, Gunn AJ, Gunning MI, Gluckman PD. Frequent episodes of brief ischemia sensitize the fetal sheep brain to neuronal loss and induce striatal injury. *Pediatr Res* 1993;33:61–65.

20. Ranck JE, Windle WF. Brain damage in the monkey *Mucacca mulatta* by asphyxia neonatorum. *Exp Neurol* 1959;1:130–154.

21. Mallard EC, Gunn AJ, Williams EJ, Johnston BM, Gluckman PD. Transient umbilical cord occlusion causes hippocampal damage in the fetal sheep. *Am J Obstet Gynecol* 1992;167:1423–1430.

22. Mallard EC, Waldvogel HJ, Williams CE, Faull RLM, Gluckman PD. Repeated asphyxia causes loss of striatal projection neurons in the fetal sheep brain. *Neuroscience* 1995;65:827–836.

23. deHaan HH, Gunn AJ, Gluckman PD. Experiments in perinatal brain injury: what have we learnt? *Prenat Neonat Med* 1996;1:16–25.

24. Mallard EC, Williams CE, Johnson BM, Gluckman PD. Increased vulnerability to neuronal damage following umbilical cord occlusion in the fetal sheep with advancing gestation. *Am J Obstet Gynecol* 1994;170:606–624.

25. Keunen H, Blanco CE, VanReempts JLH, Hassart THM. Absence of neuronal damage after cord occlusion of increasing duration in mid gestation fetal sheep. *Pedatr Res* 1995;37:381A.

26. Myers RE. Two patterns of perinatal brain damage and their conditions of occurrence. *Am J Obstet Gynecol* 1972;112:246–376.

27. Ting P, Yamaguchi S, Backer JD, Killens RH, Myers RE. Hypoxic-ischemic cerebral necrosis in mid-gestational sheep fetuses: physiopathologic correlations. *Exp Neurol* 1983;80:237–245.

28. Gunn AJ, Parer JT, Mallard EC, Williams CE, Gluckman PD. Cerebral histological and electrophysiological changes after asphyxia in fetal sheep. *Pediatr Res* 1992;31:486–491.

29. deHaan HH, vanReempts JLH, Vles JSH, deHaan J, Hassart THW. Effects of asphyxia on the fetal lamb brain. *Am J Obstet Gynecol* 1993;69:1493–1501.

30. Ikeda T, Murata Y, Qulligan EJ, Choi B, Parer JT, Doi S, Park SD. Physiological and histological changes in near term fetal lamb exposed to asphyxia by partial umbilical cord occlusion. *J Soc Gynecol Invest* 1996;3:256A.

31. Bax M, Nelson KB. Birth asphyxia: a statement. *Dev Med Child Neurol* 1993;35: 1002–1004.

32. Low JA. Intrapartum fetal asphyxia. Definition, diagnosis and classification. *AM J Obstet Gynecol* 1997;176:957–959.
33. Pelowski A, Finer NN. Birth asphyxia in the term infant. In Sinclair J, Lucey J (eds). *Effective care of the newborn infant.* Oxford: Oxford University Press, 1992;263–266.
34. Low JA, Galbraith RS, Muir DW, Killen HL, Pater EA. The relationship between perinatal hypoxia and newborn encephalopathy. *Am J Obstet Gynecol* 1985;152:256–260.
35. Gilstrap LC, Leveno KB, Burris J, Williams ML, Burris BB. Diagnosis of birth asphyxia on the basis of fetal ph, Apgar score, and newborn cerebral dysfunction. *Am J Obstet Gynecol* 1989;161:825–830.
36. Goldaber KG, Gilstrap LC, Leveno KB, Dax JS, McIntyre DD. Pathologic fetal acidemia. *Obstet Gynecol* 1997;78:1103–1106.
37. Winkler CL, Hauth JC, Tucker MJ, Owen J, Brumfield CG. Neonatal complications at term as related to the degree of umbilical artery acidemia. *Am J Obstet Gynecol* 1991;164:637–641.
38. Goodwin TM, Belai I, Hernandez P., Durance M, Paul RH. Asphyxial complications in the term newborn with severe umbilical acidemia. *Am J Obstet Gynecol* 1992;162:1506–1512.
39. Low JA, Panagiotopoulos C, Derrick EJ. Newborn complications after intrapartum asphyxia with metabolic acidosis at term. *Am J Obstet Gynecol* 1994;170:1081–1087.
40. Low JA, Panagiotopoulos C, Derrick EJ. Newborn complications after intrapartum asphyxia with metabolic acidosis in the preterm fetus. *Am J Obstet Gynecol* 1995;172:804–810.
41. Low JA, Lindsay BG, Derrick EJ. Threshold of metabolic acidosis associated with newborn complications. *Am J Obstet Gynecol* 1997;177:1391–1394.
42. Ruth VJ, Raivio KO. Perinatal brain damage: predictive value of metabolic acidosis and the Apgar score. *BMJ* 1988;297:24–27.
43. Dennis J, Johnson A, Mutch L, Yadkin P, Johnson P. Acid-base status at birth and neurodevelopmental outcome at four and one half years. *Am J Obstet Gynecol* 1989;161:213–220.
44. Fee SC, Malee, Deddish R, Minoque JP, Socol ML. Severe acidosis and subsequent neurological status. *Am J Obstet Gynecol* 1990;162:802–806.
45. Socol ML, Garcia PM, Riter S. Depressed Apgar score, acid–base status, and neurological outcome. *Am J Obstet Gynecol* 1994;170:991–999.
46. Low JA, Galbraith, RS, Muir DW, Killen HL, Pater EA, Karchmar EJ. Motor and cognitive deficits after intrapartum fetal asphyxia in the mature infant. *Am J Obstet Gynecol* 1988;158:356–361.
47. Low JA, Galbraith RS, Muir DW, Killen HL, Pater EA, Karchmar EJ. Mortality and morbidity after intrapartum asphyxia in the preterm fetus. *Obstet Gynecol* 1992;80:57–61.
48. Handley-Derry M, Low JA, Burke SO, Waurick M, Killen HL, Derrick EJ. Intrapartum fetal asphyxia and the occurrence of minor deficits in 4 to 8 year old child. *Dev Med Child Neurol* 1997;39:508–574.
49. Robertson CM, Finer NN, Grace MG. School performance of survivors of neonatal encephalopathy associated with birth asphyxia at term. *J Pediatr* 1989;114:753–760.
50. Ellis WG, Goetsman BW, Laidenberg JA. Neuropathologic documentation of prenatal brain damage. *Am J Dis Child* 1988;142:858–866.
51. Wigglesworth JS. Pathophysiology of prenatal brain damage. In Merialdi A, Vidora E (eds). *L'Ostetricia oggi il danno cerebrale feto-neonatale.* Bologna: Munduzi Editore, 1991:47–51.

52. Iida K, Takashima S, Takenchi Y. Neuropathologic study of newborns with prenatal onset of leukomalacia. *Pediatr Neurol* 1993;9:45–48.
53. Burke CJ, Tannenberg AE. Prenatal brain damage and placental infarction, an autopsy study. *Dev Med Child Neurol* 1995;37:555–562.
54. Low JA, Robertson DM, Simpson LL. Temporal relationships of neuropathologic conditions caused by perinatal asphyxia. *Am J Obstet Gynecol* 1989;160:609–614.
55. Low JA, Ludwin SK, Fisher S. Severe fetal asphyxia with neuropathology. *Am J Obstet Gynecol* 1996;175:1383–1385.

3

FETAL ADAPTIVE RESPONSES TO HYPOXIA: PHYSIOLOGICAL BASIS FOR FETAL MONITORING

Bryan S. Richardson, M.D., F.R.C.S.C.

Department of Obstetrics and Gynaecology and Department of Physiology, The Lawson Research Institute, St. Joseph's Health Centre, University of Western Ontario, London, Ontario, Canada

INTRODUCTION

The fetus lives and grows in a relatively "hypoxic" environment and yet normally exists with a surplus of oxygen for metabolic needs. When oxygenation is compromised, the fetus is capable of a number of adaptive responses, both protective and potentially pathologic, which can be categorized as those affecting fetal metabolism and those affecting fetal oxygen transport (outlined in Table 1). These adaptive responses in turn provide a physiologic basis for the monitoring techniques used in clinical practice in the assessment of fetal health. This review focuses on those metabolic and O_2 transport adaptations directly related to the clinical assessment of fetal well-being. Much of this information is based on experimental study using unanesthetized fetal sheep with chronic catheterization; however, clinical outcome data and the use of investigative techniques including

Asphyxia and Fetal Brain Damage, Edited by Dev Maulik, M.D., Ph.D.
ISBN 0-471-18427-6

Table 1. Fetal responses to hypoxemia

Fetal Metabolism
"Oxygen Margin of Safety"
Substrate alterations
Decreased growth
Behavioral state alterations
Decreased fetal movements
Fetal O_2 Transport
Increased blood O_2 capacity
Blood flow redistribution

ultrasound scanning and cordocentesis have supported the relevance of such study to the human situation.

FETAL METABOLISM AND OXYGEN TRANSPORT

Substrate consumption has been well studied in the chronically catheterized ovine fetus using Fick methodology with measurements of umbilical or cotyledonary blood flow and the venoarterial substrate difference across the placenta. Oxygen consumption rates measured by this means approximate 8 $ml{\cdot}min^{-1}{\cdot}kg^{-1}$ body weight for the ovine fetus near term (1). Glucose would appear to be the major metabolic fuel of the ovine fetus, capable of sustaining 50–70% of oxidative metabolism and representing 20% of the total caloric requirement, but with substantial uptake also of lactate and amino acids (1). Studies in the human fetus at the time of elective cesarean section again suggest glucose to be the major metabolic fuel with a slightly higher uptake relative to O_2 than in the ovine fetus (2).

This substrate consumption by the fetus serves two basic requirements: (1) provision of fuel for energy production through maintenance of oxidative metabolism; and, (2) provision of building materials for tissue growth (Figure 1). Although oxidative metabolism is the major component of total substrate needs, tissue growth requirements may not be insignificant depending on the rate of growth relative to ongoing energy requirements. For the ovine fetus near term, tissue growth requirements in fact account for approximately one-third of total substrate needs when expressed in terms of caloric equivalents (1). Furthermore, an unknown fraction of the energy produced from oxidative metabolism must fuel tissue growth. A variable "savings" in both ATP energy requirements and substrate building needs might therefore be realized with a fall-off in tissue growth when O_2 and substrate availability to the fetus becomes limited.

The transport of oxygen from the atmosphere to the fetal tissues requires a series of steps alternating bulk transport with transport by diffusion (Figure 2). The normally low fetal arterial blood partial pressure of oxygen, of approximately 20 mmHg, can be largely attributed to two aspects of this transport process: (1) the venous equi-

FETAL METABOLISM

OXYGEN CONSUMPTION

GLUCOSE CONSUMPTION

Energy Production
- Tissue maintenance
- Functional activity
- Growth

Growth

Figure 1. Fetal metabolic needs.

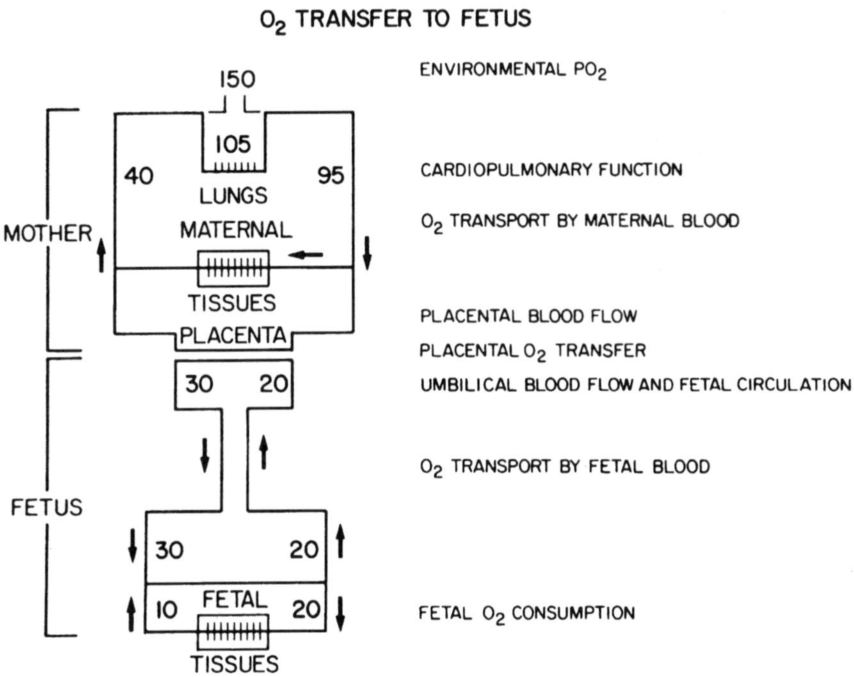

Figure 2. Maternal and fetal circulations. Numbers refer to pO_2 of each compartment (i.e., inspired air, alveolar air, maternal arterial and venous blood, umbilical venous and arterial blood, and fetal venous blood). (Modified from reference 5.)

libration of placental gas exchange whereby functionally both maternal and fetal vascular streams run in the same direction; and (2) the admixture of umbilical venous and inferior vena caval blood within the fetus, although that supplying the upper body and head region has a slightly higher pO_2 due to preferential streaming of umbilical venous blood across the foramen ovale (3,4).

In spite of the normally low arterial pO_2, the transport of oxygen to fetal tissues appears more than adequate, with no evidence for anaerobic glycolysis as a terminal source for energy production (1). This is due in part to the increased O_2 carrying capacity of fetal blood, in turn due to the higher hemoglobin concentration which increases throughout gestation (5), and to the higher oxygen affinity, which permits the saturation of fetal blood with oxygen at a lower oxygen partial pressure. A second means whereby the oxygenation of fetal tissues is maintained is the relative overperfusion of fetal organs in comparison with their O_2 requirements. The result is an oxygen concentration in fetal blood only slightly less than that in maternal blood and oxygen delivery to some organs actually in excess of their adult counterparts.

FETAL RESPONSES TO HYPOXEMIA

Interference with the transport of oxygen (and possibly of carbon dioxide) to (and from) the fetus can occur at any one of the transport steps as indicated in Table 2. However, the extent to which gas exchange is impaired covers a spectrum and may lead to mild hypoxemia alone, or to severe hypoxemia with hypercapnia and progressive metabolic acidemia. Likewise, the time course over which the impairment in gas exchange occurs may operate acutely over minutes or hours, subacutely over days, or chronically over weeks. Both the extent to which gas exchange is impaired and the duration of this impairment will come to bear on fetal adaptive responses.

Oxygen Margin of Safety (Table 3)

While interference with the transport of O_2 to the fetus can occur at any one of a number of different transport steps, ultimately this gives rise to either a lowered umbilical venous O_2 concentration or a lowered umbilical blood flow with a corresponding reduction in O_2 delivery to the fetus. With a decrease in O_2 delivery, however, the fetus is capable of a compensatory increase in fractional O_2 extraction, thus maintaining O_2 consumption (O_2 consumption = O_2 delivery × O_2 fractional extraction). Because O_2 extraction is a function of diffusion, any increase must involve an increase in the pO_2 gradient across the umbilical circulation, ultimately resulting in a drop in arterial pO_2 and thus fetal hypoxemia. The degree to which fractional O_2 extraction can increase and fetal arterial pO_2 can fall before tissue O_2 supplies are inadequate and become rate-limiting for O_2 consumption is the "oxygen margin of safety" as an indication of the oxygen reserve available to the fetus when O_2 delivery is decreased.

Studies in the ovine fetus with acute reductions in fetal oxygen delivery induced by different means (6–8) show fetal oxygen consumption to be variably maintained

Table 2. Factors decreasing O_2 transfer to the fetus

Environmental pO_2
High altitude
Maternal Cardiopulmonary Function
Cyanotic heart disease
O_2 Transport by Maternal Blood
Anemia
Cigarette smoking
Placental Blood Flow
Hypertension
Diabetes
Abruptio placenta
Uterine contractions
Placental O_2 Transfer
Abruptio placenta
Placental infarcts
Umbilical Blood Flow and Fetal Circulation
Umbilical cord occlusion
Heart disease
O_2 Transport by Fetal Blood
Anemia
Hemorrhage

Table 3. Oxygen margin of safety

Physiologic Considerations

- The O_2 margin of safety is an acute adaptive response to a limitation in oxygen availability.
- The O_2 margin of safety provides for increased tolerance of obstetrical emergencies with the fetus hypoxemic at birth, but usually without metabolic acidemia.
- The O_2 margin of safety will be lower in the IUGR and post-term fetus.

by increases in O_2 extraction until oxygen delivery is reduced by approximately 50%. That fetal O_2 consumption is maintained despite such a decrease in O_2 delivery, and thus a moderate degree of hypoxemia, is somewhat surprising since the metabolic costs of fetal movement activity and growth should diminish quickly. This suggests that other metabolic costs are increased in response to acute hypoxia which may relate to the cardiovascular and hormonal changes that occur (7,9), with increases in O_2 consumption by the myocardium, and in relation to the increase in catecholamines and possibly activated thermogenesis. The human fetus undoubtedly is also capable of this adaptive response, and this gives rise to an increased tolerance of obstetrical emergencies such as umbilical cord prolapse with the fetus at birth being hypoxemic, but usually without metabolic acidemia. However, the oxygen reserve available to the human fetus may be less than that of the ovine fetus, because the O_2 extraction with uneventful vaginal or cesarean delivery normally measures somewhat higher than that of the ovine fetus in utero (10).

With sustained hypoxemia of 24-hour duration and of a moderate degree induced by reducing uterine blood flow (11), fetal oxygen consumption continues to be maintained and O_2 extraction increased, indicating that the overall balance between decreasing and increasing metabolic costs remains unchanged. However, with prolonged reductions in fetal oxygen delivery over several days, the ovine fetus shows little change in O_2 extraction, with oxygen consumption now a linear function of oxygen delivery (12). This indicates that the fetus responds differently to long-term reductions in oxygenation (and/or other substrate deficiencies), with the decrease in oxygen-consuming processes (such as growth and perhaps certain aspects of behavioral activity) contributing to a reduction in oxygen needs over time because hormonal changes and any related increase in metabolic costs also diminish (13).

Intrauterine Growth Restriction (Table 4)

Growth is known to account for a consequential fraction of the total substrate consumption in the ovine fetus near term, as previously reviewed. With acutely induced hypoxemia of several hours' duration, protein synthesis in the ovine fetus is decreased, with a corresponding decrease in the energy requirements for growth equivalent to approximately 10% of total oxygen consumption (14). With both prolonged reduction in fetal oxygen delivery over several days (12) and induced IUGR (15,16) in the ovine fetus, total oxygen consumption is reduced approximately 20%. This decrease in fetal oxidative metabolism again represents the energy "savings" from decreased tissue growth and possibly changes in behavioral activity and associated energy requirements. The ovine fetus thus demonstrates a rapid adaptation to a limitation in substrate delivery with a decrease in growth rate (and activity) and thereby substrate needs, resulting in metabolic normalization with a variable degree of hypoxemia and usually little evidence of metabolic acidosis or anaerobic metabolism (15–17). Of note, recent studies with prolonged but gradual reductions in fetal oxygen delivery over the last 3–4 weeks of gestation induced by either chronic maternal anemia (18) or restricting uterine blood flow (19) have resulted in growth-restricted fetuses but without hypoxemia. This would suggest that when oxygenation is chronically compromised, if decreased fetal growth is sufficient, the fall-off in oxygen consumption may balance that for oxygen delivery such that fetal arterial pO_2 is in fact normalized.

Table 4. Intrauterine growth restriction

Physiologic Considerations

- IUGR is a chronic adaptive response to a limitation in substrate availability.
- Antepartum cordocentesis and umbilical cord gases at birth indicate variable hypoxemia, but usually without metabolic acidemia.
- IUGR at some point in time becomes maladaptive.

The human fetus also undergoes intrauterine growth restriction when oxygenation is compromised as seen with placental pathology and determined clinically by serial ultrasound assessment. Cordocentesis data indicate variable degrees of fetal hypoxemia (20,21), although in many instances blood gas values are within the normal range, again suggesting a degree of normalization with the fall-off in growth. However, the extent to which this mechanism is protective by decreasing substrate requirements for energy and growth, or gives rise to pathologic development of certain organ systems with time, is not known. It is possible that abnormalities in brain growth and development may contribute to the minimal cerebral dysfunction noted in follow-up studies of growth restricted infants (22).

Decreased Fetal Movements (Table 5)

Although the overall effect of behavioral state on fetal metabolic rate is minimal, at least for the ovine fetus, that of state-related biophysical parameters appears considerably greater. Neuromuscular blockade in the ovine fetus results in an approximate 20% decrease in oxygen consumption (23), presumably due in part to a decrease in breathing activity and other gross body movements. Conversely, fetal oxygen consumption is increased to a similar extent during periods of fetal breathing activity when compared to apneic periods (24). As such, a decrease in fetal movements in response to a compromise in oxygenation should reduce energy expenditure and thus oxygen requirements depending on the extent to which muscular activity is decreased.

In the near-term ovine fetus, moderate hypoxemia of short-term duration results in a marked decrease in movement activity, including forelimb, eye, and breathing movements (25–27). However, if this degree of hypoxemia is maintained in the absence of metabolic acidemia, movement activity returns toward normal after several hours (28,29). With prolonged and graded reductions in fetal oxygenation over several days, a marked decrease in fetal movement activity is only seen as the degree of hypoxemia approaches the level at which acidemia becomes apparent (30). As such,

Table 5. Decreased fetal movements

Physiologic Considerations

- Biologic as well as pathologic factors have been shown to affect fetal breathing and body movements (e.g., gestational age, behavioral state, parturition, drugs/medications).
- The preterm fetus may show less reduction in movement activity in response to hypoxemia.
- Animal studies and clinical assessment of the dynamic biophysical variables would suggest a decrease in fetal breathing movements to be an earlier indicator of fetal compromise.
- A marked decrease in fetal movement activity may only be evident with moderate to severe hypoxemia.
- The observation of the three dynamic biophysical variables, fetal breathing movements, body movements, and non-stress heart rate testing allows only for the assessment of fetal health at the time of testing.
- With IUGR, fetal movement activity is variably decreased; however, there is considerable overlap with population norms.

fetal movement assessment should be seen as a marker for moderate to severe hypoxemic change. Of note, the biophysical response of the preterm ovine fetus to induced hypoxemia is less pronounced than that of the older-gestational-aged fetus (31), which may impact on survival and have implications for the success of antenatal assessment protocols. With induced intrauterine growth restriction in the ovine fetus and variable degrees of hypoxemia, breathing movements are marginally decreased, occurring approximately 20% of the time (17). While of probable biologic importance and providing for a decrease in oxidative needs, this would not be a useful clinical marker given the effects of other influencing factors, including the diurnal and cyclic nature of breathing activity (32).

In the human fetus, movement activity has been extensively studied in the "high-risk" obstetrical patient as a component part of biophysical profile assessment (33–36). As used in the biophysical profile, fetal breathing and body movements have been scored in an "all-or-none" manner and related to a number of outcomes including subsequent intrauterine demise, fetal distress in labor requiring operative intervention, abnormal 5-minute Apgar score, abnormal umbilical cord gases and/or pH, and intrauterine growth restriction. While these endpoints differ somewhat, the physiologic basis for the use of fetal activity in the biophysical assessment of fetal health is the same; that is, with a compromise in oxygenation leading to hypoxemia with or without associated acidosis, fetal movement activity will decrease as an adaptive response whereby energy expenditure is also decreased.

As presently scored within the biophysical profile, fetal breathing movements are more likely to be falsely abnormal or positive at 26–33 weeks' gestation when compared to 34–41 weeks' gestation (37). This is in keeping with the lower incidence of breathing activity in younger fetuses (31), and it emphasizes the need to establish population norms reflecting the biological patterns and known factors affecting this activity. Likewise, non-stress testing is more likely to be falsely nonreactive prior to 32 weeks' gestation (38), again reflecting well-described maturational changes whereby the amplitude in fetal heart rate acceleration in association with body movements is normally less prior to this gestational age (39).

The negative predictive value for a normal perinatal outcome is high and similar among the three dynamic biophysical variables—fetal breathing movements, gross body movements, and non-stress heart rate testing—and is on the order of 95% with little improvement when test results are combined (33,40,41). However, the positive predictive value for an abnormal perinatal outcome is improved and the false-positive rate decreased when test results are combined. For the dynamic fetal variables, a decrease in body movements would appear to improve the positive predictive value for adverse perinatal outcome more than a decrease in breathing movements or a nonreactive non-stress fetal heart rate test (35,42). However, such comparisons are without statistical relationship to physiologic incidence data, because the unweighted and somewhat arbitrary scoring system currently used does not provide for the quantification of the dynamic fetal variables and their normal population standards (43). Conversely, blood gas data from the umbilical cord obtained immediately after biophysical assessment indicate that a nonreactive non-stress test and loss of fetal breathing are earlier signs of fetal acidosis and worsening hypoxemia than a loss of fetal movement (34,36). This would imply a hierarchy within the fetal brain for the control of these activities in response to onsetting hypoxemia and/or associated acidemia. Although this may be true, as suggested by studies in the ovine fetus (30), the clinical evidence to date shows considerable overlap of blood gas and pH values among test groupings and is again largely based on arbitrary standards without relation to normative values.

While the negative predictive value for a normal perinatal outcome is high with biophysical profile scoring, there continues to be a small number of patients with adverse perinatal outcome that is not predicted on the basis of dynamic fetal monitoring (44). This serves to emphasize that the monitoring of fetal movement activity only allows for the assessment of fetal health at the time of testing, from which a probability of continued health may be formulated. An improvement in negative predictive value might occur with more frequent testing, but the time course over which these variables become abnormal with a compromise in fetal oxygenation may well vary with different pregnancy complications and their severity. The marked decrease in fetal movement activity required for an abnormal biophysical profile score with the "all-or-none" criteria would appear to be a marker for moderate to severe hypoxemic change with onsetting acidemia as determined by related changes in umbilical cord gases and pH (34,36). This is similar to that discussed for the ovine fetus with prolonged and graded reductions in oxygenation (30); and again it suggests the need for heightened surveillance in the extremely high-risk pregnancy, perhaps with daily monitoring because metabolic deterioration may occur rapidly as acidemia worsens.

In patients with intrauterine growth restriction and presumed chronic fetal hypoxemia, fetal breathing and body movements are reported to be variably decreased and appear dependent on the severity of IUGR and the conditions and duration of study (45,46). Although of probable biologic importance with an associated decrease in energy expenditure, there is again considerable overlap with population norms, which would limit the usefulness of these parameters—at least as used clinically—as markers for intrauterine growth restriction.

Blood Flow Redistribution (Table 6)

Hypoxemia results in well-described changes within the fetal circulation, both centrally and peripherally, thus enhancing the delivery of oxygen to so-called vital organs. Acute hypoxic stress in the ovine fetus increases umbilical venous return through the ductus venosus and the preferential streaming of this blood through the foramen ovale, facilitating the delivery of the most highly oxygenated blood to the upper body and thus to the heart and brain (3,4). Peripherally, acutely induced hypoxemia results in a redistribution of cardiac output such that umbilical–placental flow is maintained, that to the heart, brain, and adrenals is increased, and that to other fetal tissues is variously maintained or decreased depending on the means by which hypoxemia is induced and the severity of the insult (47–49). In the ovine fetus, this redistribution of cardiac output results in a hyperbolic increase in that directed to the heart and brain in inverse relation to arterial O_2 content such that oxygen delivery to these tissues is well maintained (50). The mechanisms whereby these circulatory

Table 6. Blood flow redistribution

Physiologic Considerations

- Blood flow redistribution to vital organs is both an acute and chronic adaptive response to a limitation in oxygen availability.
- Blood flow redistribution in response to hypoxemia may be less effective for the preterm fetus.
- Biologic as well as pathologic factors have been shown to affect Doppler measured flow-velocity waveform indices (e.g., gestational age, behavioral state).
- Doppler measured flow-velocity waveform indices, although reflecting down-stream vascular resistance, are also affected by vascular impedance and pressure pulsatility.
- With IUGR, fetal Doppler measured indices are variably abnormal; however, there is considerable overlap with population norms dependent in part on the degree of IUGR and the etiology for such.
- Doppler waveform indices may be of clinical use in identifying placental pathology and/or associated circulatory change in response to hypoxemia; however, these measurements should represent a continuum with no "critical change" per se when worsening hypoxemia results in onsetting metabolic acidosis.

changes occur have also been well studied (3,4), and they variously reflect an interplay between local direct effects with changes in blood gases and pH, reflex effects initiated by baro- or chemoreceptors and mediated through the autonomic nervous system, and hormonal influences including catecholamines, the renin-angiotensin system, vasopressin, ACTH, and cortisol.

The protective redistribution of cardiac output is maintained in the ovine fetus when acutely induced hypoxemia is sustained for up to 48 hours by restricting uterine blood flow (51). Of note, however, whereas oxygen delivery to the brain is maintained by the increase in brain blood flow, that to heart and adrenals is substantially increased when measured after 48 hours of sustained hypoxemia. After 7 days of induced hypoxemia with chronic fetal anemia, blood flow to the brain, heart, and adrenals is again increased; however, while oxygen delivery to the heart is still increased, that to the brain and adrenals is now decreased (52). The regional distribution of blood flow in response to chronic hypoxemia can thus be seen to change over time and will again reflect the interplay between local and reflex mechanisms and changing hormonal influences, although not well studied. Underlying changes in tissue metabolic rate are also likely to be operative given the tight flow-metabolism coupling for some organs, including the brain (53) and the heart (54). While there has been limited study to date, the redistribution of blood flow to vital organs in response to hypoxic insults may be less effective for the preterm ovine fetus (55,56).

The introduction of combined real-time and pulsed Doppler ultrasound has provided a noninvasive means of monitoring the human fetal circulation. Doppler measured indices derived from velocity waveforms are assumed to be a reflection of downstream vascular resistance, and as such they may provide an indirect measure of fetal circulatory change in certain high-risk pregnancies. In patients with intrauterine growth restriction and presumed chronic fetal hypoxemia, these waveform indices are variably altered with a decrease in the cerebral circulation and an increase in the descending aorta and lower extremity (57–59) in keeping with a redistribution of blood flow to vital organs as in the ovine fetus. The ratio of the ductus venosus to umbilical blood flow has also been studied in growth-restricted fetuses and found to be increased (60) again as seen centrally with the redistribution of blood flow in the ovine fetus. However, all of these measurements show considerable overlap with population norms, since Doppler measured waveform indices are also affected by other biologic and hemodynamic factors (61–64) and growth restriction may lead to metabolic normalization. Additionally, while Doppler waveform indices may be of clinical use in identifying placental pathology leading to growth restriction and/or associated circulatory change in response to hypoxemia, thus differentiating the constitutionally small fetus, these measurements should represent a continuum with no "critical change" per se when hypoxemia is of a sufficient degree to result in onsetting metabolic acidosis.

SUMMARY

The different means of fetal surveillance that test for a compromise in oxygenation basically involve testing for causative factors (placental insufficiency with altered umbilical flow velocity waveform patterns as measured with Doppler ultrasound), testing for level of oxygen directly (umbilical cord blood gases and pH as measured with cordocentesis), and testing for reactive/adaptive responses (a decrease in growth as measured with ultrasound, decreases in fetal movement activity as measured with biophysical profile scoring and non-stress testing, and blood flow redistribution as measured with Doppler ultrasound). Whether or not these tests become abnormal will depend in part on (a) the causative role of placental insufficiency versus other factors, (b) the degree of fetal hypoxemia and onsetting acidemia, and (c) the time available for reactive/adaptive responses. Studies in the ovine fetus and with supporting evidence from the human indicate that intrauterine growth restriction is an adaptive response whereby energy expenditure is decreased and, if balanced against the compromise in oxygenation, may lead to a normalization of blood gas values. Impairments in fetal oxygenation which operate acutely over minutes or hours, or subacutely over days, will affect movement activity and circulatory patterns but will not affect growth, at least as measured clinically with serial ultrasound assessment. It is against this complex interaction between causative factors for fetal hypoxia and reactive/adaptive responses that the different means of fetal surveillance are compared, with additional consideration for the normative range of test values, the biologic factors also affecting these values, and the outcomes to be determined.

ACKNOWLEDGMENTS

The author wishes to thank Dr. Robert Gagnon and Dr. Renato Natale for their interest in this work, and he also wishes to thank Mrs. Patricia McCallum for technical assistance.

The author is supported by a Group Grant in Fetal and Neonatal Health and Development by the Medical Research Council of Canada.

REFERENCES

1. Battaglia FC, Meschia G. Principal substrates of fetal metabolism. *Physiol Rev* 1978;58:499–527.
2. Morriss FH, Makowski EL, Meschia G, Battaglia, FC. The glucose/oxygen quotient of the term human fetus. *Biol Neonate* 1975;25:44–52.
3. Rudolph AM. The fetal circulation and its response to stress. *J Dev Physiol* 1984;6:11–19.
4. Rudolph AM, Itskovitz J, Iwamoto H, Reuss, ML, Heymann M. Fetal cardiovascular responses to stress. *Semin Perinatol* 1981;5:109–121.
5. Towell ME. Fetal respiratory physiology. In Goodwin JW, Godden JO, Chance GW (eds). *Perinatal medicine*. Toronto: Longman Canada Ltd; 1976:171–186.
6. Itskovitz J, La Gamma EF, Rudolph AM. The effect of reducing umbilical blood flow on fetal oxygenation. *Am J Obstet Gynecol* 1983;145:813–818.
7. Rurak DW, Richardson BS, Patrick JE, Carmichael L, Homan J. Oxygen consumption in the fetal lamb during sustained hypoxemia with progressive acidemia. *Am J Physiol* 1990;258:R1108–R1115.
8. Wilkening RB, Meschia G. Fetal oxygen uptake, oxygenation, and acid–base balance as a function of uterine blood flow. *Am J Physiol* 1983;244:H749–H755.
9. Rurak DW, Richardson BS, Patrick JE, Carmichael L, Homan J. Blood flow and oxygen delivery to fetal organs and tissues during sustained hypoxemia. *Am J Physiol* 1990;258:R1116–R1122.
10. Rurak DW, Selke P, Fisher M, Taylor AHT, Wittman B. Fetal oxygen extraction: comparison of the human and sheep. *Am J Obstet Gynecol* 1987;156:360–366.
11. Bocking AD, White SE, Homan J, Richardson BS. Oxygen consumption is maintained in fetal sheep during prolonged hypoxaemia. *J Dev Physiol* 1992;17:169–174.
12. Anderson DF, Parks GM, Faber JJ. Fetal O_2 consumption in sheep during controlled long-term reductions in umbilical blood flow. *Am J Physiol* 1986;250:H1037–H1042.
13. Hooper SB, Coulter CL, Deayton JM, Harding R, Thorburn GD. Fetal endocrine responses to prolonged hypoxemia in sheep. *Am J Physiol* 1990;259:R703–R708.
14. Milley JR. Protein synthesis during hypoxia in fetal lambs. *Am J Physiol* 1987; 252: E519–E524.
15. Clapp JF, Szeto HH, Larrow R, Hewitt J, Mann, LI. Fetal metabolic response to experimental placental vascular damage. *Am J Obstet Gynecol* 1981;140:446–451.
16. Owens JA, Falconer J, Robinson JS. Effect of restriction of placental growth on fetal and utero-placental metabolism. *J Dev Physiol* 1987;9:225–238.
17. Worthington D, Piercy WN, Smith BT. Effects of reduction of placental size in sheep. *Obstet Gynecol* 1981;58-215–221.
18. Mostello D, Chalk C, Khoury J, Mack CE, Siddiqi TA, Clark KE. Chronic anemia in pregnant ewes: maternal and fetal effects. *Am J Physiol* 1991;261:R1075–R1083.
19. Lang U, Baker RS, Fisher UK, Clark KE. Intrauterine growth retardation following restriction of uterine blood flow: Effects on fetal oxygen delivery. 40th Annual Meeting of the Society for Gynecologic Investigation, Toronto, Ontario, 1993;Abstract 5191.

20. Pardi G, Buscaglia M, Ferrazzi E, Bazzetti P, Marconi, A, Cetin I. Cord sampling for the evaluation of oxygenation and acid-base balance in growth retarded human fetuses. *Am J Obstet Gynecol* 1987;157:1221–1228.

21. Soothill PW, Nicolaides KH, Campbell S. Prenatal asphyxia, hyperlacticaemia, hypoglycaemia, and erythroblastosis in growth retarded fetuses. *Br Med J* 1987;294:1051–1053.

22. Allen MC. Developmental outcome and followup of the small for gestational age infant. *Semin Perinatol* 1984;8:123–156.

23. Rurak DW, Gruber NC. The effect of neuromuscular blockade on oxygen consumption and blood gases in the fetal lamb. *Am J Obstet Gynecol* 1983;145:258–262.

24. Rurak DW, Gruber NC. Increased oxygen consumption associated with breathing activity in fetal lambs. *J Appl Physiol* 1983;54:701–707.

25. Boddy K, Dawes GS, Fisher R, Pinter S, Robinson JS. Foetal respiratory movements, electrocortical and cardiovascular responses to hypoxemia and hypercapnia in sheep. *J Physiol* 1974;243:599–618.

26. Koos BJ, Sameshima H, Power GG. Fetal breathing, sleep state, and cardiovascular responses to graded hypoxia in sheep. *J Appl Physiol* 1987;62:1033–1039.

27. Natale R, Clewlow F, Dawes GS. Measurement of fetal forelimb movements in the lamb in utero. *Am J Obstet Gynecol* 1981;140:545–551.

28. Bocking AD, Gagnon R, Milne KM, White SE. Behavioural activity during prolonged hypoxemia in fetal sheep. *J Appl Physiol* 1988;65:2420–2426.

29. Koos BJ, Kitanaka T, Matsuda K, Gilbert RD, Longo LD. Fetal breathing adaptation to prolonged hypoxemia in sheep. *J Dev Physiol* 1988;10:161–166.

30. Richardson B, Carmichael L, Homan J, Patrick J. Electrocortical activity, electroocular activity and breathing movements in fetal sheep with prolonged and graded hypoxemia. *Am J Obstet Gynecol* 1992;167:553–558.

31. Matsuda J, Patrick J, Carmichael L, Challis J, Richardson B. Effects of sustained hypoxemia on the sheep fetus at midgestation: endocrine, cardiovascular, and biophysical responses. *Am J Obstet Gynecol* 1992;167:531–540.

32. Dawes GS, Fox HE, Leduc BM, Liggins M, Richards RT. Respiratory movements and rapid eye movement sleep in the foetal lamb. *J Physiol* 1972;220:119–143.

33. Manning FA, Platt LD, Sipos L. Antepartum fetal evaluation: development of a fetal biophysical profile. *Am J Obstet Gynecol* 1980;136:787–795.

34. Manning FA, Snijders R, Harman CR, Nicolaides K, Menticoglou S, Morrison I. Fetal biophysical profile score. VI. Correlation with antepartum umbilical venous fetal pH. *Am J Obstet Gynecol* 1993;169:755–763.

35. Vintzileos AM, Campbell WA, Ingardia CJ, Nochimson DJ. The fetal biophysical profile and its predictive value. *Obstet Gynecol* 1983;62:271–278.

36. Vintzileos AM, Gaffney SE, Salinger LM, Kontopoulos VG, Campbell WA, Nochimson DJ. The relationship among the fetal biophysical profile, umbilical cord pH, and Apgar scores. *Am J Obstet Gynecol* 1987;157:627–631.

37. Baskett TF. Gestational age and fetal biophysical assessment. *Am J Obstet Gynecol* 1988;158:332–334.

38. Vintzileos AM, Feinstein SJ, Lodeiro JG, Campbell WA, Weinbaum PJ, Nochimson DJ. Fetal biophysical profile and the effect of premature rupture of the membranes. *Obstet Gynecol* 1986;67:818–823.

39. Natale R, Nasello-Paterson C, Turliuk R. Longitudinal measurements of fetal breathing, body movements, heart rate, and heart rate accelerations and decelerations at 24–32 weeks of gestation. *Am J Obstet Gynecol* 1985;151:256–263.
40. Schifrin BS, Guntes V, Gergely RC, Eden R, Roll K, Jacobs J. The role of real-time scanning in antenatal fetal surveillance. *Am J Obstet Gynecol* 1981;140:525–530.
41. Baskett TF, Gray JH, Prewett SJ, Young LM, Allen AC. Antepartum fetal assessment using a fetal biophysical profile score. *Am J Obstet Gynecol* 1984;148:630–633.
42. Platt LD, Eglinton GS, Sipos L, Broussard PM, Paul RH. Further experience with the fetal biophysical profile. *Obstet Gynecol* 1983:61:480–485.
43. Devoe LD, Castillo RA, Searle N, Searle JS. Prognostic components of computerized fetal biophysical testing *Am J Obstet Gynecol* 1988;158:1144–1148.
44. Manning FA, Morrison J, Harman CR, Lange IR, Menticoglou S. Fetal assessment based on fetal biophysical profile scoring. Experience in 19,221 high-risk pregnancies. II. An analysis of false-negative fetal deaths *Am J Obstet Gynecol* 1987;157:880–884.
45. Bekedam DJ, Mulder EJH, Snijders RJM, Visser GHA. The effects of maternal hyperoxia on fetal breathing movements, body movements and heart rate variation in growth retarded fetuses. *Early Hum Dev* 1991;27:223–232.
46. Gagnon R, Hunse C, Vijan S. The effect of maternal hyperoxia on behavioural activity in growth-retarded human fetuses. *Am J Obstet Gynecol* 1990;163:1894–1899.
47. Cohn HE, Sacks EJ, Heymann MA, Rudolph AM. Cardiovascular responses to hypoxemia and acidemia in fetal lambs. *Am J Obstet Gynecol* 1974;120:817–824.
48. Iskovitz J, La Gamma EF, Rudolph AM. Effects of cord compression on fetal blood flow distribution and O_2 delivery. *Am J Physiol* 1987;252:H100–H109.
49. Peeters LLH, Sheldon RE, Jones MD, Makowski EL, Meschia G. Blood flow to fetal organs as a function of arterial oxygen content. *Am J Obstet Gynecol* 1979;135:637–646.
50. Sheldon RE, Peeters LLH, Jones MD, Makowski EL, Meschia G. Redistribution of cardiac output and oxygen delivery in the hypoxemic fetal lamb. *Am J Obstet Gynecol* 1979;135:1071–1078.
51. Bocking AD, Gagnon R, White SE, Homan J, Richardson BS. Circulatory responses to prolonged hypoxemia in fetal sheep. *Am J Obstet Gynecol* 1988;159:1418–1424.
52. Davis LE, Hohimer AR. Hemodynamics and organ blood flow in fetal sheep subjected to chronic anemia. *Am J Physiol* 1991;261:R1542–1548.
53. Sokoloff L. Relationships among local functional activity, energy metabolism and blood flow in the cerebral nervous system. *Fed Proc* 1981;40:2311–2316.
54. Berne RM, Knabb RM, Ely SW, Rubio R. Adenosine in the local regulation of blood flow: a brief overview. *Fed Proc* 1983;42:3136–3142.
55. Iwamoto HS, Kaufman T, Kell LC, Rudolph AM. Responses to acute hypoxemia in the fetal sheep at 0.6–0.7 gestation. *Am J Physiol* 1989;256:H613–H620.
56. Richardson B, Korkola S, Asano H, Challis J, Polk D, Fraser M. Regional blood flow and the endocrine response to sustained hypoxemia in the preterm ovine fetus. *Pediatr Res* 1996;40:337–343.
57. Hadjiev C, Ishikawa M, Sasaki K, Sengoku K, Shimizu T. Pulsatility indexes of the fetal middle cerebral, umbilical, internal iliac, and femoral arteries as predictors of intrauterine growth retardation. *J Matern Fetal Invest* 1992;1 :271–275.
58. Groenenberg IAL, Wladimiroff JW, Hop WCJ. Fetal cardiac and peripheral arterial flow velocity waveforms in intrauterine growth retardation. *Circulation* 1989;80:1711–1717.

59. Stewart PA, Wladimiroff JW, Stijnen I. Blood flow velocity waveforms from the fetal external iliac artery as a measure of lower extremity vascular resistance. *Br J Obstet Gynaecol* 1990;97:425–430.

60. Todros T, Sciarrone A, Ai H, Sorbill E. Umbilical blood flow distribution in normal and growth retarded fetuses. 23rd Annual Meeting of the Fetal and Neonatal Physiological Society, Arica, Chile, 1996, Abstract #24.

61. Van Eyck J, Wladimiroff JW, Van Den Wijngaard JAGW, Noordam MJ, Prechtl HFR. The blood flow velocity waveform in the fetal internal carotid and umbilical artry; its relation to fetal behavioural states in normal pregnancy at 37–38 weeks. *Br J Obstet Gynaecol* 1987;94:736–741.

62. Connors G, Gillis S, Hunse C, Gagnon R, Richardson B. The interaction of behavioural state, heart rate and resistance index in the human fetus. *J Dev Physiol* 1991;15:331–336.

63. Schulman H, Winter D, Farmakides G, Ducey J. *Normal umbilical artery velocity waveforms and umbilical vein flow.* Ithaca, NY: Perinatology Press, 1987:133.

64. Adamson SL, Langille BL. Factors determining aortic and umbilical blood flow pulsatility in fetal sheep. *Ultrasound Med Biol* 1992;18:255–266.

4

THE MOLECULAR MECHANISMS OF FETAL BRAIN INJURY: THE ROLE OF OXYGEN FREE RADICALS

Dev Maulik, M.D., Ph.D.

Department of Obstetrics and Gynecology, Winthrop-University Hospital, Mineola, New York

INTRODUCTION

Perinatal neurologic compromise constitutes a wide spectrum of disorders ranging from severe cerebral palsy to relatively minor forms of neurologic dysfunction such as learning disabilities. The incidence of cerebral palsy which is often attributed to perinatal asphyxia has remained constant over the last two decades despite immense changes in the management of high-risk obstetrics including the widespread use of fetal surveillance tests and increased cesarean deliveries for fetal indications (1). The needs for clinical and supportive care, as well as the human dimensions of this problem, are simply enormous. This is also reflected in the cost of care of the individuals

Asphyxia and Fetal Brain Damage, Edited by Dev Maulik, M.D., Ph.D.
ISBN 0-471-18427-6

suffering from cerebral palsy and other perinatal neurologic compromises (2). Fetal brain damage is the most frequent primary allegation for obstetrical malpractice (3).

Fetal brain injury has multiple potential or proven etiologies which include perinatal asphyxia, sepsis, substance abuse, and other conditions. Of these, perinatal hypoxia-ischemia has long been recognized as one of its significant causes. At the molecular level, there is emerging evidence that oxygen free radicals may be critically involved in the mechanism of hypoxic-ischemic brain damage. This is not a novel hypothesis. Flamm, Demopoulos, and associates (4) suggested two decades ago that free radicals may be important mediators of ischemic brain injury. Increased free radical generation has also been implicated in the mechanism of other proven or suggested clinical preconditions of perinatal neurologic injury. For example, it has long been known that Down's syndrome is the most frequent genetic cause of mental retardation. However, recent evidence suggests that neurons from Down's syndrome fetuses have altered oxygen free radical metabolism resulting in programmed neuronal death which may contribute to mental retardation (5). Similarly, experimental data implicate oxygen free radicals in fetal neuronal injury from prenatal alcohol exposure and sepsis (6,7). It is noteworthy that fetal alcohol syndrome is a significant cause of mental retardation and that recent epidemiologic evidence suggests perinatal sepsis as an important cause of cerebral palsy (8).

Obviously, it is imperative that the molecular mechanisms of fetal brain injury, particularly the role of oxygen free radicals, should be elucidated so that strategies may be developed to limit or even prevent its harmful consequences. However, there is a great paucity of data on this subject. This can be partly explained by the ethical considerations and technical limitations of conducting fetal research. Most of the information on brain injury pertains to the adult brain and, to a limited extent, the neonatal brain. Most of the experimental data are based on the cell, tissue, or animal models of neuronal injury and are potentially applicable to fetal neurological compromise. Caution, however, must be exercised for such extrapolations because of ontogenic variance in the neuronal response to these insults and species differences in brain development. However, they provide a hypothetical framework for designing fetus-specific experimental investigations in this area.

This chapter presents a brief review of the molecular mechanisms of free radical mediated hypoxic-ischemic fetal neuronal injury. The chapter begins with a brief introduction to oxygen free radicals which is followed by a discussion of the proven as well as the proposed mechanisms of hypoxia-ischemia induced and radical mediated neuronal injury. This is followed by a review of the current information on the role and prenatal ontogeny of these mechanisms in mediating hypoxic-ischemic fetal neuronal compromise.

OXYGEN FREE RADICALS AND OXIDATIVE STRESS

An atom is structurally comprised of a central nucleus of positively charged protons and neutral neutrons with the negatively charged electrons spinning in space orbitals around the nucleus. Electrons exist in pairs which move in their own specific orbitals.

A free radical is any atomic or molecular species capable of free existence with one or more unpaired electrons (9). In a molecular free radical, one or more of the constituent atoms have unpaired electrons. Free radicals are reactive because they must either donate or accept additional electrons in order to balance the unpaired ones. If the radical reacts with a nonradical biological molecule, a compound with unbalanced electrons (i.e., a new free radical) is generated which then reacts with another biological compound. Thus a chain reaction is initiated. Lipid peroxidation offers an important example of such a chain reaction. The only way a free radical either accepts or donates an electron without creating another radical is by reacting with another free radical.

Oxygen free radicals are redox intermediaries of molecular oxygen or dioxygen (O_2), produced during the reduction of oxygen to water occurring as an integral part of the energy regenerating process of oxidative phosphorylation. An oxygen molecule, although a free radical because of the presence of two unpaired electrons, is only modestly reactive. However, highly reactive oxygen free radicals such as a hydroxyl radical and nonradical intermediates such as hydrogen peroxide are generated by mitochondrial respiration and also by various metabolic pathways (10–13). These radical and nonradical products are often collectively called reactive oxygen species. The high affinity for biological compounds displayed by these oxidants is the basis of the oxidative stress which may be defined as the generation of oxygen free radicals and other reactive oxygen species in excess of the antioxidant defense mechanisms (14). The reactive oxygen species commonly encountered in biological systems are listed in Table 1.

The reduction of oxygen to water involves a sequence of four reactions (Figure 1). During each reaction, an electron is added and in the overall reaction, one molecule of O_2 combines with four electrons (e^-) and four hydrogen ions (H^+) to produce two molecules of water. The conversion of hydrogen peroxide to hydroxyl radical is catalyzed by the presence of trace transitional metal iron (Fe^{2+}) and is called the Fenton reaction. The entire process of reduction of oxygen sequentially yields superoxide, perhydroxyl, and hydroxyl radicals. Of these, the hydroxyl radical is the most reactive while the superoxide radical is the least reactive. Hydroxyl radicals are also generated by other mechanisms such as the Haber–Weiss reaction in which

Table 1. Biologically significant reactive oxygen species

Radical	
Superoxide anion	$O_2^{\bullet -}$
Hydroxyl radical	$OH\bullet$
Lipid peroxyl radical	$LOO\bullet$
Lipid alkoxyl radical	$LO\bullet$
Nitric oxide	$NO\bullet$
Nonradical	
Hydrogen peroxide	H_2O_2
Singlet oxygen	$^1O_2$
Hypochloric acid	HOCl

Oxygen Reduction During Oxidative Phosphorylation

Overall Reaction

$$O_2 + 4e^- + 4H^+ = 2H_2O$$

Steps of Reaction

Step 1.	$O_2 + e^- = O_2^{\bullet -} \ (+ H^+ = HO_2^{\bullet})$
Step 2.	$O_2^{\bullet -} + e^- = O_2^{2-} \ (+ 2H^+ = H_2O_2)$
Step 3.	$H_2O_2 + e^- \ (+Fe^{2+}) = HO^{\bullet} + OH^-$
Step 4.	$HO^{\bullet} + e^- = OH^- \ (+ H^+ = H_2O)$

Figure 1. Reduction of molecular oxygen (O_2) to water (H_2O) during oxidative phosphorylation. The upper panel shows overall reaction of one molecule of O_2 with four electrons (e^-) to yield two molecules of H_2O. The lower panel shows sequential stepwise reactions. Please note that step 3 represents the Fenton reaction (see the text). e^- = unpaired electron; $O_2^{\bullet -}$, superoxide radical; $HO_2^{\bullet}$, perhydroxyl radical; O_2^{2-}, peroxide ion; H_2O_2, hydrogen peroxide; $HO^{\bullet}$, hydroxyl radical; HO^-, hydroxyl ion; Fe^{2+}, ferrous iron.

superoxide radicals interact with hydrogen peroxide, yielding hydroxyl radicals (15). This reaction is slow but is accelerated by the catalytic action of Fe^{2+}. Another transitional metal, Cu^{2+}, also facilitates radical production. Hydroxyl radicals are also produced by the degradation of peroxynitrite which is generated by nitric oxide reacting with superoxide radicals (16).

HYPOXIA-ISCHEMIA AND NEURONAL INJURY

There is substantial experimental evidence that oxygen (O_2) deprivation at the cellular level initiates a series of molecular events which lead to neuronal dysfunction and death. Of the different types of hypoxia, the ischemic variety occurs most frequently and poses the gravest risk because it results in simultaneous energy failure, substrate deprivation, and waste accumulation. Perfusion may be insufficient or completely cease, which may be limited to an area or include the whole brain. The former is known as focal ischemia and the latter is known as global ischemia (17). This terminology, however, may be misleading because cerebral lesions resulting from global ischemia are distributed not globally but regionally. This distribution depends on several factors including (a) severity and duration of the insult and (b) neuronal metabolic state and maturity. The relative preponderance of hypoxia or hypoxia-ischemia in the causation of fetal brain injury is unknown. Based on our current knowledge on fetal circulatory response, one may reasonably speculate that fetal brain injury from only oxygen deprivation without any compromise in brain perfusion is an unlikely clinical event. Moreover, secondary perfusion failure may also occur because of microvascular dysfunction triggered by upregulation of cytokines, expression of adhesion receptors, leukocyte adhesion, platelet aggregation, inflammatory response, and capillary or venule occlusion (18). In neonates, hypoxia-ischemia seems to be critical in the causation of encephalopathy (19). There is significant evidence from animal models demonstrating the critical role of hypoxemia and ischemia in causing cerebral injury in the primate fetus (20). By limiting the availability of O_2 and glucose, the two obligatory substrates for brain energy metabolism, hypoxia-ischemia has the greater potential for neuronal injury than hypoxia alone. This issue has been comprehensively reviewed recently (21). There appears to be two perfusion thresholds for neuronal compromise (22–24), one for the cessation of electrical activity and the other at a lower level for the loss of ionic homeostasis which also serves as a threshold at which neuronal energy failure occurs. The latter is of significance because the ultimate pathway for neuronal hypoxic injury consists of varying degrees of energy failure and its sequelae.

NEURONAL ENERGY REQUIREMENT AND PRODUCTION

Neurons have a high energy demand driven by continuous activities essential for cellular function and survival, but they possess inadequate reservoirs of oxygen and substrates for energy production (25). This renders neurons uniquely vulnerable to hypoxic-ischemic injury. The energy-dependent neuronal functions include plasma membrane and mitochondrial ion fluxes, intraneuronal transport of materials needed for gene expression, synthesis of proteins and other macromolecules, and repair and restoration of various membranes and intracellular structures (26). This high activity level is reflected by the relatively high level of oxygen utilization by the human brain which even at rest consumes one-fifth of the total available O_2 in the body although it weighs only one-tenth of the body weight.

Because neurons do not contain any glycogen or fat, they exclusively depend on a continuous supply of glucose to fulfill their energy needs. In the neuronal cytosol, glycolysis generates pyruvate which is further metabolized in the mitochondrial matrix to form the acetyl group of the acetyl coenzyme A. The latter enters the Krebs cycle to yield carbon dioxide and high-energy electrons which are then carried by the reduced nicotine adenine dinucleotide (NADH) and reduced flavin adenine dinucleotide (FADH2) to enter the final step of oxidative phosphorylation. During this last step, electrons released from NADH and FADH2 are transported by a complex system of electron carriers in the mitochondrial inner membrane called the respiratory chain, and they are eventually combined with the molecular O_2 at the end of the chain. During this transport, an enormous amount of energy is unleashed which is chemically stored by the formation of adenosine triphosphate (ATP) which is derived from adenosine diphosphate (ADP) and inorganic phosphate. The reaction depends on the activity of ATP synthase, which is a large enzyme complex in the mitochondrial inner membrane.

ATP is the principal source of energy in a cell. Another high-energy phosphate compound, phosphocreatine (PCr), is also an important source of energy. In the mammalian brain, the approximate level of ATP is 3 μmol per gram of wet brain tissue and that of PCr is 5 μmol per gram of wet brain tissue (27). Most of the high-energy phosphates reside in the cytosol in free form, which is the amount available for cellular energy needs. Under normoxic resting conditions, the brain generates 25–32 μmol of ATP per gram of wet tissue per minute (3). Oxidative phosphorylation is the primary ATP-generating mechanism of the brain and is responsible for 95% of the ATP production. The process involves the Krebs cycle and the electron transport mechanisms of the mitochondrial respiratory chain and requires O_2. From the combustion of one molecule of glucose, oxidative phosphorylation generates 36 molecules of ATP whereas anaerobic glycolysis, the alternative pathway, yields only two molecules of ATP. Thus oxidative phosphorylation is approximately 16–17 times more efficient in replenishing cellular energy supply.

CONSEQUENCES OF NEURONAL ENERGY FAILURE

Neurons exposed to hypoxia-ischemia have a variable but limited time window before energy failure ensues. The energy failure, in turn, unleashes a series of events which threaten neuronal integrity and survival. The underlying cellular events are complex (26,28) and include failure of ionic pumps, efflux of potassium (K^+) and influx of sodium (Na^+) and chloride (Cl^-), neuronal membrane depolarization, activation of excitatory amino acid receptor systems, rise in the intracellular calcium (Ca^{2+}), activation of enzyme systems, and generation of free radicals. The spectrum of response extends from complete recovery to immediate necrotic or delayed programmed death and is determined by many factors including (a) the severity and duration of hypoxic-ischemic insult and (b) the neuronal maturity and metabolic state.

Sustained Anoxia-Ischemia

In complete and sustained ischemia and anoxia, energy failure and its fatal consequences are rapidly set in motion (26,28,29). There is cessation of regeneration of ATP, but its hydrolysis continues resulting in the elevation of ADP level. Neuronal energy supply is maintained during the first minute by the conversion of PCr and ADP to ATP by the enzyme creatine kinase. Following the consumption of PCr store, ATP is depleted within the next 3–4 minutes. This initiates a rapid cascade of changes leading to cell dysfunction and eventual death. Energy-dependent maintenance of transmembrane ionic conductance is profoundly perturbed, leading to extrusion of K^+ from the cell and uptake of Na^+, Ca^{2+} and Cl^- into the cell. This is associated with concomitant osmotic movement of water into the cell, resulting in cellular edema and disruption. With the loss of ionic homeostasis, depolarization of the neuronal membrane occurs along with excitotoxic neurotransmitter release, activation of Excitatory Amino Acid receptor, and Ca^{2+} entry into the cell. With the collapse of all the mechanisms for survival, the cell ultimately dies a necrotic death. It has been demonstrated, however, that in acute anoxic insult the critical event for neuronal death may be the intraneuronal elevation in the levels of Na^+ rather than that of Ca^{2+} (29).

Partial Hypoxia-Ischemia

When the ischemia and oxygen deprivation are incomplete, the high-energy phosphates are depleted at a rate less consistent with the duration and intensity of the insult. The neuronal response in this situation may be considered as being triphasic (30). The first phase consists of hypoxia-ischemia induced swiftly developing neuronal energy depletion, altered membrane function including the receptor activity especially of Na^+K^+-ATPase, consequent loss of transmembrane ionic homeostasis, and membrane depolarization. The energy deficit also affects various cellular synthetic processes including protein synthesis and gene expression, and it results in degradation of various macromolecules including phospholipids, proteins, and deoxyribonucleic acid (DNA). The phenomenon is associated with generation of reactive oxygen species which further aggravates the deterioration of cellular function and structure. The sources of radical generation at this stage include predominantly the mitochondrial electron transport chain and also the radical generating enzymatic pathways activated by high cytosolic Ca^{2+} level secondary to glutamate receptor stimulation and other mechanisms (see below).

REPERFUSION-REOXYGENATION

Cessation of the insult with reperfusion and reoxygenation is characterized by the resumption of cellular energy status via ATP generation and the restoration of various aspects of neuronal function including repolarization of the neuronal membrane. Paradoxically, this phase is also characterized by enhanced oxidative stress (31). Resumption of O_2 supply to the damaged tissue leads to the generation of free radicals from multiple sources. These include markedly increased mitochondrial radical generation and production of free radicals by the various enzymatic pathways such as xanthine oxidase (see below). Hypoxia also leads to depletion of local antioxidants (e.g., the glutathione system), thus further exacerbating the stress. The increased radical generation during the reoxygenation initiates the cascade of processes which involve continued intracellular Ca^{2+} excess and activation of the various oxygen free-radical-generating pathways (see below), which may lead to the next phase of delayed neuronal death. Neurons slow to recover are particularly susceptible to this outcome. There is emerging information that this third phase is associated with the secondary failure of mitochondrial respiratory function and the formation of mitochondrial permeability transition pores in the mitochondrial inner membrane (32). The latter may be causally related to mitochondrial Ca^{2+} overload secondary to cytosolic Ca^{2+} abundance. Permeability transition pore formation further aggravates the intracellular Ca^{2+} overload and accentuates the oxidative stress. Recent evidence suggests that this process may be a critical triggering mechanism for neuronal apoptosis (33).

MECHANISMS OF OXYGEN FREE RADICAL GENERATION

Cells generate reactive oxygen species during normal respiratory and metabolic activities. However, the production is enhanced during hypoxia-ischemia, but more so during reperfusion-reoxygenation (25). The mechanisms suggested for free radical generation include radical leakage from the neuronal mitochondrial respiratory chain and from the various metabolic processes which include the excitatory amino acid receptor activation, the xanthine oxidase pathway, and the arachidonic acid pathway. These are summarized below (Figure 2).

Mitochondrial Respiratory Chain

Mitochondrial respiration is a major source of oxygen free radical generation during hypoxia-ischemia, subsequent reperfusion-reoxygenation and excitotoxic exposure (34–36). As mentioned previously, the critical process of ATP regeneration involves sequential transfer of electrons from NADH to molecular O_2 by a system of carriers located in the mitochondrial inner membrane and consisting of three major enzyme systems: the NADH, cytochrome b-c_1, and cytochrome oxidase complexes. The NADH complex accepts electrons from NADH and transfers them via ubiquinone to the cytochrome b-c_1 complex which then transfers the electrons via cytochrome c to the cytochrome oxidase complex. Cytochrome oxidase removes electrons from the cytochrome ferrous-hem combination and donates these electrons, one at a time, to O_2. Leakage of electrons during the transfer leads to their interaction with oxygen and consequent generation of superoxide radicals. Cytochrome oxidase avidly interacts with O_2 and is highly efficient in binding oxygen free radicals and reactive intermediaries, en-

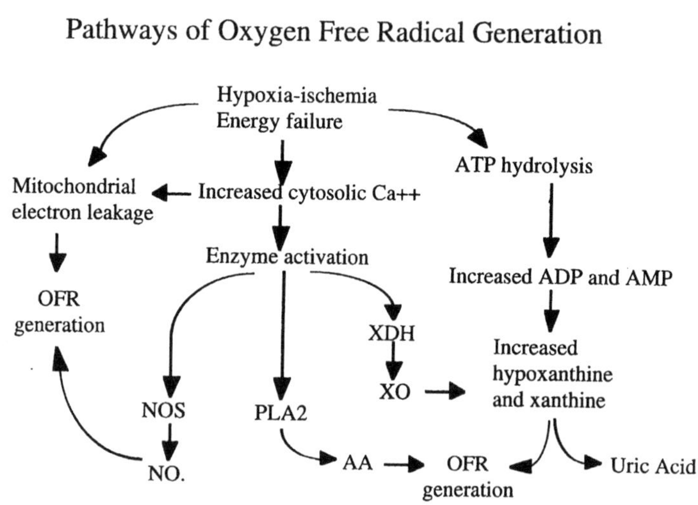

Figure 2. Hypoxia-ischemia and mechanisms of oxygen free radical generation. ATP, adenosine triphosphate; ADP, adenosine diphosphate; ATP, adenosine monophosphate; OFR, oxygen free radical; XDH, xanthine dehydrogenase; XO, xanthine oxidase; PLA2, phospholipase A2; AA, arachidonic acid; NO•, nitric oxide.

suring that these reactive species remain bound within the system. Under normal circumstances, only 1% of total utilized O_2 ends up generating oxygen free radicals. Both decreased and increased O_2 supply to mitochondria are associated with increased electron leakage and greater radical production. During hypoxia-ischemia, oxygen deficiency leads to decreased electron acceptance at the cytochrome oxidase level, which results in the reduced state of the components of the mitochondrial respiratory chain. Thus there is an abundance of electron donors at the proximal level in the respiratory chain, which leads to a greater leakage of electrons and an increased production of superoxides (37). Increasing O_2 supply to mitochondria results in more electron leakage and consequent radical production. The ubiquinone-cytochrome b-c_1 site of the chain appears to be the major source of superoxide radical generation in mitochondria (38,39).

Excitotoxic Receptor Activation and Altered Calcium Homeostasis

Hypoxia-induced abnormalities of Ca^{2+} homeostasis play a significant role in free radical generation (40,41). Hypoxia-ischemia and the consequent failure leads to perturbed ionic conductance and membrane depolarization. This leads to the release of excitatory amino acids, particularly glutamate, from presynaptic vesicles. The profound perinatal implications of this excitotoxic response are reviewed in depth in Chapter 6. Other ATP-dependent ion channels are also involved in this (42). Extracellular glutamate rise results in the activation of *N*-methyl D-aspartate (NMDA) receptors in the neuronal membrane and entry of Ca^{2+} into the cell. The entry is facilitated by the removal of a Mg^{2+} block from inside the NMDA receptor ion channel by membrane depolarization. The net result is an enormous increase in the intracellular Ca^{2+} level, which is aggravated further by the release of Ca^{2+} from intracellular stores (Figure 3). The latter is mediated by the second messenger system involving the activation of phospholipase C and consequent increase in inositol 1,4,5-triphosphate (43). One of the effects of intracellular Ca^{2+} elevation is the activation of a variety of enzyme systems such as lipases, proteases, and endonucleases with grave consequences for the cell survival (44). Some of these enzymes such as phospholipase A2 and xanthine oxidase participate in the metabolic pathways for reactive oxygen species generation and are discussed below.

Enzymatic Pathways

During hypoxia, there is increased hydrolysis of ATP resulting in accumulation of AMP which is converted through several intermediary products to hypoxanthine and xanthine. Hypoxia also causes Ca^{2+}-induced conversion of xanthine dehydrogenase to xanthine oxidase, which catalyzes the metabolic degradation of xanthine and hypoxanthine to uric acid and leads to consequent generation of reactive oxygen species in the presence of O_2 (30). This process becomes a critical source of radical generation with the increased availability of O_2 during reperfusion-reoxygenation. Intraneuronal Ca^{2+} influx also activates phospholipase A2 enzyme, leading sequentially to hydrolysis of the membrane phospholipids, release of arachidonic acid, stimulation of lipo-oxygenase and cyclo-oxygenase enzymes, production of prostaglandins and leucotrienes, and generation of free radicals (45). Increased Ca^{2+} also activates neuronal nitric oxide synthase, which results in the synthesis of nitric oxide, a gaseous

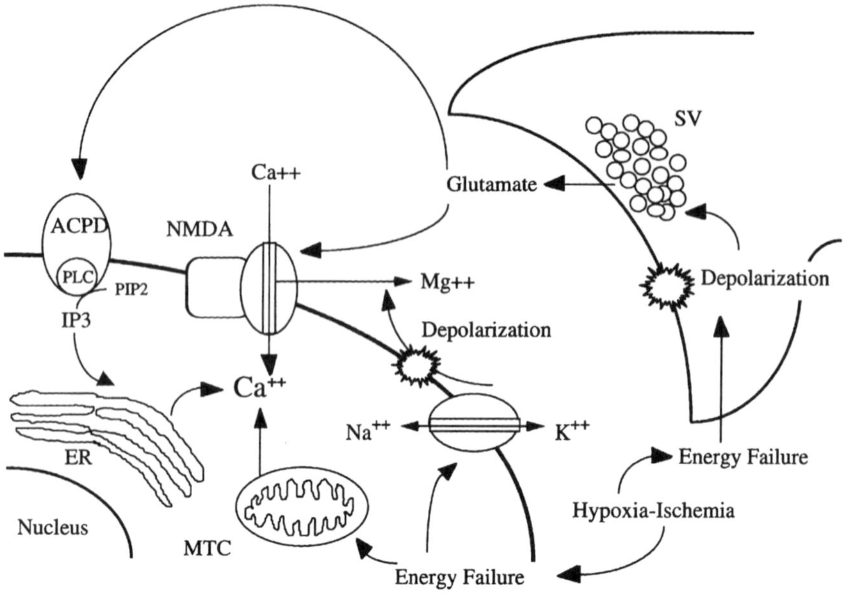

Figure 3. Graphic depiction of hypoxia-ischemia induced changes in calcium metabolism. SV, synaptic vesicles; NMDA, *N*-methyl D-aspartate receptor; ACPD, 1-amino-cyclopentyl-1,3-dicarboxylate receptor; PLC, phospholipase C; PIP2, phosphatidyl-inositol-4,5-biphosphate; IP3, inositol-l,4,5-triphosphate; MTC, mitochondria; ER, endoplasmic reticulum.

free radical. The latter reacts with the superoxide radical to produce peroxynitrate which then converts to the highly destructive hydroxyl radical (46). This reaction is facilitated by the presence of transitional metal ion, Fe^{2+}.

Other Sources

An additional mechanism of free radical generation in the brain may involve inflammatory and immunological reactions triggered by hypoxic-ischemic events and sepsis. The resultant expression of adhesion molecules such as intercellular adhesion molecule-1 stimulates polymorphonuclear leukocytes to generate oxygen free radicals and nonradical reactive species (47). Finally, cerebrovascular endothelial cells may also contribute to the neuronal hypoxic-ischemic damage because they are capable of generating reactive oxygen species including hydroxyl and superoxide radicals.

ANTIOXIDANT HOMEOSTASIS

In order to protect the cellular and extracellular targets from oxidative injury, elaborate enzymatic and nonenzymatic defense systems have evolved in the intra- and extracellular domains. Antioxidants of biological significance are listed in Table 2.

Table 2. Biologically significant antioxidants

Enzymatic
Manganese superoxide dismutase
Copper zinc superoxide dismutase
Glutathione and glutathione peroxidase
Catalase
Nonenzymatic
α-Tocopherol
Ascorbate
Carotenes
Ubiquinone
Selenium
Uric acid

Under physiological circumstances, there is a balance between the background oxygen free radical production and the antioxidant defense mechanisms. Under various pathological conditions, this balance is disturbed in favor of the oxidative stress because of either excessive free radical generation or deficient antioxidant activity. Oftentimes both mechanisms occur simultaneously. A brief description of these defense mechanisms is given below.

Enzymatic Antioxidant

The major antioxidant enzymes distributed within the cell include superoxide dismutase (SOD), the glutathione system (glutathione, glutathione peroxidase, glutathione reductase, and others), and catalases. Of these, the catalase is relatively scant in the brain tissue. Superoxide dismutase rapidly reduces superoxide radicals to H_2O_2 and is one of the most important free radical scavengers in the body. The manganese form of SOD is present in the mitochondria, one of the major sources of free radical production in a cell; the copper-zinc SOD exists in the cytosol. Although SOD degrades superoxide, the resultant H_2O_2 is a major source of subsequent more lethal hydroxyl radical generation. Neutralization of H_2O_2 to water is accomplished by glutathione and glutathione peroxidases. Because H_2O_2 is not a free radical but a reactive oxygen species, glutathione system is not a free radical scavenger. The enzymatic intracellular defense mechanisms also include enzymes for repairing DNA injury incurred by the free radicals and also for removing altered proteins.

Nonenzymatic Antioxidant

Nonenzymatic antioxidants include alpha-tocopherol, ascorbate, carotenoids, and other substances. Alpha-tocopherol is the most important lipid-soluble free radical scavenger capable of terminating radical generating chain reactions and is found bound to lipoproteins. It is the principal radical scavenger of the cell membrane. Ascorbate is the most important water-soluble scavenger, and it probably acts synergistically with alpha-tocopherol by regenerating the latter. It reacts with hydroxyl, superoxide, and other radicals and also protects against lipid free radicals such as peroxyl radicals. Caroteinoids are radical scavengers effective against singlet oxygen and peroxyl radicals. A comprehensive review of these and other antioxidant defense mechanisms can be found elsewhere (48). The ontogeny of antioxidant defenses in the fetus is discussed later in this review.

MECHANISMS OF FREE-RADICAL-MEDIATED NEURONAL INJURY

Oxygen free radicals avidly interact with the constituent organic molecules of a cell including lipid, proteins, and DNA constituents of neurons. Consequent to these reactions, free radicals affect cellular and extracellular constituents of neural tissue, profoundly alter its functions, and may lead to immediate necrotic or delayed programmed death of the neurons. This forms the basis for neuronal oxidative stress. The free radical reactivity involving specific organic molecules and its effect on the cellular structure and function are briefly discussed below and summarized in Figure 4.

Organic Molecules

The phospholipid bilayer in the neuronal cell membrane is rich in polyunsaturated fatty acids, thereby increasing the susceptibility of the neurons to peroxidative damage. The presence of unsaturated carbon-to-carbon bonds in the lipids enhances their roles as electron donors. The higher the unsaturation of these fatty acids, the greater

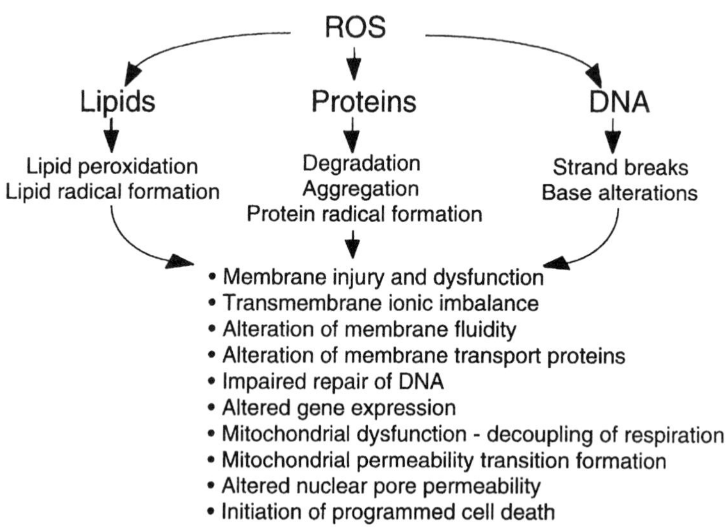

Figure 4. Graphic summarization of the adverse effects of oxidative stress on neuronal survival. ROS, reactive oxygen species; DNA, deoxyribonucleic acid.

the propensity of oxidative reaction with the free radicals. The process is known as lipid peroxidation. The initial electron donation by the membrane lipids results in forming a carbon-centered radical which stabilizes by bond rearrangement into conjugated dienes. The dienes combine with oxygen to form the peroxyl radical, which then reacts with additional fatty acid side chains in the cell membrane to form lipid hydroperoxides. The latter propagate the process into an ever-expanding chain reaction aided by transitional metals and metal complexes and generating lipid peroxyl and alkoxyl radicals. These radicals attack more lipids and proteins locally, and they also diffuse out of their site of generation and produce distant effects. The extent of the chain reaction depends on the preponderance of lipids in the membrane and the presence of chain-breaking antioxidant systems in the membrane (49). The importance of lipid peroxidation lies with its role in mediating and extending oxidative neuronal injury (21). Consequent to the peroxidative consumption, the polyunsaturated fat content of the neuronal membrane declines, resulting in loss of fluidity and permeabilitiy of the membrane. In addition, alterations occur in the membrane-bound receptors, such as Na^+, K^+-ATPase or Ca^{2+}-ATPase, leading to altered ionic homeostasis. Although lipid peroxidation is a significant destructive event associated with free radical generation, alterations in proteins, DNA, and intracellular homeostasis may be more critical for initiating the destructive cascade of events leading to neuronal death (49).

One of the major mechanisms by which free radicals mediate cellular injury is their affinity for proteins. Protein damage is induced by free radicals generated either primarily by neuronal energy failure and reoxygenation or as a consequence of lipid peroxidation. Although many radicals participate in the process, hydroxyl radical is especially important for protein damage because it reacts avidly with the majority of the amino acid constituents of the various protein molecules. The radicals react at several locations in the protein molecule, oxidize the disulfide links, and may cause formation of protein free radicals which can move to other locations within the protein molecule and cause further reactions (50). The presence of ferrous or cuprous ions in proteins catalyzes the reactivity. Free radical damage to the protein structure results in the formation of cross linkage, aggregation, degradation, and fragmentation. Moreover, proteins damaged by free radicals are more prone to hydrolytic degradation.

Free radicals can inflict substantial damage to DNA structure (51). The effect may be mediated primarily by the direct reaction of free radicals, particularly hydroxyl radicals, with the DNA structure, or secondarily by the effect of proteases and endonucleases activated by the free-radical-induced intracellular Ca^{2+} excess. The effects include purine and pyrimidine base alterations, damage to deoxyribose, and single or double strand breakage of the double helix backbone of the DNA structure (51). The damage inflicted by the free radicals on DNA has far reaching consequences for neuronal function and survival.

Neuronal Structure and Function

Because of their reactivity against the basic building blocks of a cell, free radicals can cause widespread damage to neuronal structure and function. Radical generation is associated with dysfunction of various components of the cell membrane including alteration of membrane fluidity. This can lead to further deterioration of ionic homeostasis and more radical generation, thus creating a vicious cycle. The deleterious effects of free radicals on cellular proteins can have a wide spectrum of adverse effects such as alterations of membrane transport proteins and various enzyme systems including those responsible for DNA repair which may significantly compromise cellular structural and functional integrity. Arachidonic acid liberated by the radical activity on lipids not only acts as the substrate for the prostanoid pathway further fueling radical generation, it also decouples mitochondrial respiration. Free radicals may also be involved in cerebral microvascular dysfunction, and the resulting increased permeability and the consequent damage to blood–brain barrier may lead to cerebral edema and neuronal injury.

Programmed Cell Death

Radical reactivity contributes to mitochondrial dysfunction and further free radical generation. These effects combined with the slow development of mitochondrial Ca^{2+} overload may contribute to delayed neuronal death by apoptosis (52). Although programmed cell death or apoptosis is an essential process in the development and differentiation of the central nervous system, it also occurs in various pathological disorders involving the generation of reactive oxygen species. Apoptotic neuronal death has been demonstrated in hypoxic-ischemic perinatal brain injury (53). It has been suggested that the development of mitochondrial permeability transition pores may be a critical link in this process (32,33). Alterations in the nuclear pore permeability may also play a significant role in this phenomenon by altering Ca^{2+} transport across the nuclear membrane, thereby affecting several critical intranuclear processes including the induction of Ca^{2+}-dependent enzymes such as endonucleases (54). These events may initiate or execute the apoptotic trigger. There is considerable evidence correlating oxidative stress, gene expression, and induction of neuronal apoptosis. Hockenbery et al. (55) demonstrated progressive lipid peroxidation following an apoptotic signal and complete suppression of the peroxidative response by the overexpression of Bcl-2, an anti-apoptotic gene. The authors hypothesized that Bcl-2 may regulate an antioxidant pathway at sites of free radical generation. Busciglio and Yankner (5) reported that cortical neurons from fetal Downs syndrome undergo apoptotic death which is preceded by a substantial rise in the reactive oxygen species and which can be prevented by antioxidant treatment.

OXIDATIVE STRESS IN THE FETAL BRAIN

It is reasonable to assume that the physiology and pathology of oxidative stress in the fetal brain would involve the same fundamental processes as in the adult or the neonatal brain. Differences exist, however, in the circumstances of the stress because of the uniqueness of fetal intrauterine existence and also because of the ontogenic differences in the various mechanisms of, and responses to, radical generation. Although the effects of hypoxia and hypoxia-ischemia on the developing brain have been extensively investigated, these studies address mostly postnatal ontogeny.

As expected from the previous discussions in this chapter, the triggering mechanism for neuronal response to hypoxia is energy deficit. The fetus is no exception. Exposed to maternal hypoxia (7% of O_2 in the inhaled air for 60 min), ATP and PCr levels in the guinea pig fetal brain decline precipitously (90% of the normoxic levels). Evidence for free radical mediated hypoxic-ischemic brain injury is examined below. Specifically, the following issues will be addressed: ontogeny of excitotoxic receptor activation in the fetal brain; evidence for free radical generation in the fetal brain; and the ontogeny of antioxidant defense.

Ontogeny of Excitotoxic Receptor System in the Fetus

Hypoxia-ischemia-induced excitotoxic receptor activation constitutes an essential link in the cascade of events that include free radical generation and culminates in neuronal injury. Developmental changes in the excitatory amino acid receptors have been comprehensively investigated in postnatal animals. As reviewed by McDonald and Johnston (56), overexpression of synaptic NMDA and other excitatory amino acid pathway markers occurs transiently in various brain areas in postnatal animals and relates to synaptic and neuronal plasticity such as long-term potentiation. This ontogenic overexpression increases the vulnerability of the brain to excitotoxic injury which contributes to the initiation of the neurotoxic cascade leading to neuronal injury and death. Hypoxia-induced modifications in the excitatory amino acid receptor systems in the fetal brain have been described in a guinea pig fetal model (57). Term fetuses (60 days) demonstrate significant increases in the quantity and the affinity of NMDA receptors when exposed to maternal hypoxia. In the developing fetus, the NMDA system shows distinctive ontogenic characteristics (58). The receptors increase in number approximately threefold from mid- to term gestation, whereas the apparent affinity of the receptors shows a biphasic pattern with decline near term (45–50 days) and increase toward the end of gestation. These developmental changes most probably indicate a role for the NMDA receptor during the proliferation period of brain development. They may also play a critical role in determining the differential response of the fetal brain to hypoxic-ischemia in the various stages of gestation.

Hypoxia-Induced Free Radical Generation in the Fetal Brain

The evidence of oxygen free radical injury to the fetal brain has been investigated mostly indirectly by measuring the effects of injury such as lipid peroxidation or alterations in the membrane function. More recently, preliminary reports have been presented for the generation of oxygen free radicals by direct measurement utilizing electronic spin resonance spectroscopy. Excitotoxic response in the fetal brain has also been described. Furthermore, ontogeny of these mechanisms and also that of the antioxidant enzyme defense system have been described. Interestingly, evidence for higher susceptibility of the brains of experimentally growth restricted fetuses have also been described. These are further discussed below.

EVIDENCE OF OXIDATIVE STRESS IN THE FETAL BRAIN

Animal Studies

The importance of peroxidation of neuronal membrane lipids in mediating and perpetuating oxidative stress has been discussed previously in this chapter. The phenomenon is assessed by measuring the metabolic degradation products of lipid peroxidation such as conjugated dienes, fluorescent labeled compounds, and thiobarbituric acid (TBA)-reactive substances. The *guinea pig fetal brain* at term demonstrates significant increases in lipid peroxidation when challenged by hypoxia (Figure 5). Lipid peroxidation under normoxic conditions in the fetal guinea pig brain peaks just after midgestation, but it declines thereafter reaching a plateau by the last quarter of pregnancy, and continues at that level until term (63 days) (Figure 6) (59). The greater lipid peroxidation under normoxic conditions in early gestation may result from either an immature antioxidant defense system, or more intense peroxidation in preterm brains. This is a highly relevant issue and is further discussed later. Hypoxia-induced increased lipid peroxidation was also reported by other investigators (60). A time-dependent significant rise in the levels of TBA-reactive substances is observed in the fetal brain following complete cessation of maternal–fetal blood supply for up to 30 min. Lipid peroxidation-associated functional compromise in the fetal neuronal membrane has also been reported (61). Following maternal hypoxia, the activity of Na^+, K^+-ATPase in the brain declines by 50% in the term guinea pig fetus, whereas the preterm (50 days) brain activity remains unaffected. The high sensitivity of Na^+,

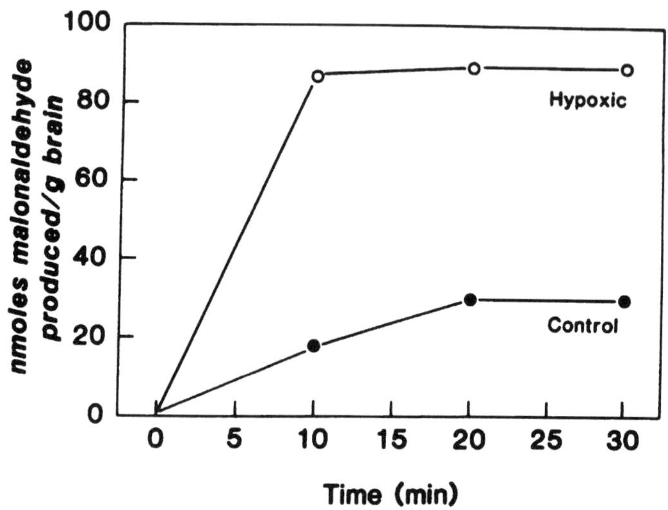

Figure 5. The time course of formation of TBA-reactive substances in control and hypoxic term fetal brain. Each point represents the mean of four experiments conducted in duplicate with standard deviations ranging from 5% to 10% of the mean. (Reproduced with permission from reference 59.)

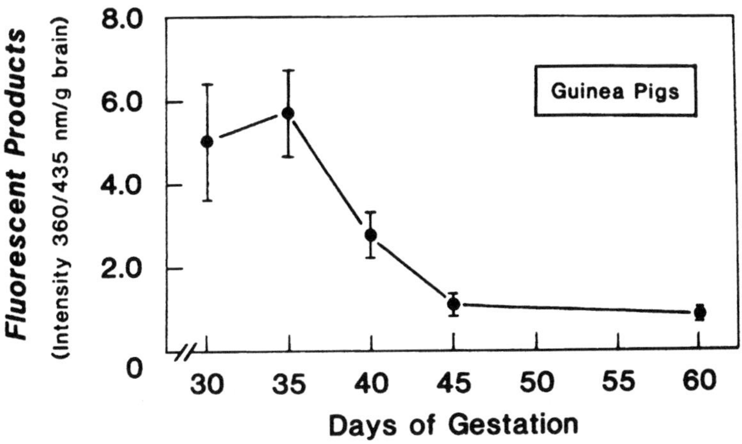

Figure 6. Evidence of lipid peroxidation in fetal brain. Level of fluorescent compounds in guinea pig fetal brain at different ages of gestation. Values are expressed as fluorescent intensity at 360/435 nm per g brain. Each point represents the mean ± SD of 12 animals. (Reproduced with permission from reference 59.)

K^+-ATPase activity to hypoxia in the guinea pig brain at term suggests that the cell membrane functions of the fetal brain may be more susceptible to hypoxia at term than it is earlier in gestation.

de Haan et al. (62) studied in a lamb model the effect of fetal asphyxia on the release of hypoxanthine and xanthine in cerebrospinal fluid and on brain histologic characteristics. Fetal asphyxia was induced by restriction of uterine blood flow. Limited microscopically detectable brain damage were observed mostly in the cerebellum. Cerebrospinal fluid hypoxanthine and xanthine levels peaked in the normoxemic recovery phase, which is consistent with reperfusion-reoxygenation induced oxidative stress.

Direct Evidence

Although these studies strongly suggest free radical generation in the fetal brain following hypoxia, there has been a dearth of investigation involving direct demonstration and characterization of these compounds. In contrast to the indirect techniques, electron spin resonance (ESR) spectroscopy allows direct quantification and identification of oxygen free radicals. The technique is based on the principle that when a free radical containing sample is placed in a magnetic field and radiant microwave energy is applied, the resonant absorption characteristics of the energy by the sample allow direct quantification as well as structural identification of the free radicals present in the sample. As free radicals possess an extremely short life span, spin traps such as nitrones are used to conjugate the radicals and the resultant adduct significantly extends longevity of the radicals which permits their spectroscopic measurement and identification. ESR spectroscopy has been employed to demonstrate hypoxia and ischemia-reperfusion induced free radical generation in the heart (63) and in the postnatal brain (64–66). Recently, a preliminary report has described the utilization of this technique with phenyl butyl nitrone spin trapping in the guinea pig fetal bain (67). The mothers in the experimental group were exposed to 7% oxygen for 60 minutes, whereas the control group inhaled 21% oxygen. In comparison with the normoxic group, the hypoxic fetuses demonstrated significant increases (average of 71%) in oxygen free radical generation in the brain tissue. Concomitant measurements also confirmed significantly increased lipid peroxidation and decreased Na^+, K+-ATPase activity, indicating deleterious effects of the free radicals on the fetal neuronal membrane function.

Human Experience

Significantly, association between perinatal pathology and activation of the free-radical-generating pathways with lipid peroxidation has been shown in human infants. Zhou et al. (68) observed significant ($P = 0.01$) lipid peroxidation and prostanoid activation in the neonates suffering from severe asphyxia in comparison with the control groups of normal neonates and those with only mild asphyxia. However, no significant difference was noted between the mild asphyxia group and the normal control group. The authors hypothesized that cerebral ischemia and hypoxia contributes to the augmented production of prostaglandins and free radicals which may enhance brain damage in intrauterine asphyxia. Russell et al. (69) measured hypoxanthine by high-performance liquid chromatography in 116 preterm (<32 weeks) infants at risk of periventricular leucomalacia. Periventricular leucomalacia was detected by ultrasound. In comparison with the unaffected infants, those with cavitating periventricular leucomalacia demonstrated a fourfold increase in median plasma hypoxanthine concentration (7.8 μmol/liter versus 31.9 μmol/liter). Cavitating periventricular leucomalacia was significantly dependent only on hypoxanthine when controlling for the effects of weight and gestation. The authors speculated that peripartum hypoxia-ischemia may be one of the etiologic factors in cavitating periventricular leucomalacia.

ONTOGENY OF ANTIOXIDANT DEFENSE IN THE FETAL BRAIN

Information on fetal cellular and extracellular defense mechanisms against neuronal oxidative stress is rather scarce. Although most of the data pertaining to antioxidant defense in the developing brain is limited to postnatal animals, there is emerging information pertaining to the fetal brain. The levels of most of the enzymatic antioxidants increase in the developing brain through the perinatal period. However, the developmental changes in the nonenzymatic antioxidants in fetal life remain unclear. This is further discussed below.

In the guinea pig fetal brain, the ontogeny of intracellular antioxidant enzymes has been characterized (70). Glutathione peroxidase, glutathione reductase, catalase, and glucose-6-phosphate dehydrogenase remain unchanged until 45 days and thereafter increase to mature levels at term, indicating an increased ability of the fetal brain to defend against oxidative stress by reinforcing the glutathione system (Figures 7–9). In contrast, superoxide dismutase remains unchanged throughout the gestation (Figure 10). Paradoxically, the enzyme activities did not respond to maternal hypoxia (inspired oxygen, 7% for 40 minutes) which raises questions regarding the actual effectiveness of these defense mechanisms. Moreover, these mechanisms are underdeveloped during early gestation during which the fetal brain may be at an increased risk for free radical injury. In comparison with the neonates, a higher oxidative stress in conjunction with lower levels of copper and zinc superoxide dismutase and glutathione peroxidase are also observed in the non-neural tissues of fetal rats (71).

Regarding the nonenzymatic antioxidants, a relatively stable alpha-tocopherol level is observed in the fetal guinea pig brain during the final period of gestation and early neonatal life (72). Similarity of the ontogeny of alpha-tocopherol in brain, lung and erythrocytes have been reported. Glozman and Yavin (73) observed a 50% reduction in the fetal rat brain tissue alpha-tocopherol levels following a five minute complete cessation of maternal–fetal blood supply suggesting consumption from oxidative stress. However, the results indicated only a limited role for the lipid soluble antioxidants in protecting the brain against oxidative stress of short duration. In contrast, Iwasa et al. (74) showed the effectiveness of tocopherol supplementation in

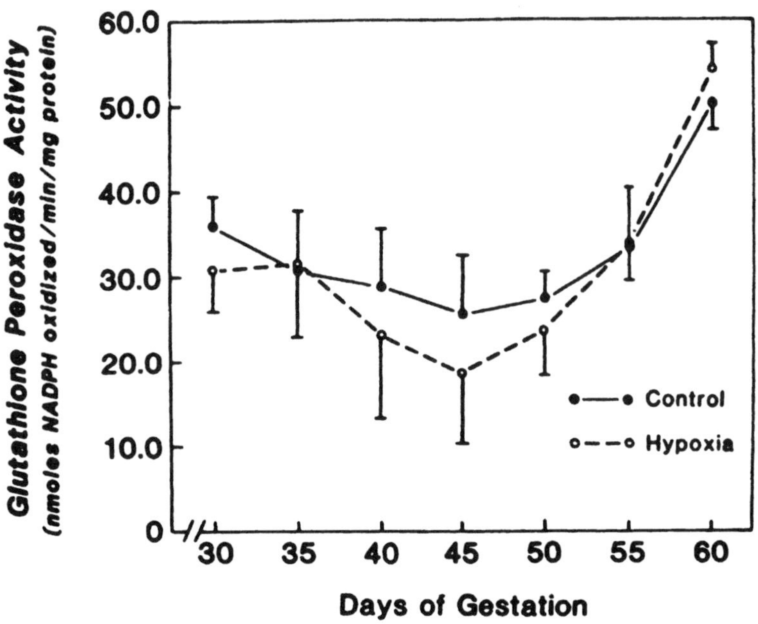

Figure 7. Glutathione peroxidase activity in fetal guinea pig brain during gestation. The enzyme activity is expressed as nmol NADPH oxidized/min/mg protein. Each point represents mean ± SD of 12 fetuses; 12 control and 12 hypoxic fetuses were used at each age. Hypoxia samples were not significantly different from their corresponding controls (p values were >0.50). (Reproduced with permission from reference 70.)

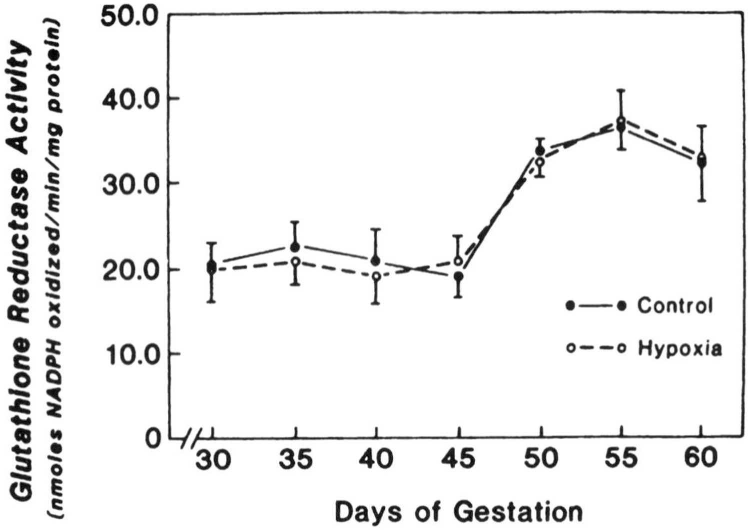

Figure 8. Glutathione reductase activity in fetal guinea pig brain during gestation. The activity is expressed as nmol NADPH oxidized/min/mg protein. Each point represents mean ± SD of 12 fetuses; 12 control and 12 hypoxic fetuses were used at each age. Hypoxia samples were not significantly different from their corresponding controls (p values were >0.50). (Reproduced with permission from reference 70.)

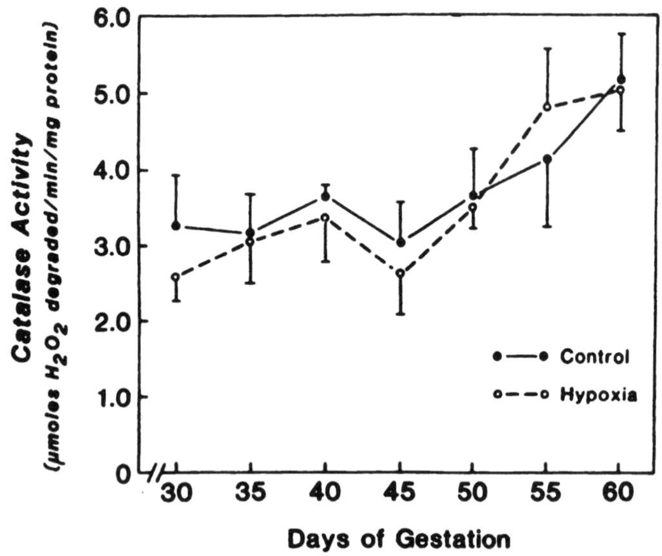

Figure 9. Catalase activity in guinea pig brain during gestation. The enzyme activity is expressed in μmol H_2O_2 degraded/min/mg protein. Each point represents mean ± SD of 12 fetuses; 12 control and 12 hypoxic fetuses were used at each age. Hypoxia samples were not significanty different from their corresponding controls (p values were >0.50). (Reproduced with permission from reference 70.)

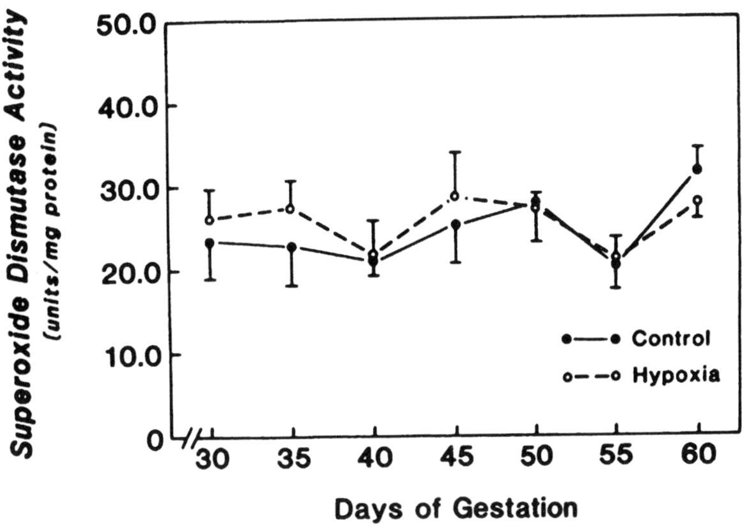

Figure 10. Superoxide dismutase activity in fetal guinea pig brain during gestation. The activity is expressed as units/mg protein. Each point represents mean ± SD of 12 fetuses; 12 control and 12 hypoxic fetuses were used at each age. Hypoxia samples were not significantly different from their corresponding controls (p values were >0.50). (Reproduced with permission from reference 70.)

preventing ischemia-reperfusion-induced lipid peroxidation in the fetal rat brain. Nakajima et al. (75) observed that the addition of this agent significantly prolonged the survival of fetal rat neurons in tissue cultures. A more specific evidence for perinatal neuroprotective effect of alpha-tocopherol is available from controlled experiments involving a neonatal piglet hypoxia model (76). This study suggests that alpha-tocopherol may protect brain cell membranes in newborn piglets from hypoxia induced lipid peroxidative damage by its inclusion in the neuronal cell membrane and also as a circulating antioxidant. There is limited data regarding fetal brain ascorbic acid level and activity. In the fetal rat brain a significant rise in ascorbic acid level is found during late pregnancy (77). The level peaks at birth and declines thereafter to the adult level. In contrast to the animal fetal data, information on the ontogeny of the human fetal antioxidant defense is scant. As mentioned before, caution should be exercised in extrapolating the animal data to the human fetus.

CONCLUSION

Significant progress has been made in recent years in elucidating the molecular mechanisms of hypoxic-ischemic brain injury. The primary initiator appears to be neuronal energy failure which initiates a complex cascade of interacting events which include generation of reactive oxygen species and its consequences. The latter is known as oxidative stress, which is paradoxically prominent during reperfusion-reoxygenation following the initial insult. The mechanisms of neuronal injury include glutamate receptor activation, loss of ionic homeostasis, elevation of intracellular Ca^{2+} level, generation of free radicals, and consequent deleterious effects on organic molecules and neuronal structure and function. In order to counteract oxidative stress, the body has developed elaborate antioxidant defense mechanisms. The spectrum of neuronal response ranges from complete recovery to delayed programmed death or immediate necrotic death, depending on factors such as (a) severity and duration of the insult and (b) neuronal maturity. The delayed response, which offers a potential window of therapeutic intervention, is mediated by secondary energy failure, formation of mitochondrial permeability pore, and triggering of the apoptotic pathway. Although most of the above information and concepts are based on adult and neonatal animal models and clinical investigations, there is emerging evidence that similar mechanisms may also be operating in the fetus despite developmental differences. There is indirect and direct evidence of oxygen free radical generation in the fetal brain in response to hypoxia and in experimentally induced fetal growth restriction. The excitatory amino acid receptor systems demonstrate overexpression at term gestation and during the immediate postnatal life which may modulate the response of the fetal brain to hypoxia-ischemia. The ontogeny of antioxidant defense in the fetal brain indicates variable progression to maturity. In spite of the recent significant advances, our knowledge on the mechanisms of fetal brain injury remains fragmentary and is often hypothetical. However, the development of any successful strategy for effective perinatal therapeutic intervention essentially depends on elucidation of these mechanisms. Obviously, this provides the most powerful rationale for further investigations in this area.

REFERENCES

1. Scheller JM, Nelson KB. Does cesarean delivery prevent cerebral palsy or other neurologic problems of childhood? *Obstet Gynecol* 1994;83:624–630.
2. MMWR Weekly Report. Economic costs of birth defects and cerebral palsy. 1995;44(37).
3. The American College of Obstetricians and Gynecologists. *Professional liability and its effects: report of a 1992 survey of ACOG's membership.* 1992.
4. Flamm ES, Demopoulos HB, Seligman ML, Posner SR, Ransohoff J. Radicals in cerebral ischemia. *Stroke* 1978;9:445–447.
5. Busciglio J, Yankner BA. Apoptosis and increased generation of reactive oxygen species in Down's syndrome neurons in vitro. *Nature* 1995;378(6559):776–779.
6. Henderson GI, Devi BG, Perez A, Schenker S. In utero ethanol exposure elicits oxidative stress in the rat fetus. *Alcohol Clin Exp Res* 1995;19:714–720.
7. McKnight AA, Keyes WG, Hudak ML, Jones MD Jr. Oxygen free radicals and the cerebral arteriolar response to group B streptococci. *Pediatr Res* 1992;31:640–644.
8. Grether JK, Nelson KB. Maternal infection and cerebral palsy in infants of normal birth weight. *JAMA* 1997;278:207–211.
9. Gutteridge JMC, Halliwell B. *Antioxidants in nutrition, health and disease.* New York: Oxford University Press, 1994:7.
10. Fridovich I. The biology of oxygen radicals. *Science* 1978;201:875–880.

11. Chance B, Sies H, Boveris H. Hydroperoxide metabolism in mammalian organs. *Physiol Rev* 1979;59:527–605.
12. Fridovich I. Superoxide radical: an endogenous toxicant. *Am Rev Pharmacol Toxicol* 1983;23:239–257.
13. Halliwell B. Reactive oxygen species and the central nervous system. *J Neurochem* 1992;59:1609–1623.
14. Gutteridge JMC, Halliwell B. Oxidative stress. In *Antioxidants in nutrition, health and disease.* New York: Oxford University Press, 1994:90–102.
15. Halliwell B, Gutteridge JMC. *Mol Aspects Med* 1985;8:89–193.
16. Beckman JS. The double edge role of nitric oxide in brain function and superoxide mediated injury. *J Dev Physiol* 1991;15:53–59.
17. Siesjö BK, Ekholm A, Katsura K, Memezawa H, Ohta S, Smith ML. The type of ischemia determines the pathohysiology of brain lesions and the therapeutic response to calcium channel blockade. In Kriegelstein J, Oherpichler H (eds). *Pharmacology of cerebral ischemia.* Stuttgart: Qissenschaftliche Verlagaagesselsch GnBH, 1990:79–88.
18. del Zoppo GJ. Microvasculur response to cerebral ishcemia/inflammaiton. *Ann NY Acad Sci* 1997;823:132–147.
19. Johnston MV. Hypoxic and ischemic disorders of infants and children. *Brain Dev* 1997;19:235–239.
20. Brann AW, Myers RE. Central nervous system findings in the newborn monkey following severe in utero partial asphyxia. *Neurology* 1975;25:327–338.
21. Vanucci R. Heterogeneity of hypoxic-ischemic thresholds in experimental animals. In Lou HC, Greisen G, Larsen JF (eds). *Brain lesions in the newborn: hypoxic and haemodynamic pathogenesis.* Copenhagen: Munksgaard, 1994:192–204.
22. Branston NM, Symon AJ, Crockard HA. Relationship between the cortical evoked potential and local cortical blood flow following acute middle cerebral artery occlusion in the baboon. *Exp Neurol* 1974;45:195–208.
23. Heiss WD, Hayakawa T, Waltz AG. Cortical neuronal function during ischemia. Effects of occlusion of on middle cerebral artery on single unit activity in cats. *Arch Neurol* 1976;33:813–820.
24. Siesjö BK. Pathophysiology and treatment of focal cerebral ischemia. Part I: Pathophysiology. *J Neurosurg* 1992;77:169–184.
25. Seisjö BK. *Brain energy metabolism.* New York: John Wiley, 1978.
26. Seisjö BK. Cell damage in the brain: a speculative systhesis. *J Cereb Blood Flow Metab* 1981;1:155–185.
27. Erecinska M, Silver IA. ATP and Brain function. *J Cereb Blood Flow Metab* 1989;9:2–19.
28. Hansen AJ. Effect of anoxia on ion distribution in the brain. *Physiol Rev* 1985;65:101–148.
29. Friedman JE, Haddad GG. Major differences in Ca_i^{2+} response to anoxia between neonatal and adult rat CA1 neurons: role of Ca_o^{2+} and Na_o^+. *J Neurosci* 1993;13:63–72.
30. Siesjö BK, Zhao Q, Pahlmark K, Siesjo P, Katsura K, Folbergrova J. Glutamate, calcium, and free radicals as mediators of ischemic brain damage. *Ann Thorac Surg* 1995;59:1316–1320.
31. McCord JM. Oxygen-derived free radicals in postischemic tissue injury. *N Engl J Med* 1985;312:159–63.
32. Kristian T, Siesjö BK. Calcium-related damage in ischemia. *Life Sci* 1996; 59:357–367.

33. Hirsch T, Marzo I, Kroemer G. Role of the mitochondrial permeability transition pore in apoptosis. *Biosci Rep* 1997;17:67–76.

34. Ambrosio G, Zweier J, Duilio C, Kuppusamy P, Santoro G, Elia P, Tritto I, Cirrillo P, Condorelli M, Chiariello M, Flaherty J. Evidence that mitochondrial respiration is a source of potentially toxic oxygen free radicals in intact rabbit heart subjected to ischemia and reflow. *J Biol Chem* 1993;25:18532–18541.

35. Dugan L, Sensi S, Canzoniero L, Handran X, Rothman S, Lin TS, Goldberg M, Choi D. Mitochondrial production of reactive oxygen species in cortical neurons following exposure to *N* methhyl-D-aspartate. *J Neurosci* 1995;15:6377–6388.

36. Piantadosi C, Zhang J. Mitochondrial generation of reactive oxygen species after brain ischemia in the rat. *Stroke* 1996;27:327–332.

37. Flamm ES, Demopoulos HB, Seligman ML, Poser RG, Ransohoff J. Free radicals in cerebral ischemia. *Stroke* 1978;445–447.

38. Forman HJ, Boveris A. Superoxide radical and hydrogen peroxide in mitochondria. In Pryor WA (ed). *Free radicals in biology,* vol 5. New York: Academic Press, 1982:65–90.

39. Turrens JG, Alexandre A, Lehninger. Ubisemiquinone is the electron donor for superoxide formation by complex III of heart mitochondria. *Arch Biochem Biophys* 1985;237: 408–414.

40. Siesjö BK. Historical overview: calcium, ischemia and death of brain cells. *Ann NY Acad Sci* 1988;522:638–661.

41. Choi DW. Calcium mediated neurotoxicity: relationship to specific channel types and role in ischemic damage. *Trends Neurosci* 1988;11:465–469.

42. Haddad GG, Jiang C. Mechanisms of anoxia induced depolarization in brain stem neurons: in vitro current and voltage clamp studies in adult rat. *Brain Res* 1993; 625:261–268.

43. Berridge MJ, Irvine RF. Inositol phosphate and cell signalling. *Nature* 1989;341:197–205.

44. Orrenius S, McConkey DJ, Bellomo G, Nicotera P. Role of Ca^{2+} in toxic cell killing. *TIPS* 1988;10:281–285.

45. Choi DW. The role of glutamate neurotoxicity in hypoxic-ischemic neuronal death. *Annu Rev Neurosci* 1990;13:171–182.

46. Beckman JS. The double-edge role of nitric oxide in brain function and speroxide mediated injury. *J Dev Physiol* 1991;15:53–59.

47. Winn RK, Sharar SR, Vedder NB, Harlan JM. Leukocytes and endothelial adhesion molecules in ischemia/reperfusion injuries. In *Cell adhesion and human disease.* Chichester Ciba Foudation Symposium, 189. New York: Wiley, 1995:63–76.

48. Gutteridge JMC, Halliwell B. *Antioxidants in nutrition, health and disease.* New York: Oxford University Press, 1994.

49. Halliwell B, Chirico S. Lipid peroxidation: its mechanism, measurement, and significance. *Am J Clin Nutr* 1993;57(suppl):715S–725s.

50. Butler J, Hoey BM, Lea JS. In Rice-Evans _, Halliwell B (eds). *Free radicals, methodology and concepts.* London: Richelieu Press, 457–479.

51. Halliwell B, Aruoma OI. DNA damage by oxygen derived species: its mechanism and measurement in mammalian systems. *FEBS Lett* 1991;281:9–19.

52. Kuroda S, Siesjö BK. Reperfusion damage following focal ischemia: pathophysiology and therapeutic windows. *Clin Neurosci* 1997;8:199–212.

53. Edwards AD, Mehmet H. Apoptosis in perinatal hypoxic-ischaemic cerebral damage. *Neuropathol Appl Neurobiol* 1996;22:494–498.

54. Nicotera P, Rossi AD. Nuclear Ca^{2+}: physiological regulation and role in apoptosis. *Mol Cell Biochem* 1994;135:89–98.

55. Hockenbery DM, Oltvai ZN, Yin XM, Milliman CL, Korsmeyer SJ. Bcl-2 functions in an antioxidant pathway to prevent apoptosis. *Cell* 1993;75:241–251.

56. McDonald JW, Johnston MV. Physiological and pathophysiological roles of excitatory amino acids during central nervous system development. *Brain Res Rev* 1990;15:41–70.

57. Mishra OP, Delivoria-Papadopoulos M. NMDA receptor modification in the fetal guinea pig brain during hypoxia. *Neurochem Res* 1992;17:1211–1216.

58. Mishra OP, Delivoria-Papadopoulos M. Modification of modulatory sites of NMDA receptor in the fetal guinea pig brain during development. *Neurochem Res* 1992;17: 1223–1228.

59. Mishra OP, Delivoria-Papadopoulos M. Lipid peroxidation in developing fetal guinea pig brain during normoxia and hypoxia. *Brain Res Rev* 1989;45:129–135.

60. Glozman S, Yavin E. Lipid peroxides are generated by the fetal rat brain after episodes of global ischemia in utero. *Neurochem Res* 1997;22:201–208.

61. Mishra OP, Delivoria-Papadopoulos M. Na^+, K^+-ATPase in developing fetal guinea pig brain and the effect of maternal hypoxia. *Neurochem Res* 1988;13:765–770.

62. de Haan HH, Van Reempts JL, Vles JS, de Haan J, Hasaart TH. Effects of asphyxia on the fetal lamb brain. *Am J Obstet Gynecol* 1993;169:1493–1501.

63. Zweir JL, Flaherty JT, Weisfeldt ML. Direct measurement of free radical generation following reperfusion of ischemic myocardium. *Proc Natl Acad Sci USA* 1987;84:1404–1407.

64. Sakamoto A, Ohnishi ST, Ohnishi T, Ogawa R. Relationship between free radical production and lipid peroxidation during ischemia-reperfusion injury in the rat brain. *Brain Res* 1991;554:186–192.

65. Sakamoto A, Ohnishi ST, Ohnishi T, Ogawa R. Protective effect of a new anti-oxidant on the rat brain exposed to ischemia-reperfusion injury: inhibition of free radical formation and lipid peroxidation. *Free Radic Med Biol* 1991;11:385–389.

66. Kramer JH, Misik V, Weglicki WB. Magnesium deficiency potentiates free radical production associated with postischemic injury to rat hearts: vitamin E affords protection. *Free Radic Biol Med* 1993;16:713–723.

67. Maulik D, Numagami Y, Ohnishi ST, Mishra OP, Farmakides G, Delivoria-Papadopoulos M. Identification of oxygen free radical generation during in-utero hypoxia in the fetal guinea pig brain. *J Soc Gynecol Invest* 1996;3:16A.

68. Zhou S, Yao Y, Li W, Tang Z. The changes in free radical and prostaglandin metabolism in newborn infants with asphyxia. *Hua Hsi I Ko Ta Hsueh Hsueh Pao* 1993;24:219–221.

69. Russell GA, Jeffers G, Cooke RW. Plasma hypoxanthine: a marker for hypoxic-ischaemic induced periventricular leucomalacia? *Arch Dis Child* 1992;67:388–392.

70. Mishra OP, Delivoria-Papadopoulos M. Anti-oxidant enzymes in fetal guinea pig brain during development and the effect of maternal hypoxia. *Dev Brain Res* 1988;470:173–179.

71. Gunther T, Hollriegl V, Vormann J. Perinatal development of iron and antioxidant defense systems. *Trace Elem Electrolytes Health Dis Mar* 1993;7:47–52.

72. Kelly FJ, Safavi M, Cheeseman KH. Tissue alpha-tocopherol status during late fetal and early neonatal life of the guinea-pig. *Br J Nutr* 1992;67:457–462.

73. Glozman S, Yavin E. Lipid peroxides are generated by the fetal rat brain after episodes of global ischemia in utero. *Neurochem Res* 1997;22:201–208.

74. Iwasa H, Aono T, Fukuzawa K. Protective effect of vitamin E on fetal distress induced by ischemia of the uteroplacental system in pregnant rats. *Free Radic Biol Med* 1990;8:393–400.
75. Nakajima M, Kashiwagi K, Hayashi Y, Saito M, Kawashima T, Furukawa S, Kobayashi K. Alpha-tocopherol supports the survival and neurite extension of neurons cultured from various regions of fetal rat brain. *Neurosci Lett* 1991;133:49–52.
76. Shin SM, Razdan B, Mishra OP, Johnson L, Delivoria-Papadopoulos M. Protective effect of alpha-tocopherol on brain cell membrane function during cerebral cortical hypoxia in newborn piglets. *Brain Res* 1994;653:45–50.
77. Wilson JX. Regulation of ascorbic acid concentration in embryonic chick brain. *Dev Biol* 1990;139:292–298.

5

PERINATAL ASPHYXIA AND PLACENTAL PATHOLOGY

Carolyn M. Salafia, M.D.
Department of Pathology, Montefiore Medical Center, Bronx, New York

INTRODUCTION

Studies of human infants have identified maternal, fetal, and neonatal factors related to an increased risk of long-term neurologic compromise (1,2). Animal models have further elucidated pathophysiology(ies) which may be causal to antenatal brain damage (3,4). Current clinical risk factors are too poorly specific to permit effective obstetric intervention. Also, risk factors may not mark risk for *future* damage, but may instead indicate fetal damage that has already occurred. For example, decreased fetal movement in the mid-trimester is a "risk factor" for cerebral damage, but it may mean that cerebral damage has already occurred and, more seriously, that intervention at this point may be too late.

There are three major clinical factors which, alone or in combination, have been identified as important antecedents to fetal cerebral injury: systemic acidosis, hypotension, and anoxemia/hypoxemia. Severe systemic acidosis has been associated with a pattern of multiorgan system failure in the perinatal period (5,6), and it may be coincident with systemic hypotension (7) and with neuronal death (8). Sustained hypotension alone has been isolated as an important factor in the genesis of cerebral

Asphyxia and Fetal Brain Damage, Edited by Dev Maulik, M.D., Ph.D.
ISBN 0-471-18427-6

injury (9). Penning et al. (10) demonstrated that prolonged fetal hypoxemia without severe acidosis or hypotension may be associated with predominantly white matter damage similar to that seen in periventricular leukomalacia Windle and co-workers (11,12) suggested that if complete anoxia is applied to the fetus, then insults of less than 8-min duration variably cause brain damage, insults of greater than 10 min invariably cause neuropathology, and fetal death will ensue after 20–25 min of anoxia. In contrast, the duration of exposure to hypoxia required to produce neuropathology may vary from 1 to 3 hours depending upon the severity of the hypoxia (13). The ability of the fetus to compensate, especially in terms of adaptation of the fetal cardiovascular system to maintain cerebral oxygenation during the course of the hypoxic event(s), is critical to the cerebral outcome.

When in gestation the potentially asphyxiating fetal injury occurred is also important in determining what may be the final (if any) fetal effect. Two features of timing need to be considered: the timing relative to delivery (information which can be provided through placental examination) and whether the event was a single injurious event or a multiple repetitive or intermittent stressor. The latter feature can be more difficult to distinguish by gross and microscopic placental examination. Timing of injury during gestation helps determine fetal effect; developmental windows of vulnerability (shaped by cellular and vascular maturational factors) in gray and white matter correlate with location of brain injury and the clinical pattern of neurologic deficit (14). In order to assess peripartum events which may cause fetal injury, neuropathologic criteria have been developed which allow approximation of the time of onset of injury within the range of 18 to greater than 96 hours before death (15). These criteria have been applied to a series of perinatal deaths; in one such series of 208 perinatal deaths, 30 (14%) had evidence of white matter or neuronal necrosis due to asphyxia. The neuropathology suggested that asphyxia may occur at any time in the last half of pregnancy; in most instances, the neuropathology dated the time of fetal injury to before the time clinical markers of fetal well-being became abnormal. Fifty percent of the cases with histologic neurologic injury had no clinical risk factors; routine periodic fetal assessment failed to identify the asphyxial episodes (16).

Multiple, repetitive brief episodes of ischemia, which individually would not cause brain damage, will serially sensitize the brain and lead to neuronal injury (17), possibly through repeated episodes of cerebral hypoperfusion/reperfusion (18). Intermittent reduction of uteroplacental blood flow in the mid-gestational sheep fetus to the point of causing fetal heart rate tracings reminiscent of variable decelerations has been associated with white matter injury (19). Such processes are a particular challenge to the perinatal pathologist, because it is often extremely difficult to differentiate *histologically* between single and multiple events such as, for example, passage of meconium or umbilical cord trauma. Once the histopathology due to a certain process is present, it can be difficult to identify additional/subsequent events that would be expected to generate the same histopathology. The distinction between a large single event (such as passage of a large volume of meconium, leading to the tissue response of a large number of meconium laden cells) and several moderate events (which may lead eventually to passage of the same volume of meconium, and, with time, the same burden of meconium laden cells) can be subtle. Clinically, intermittent, subcatastrophic stressors may be particularly difficult to detect; while a single pathologic feature may not determine the precise time characteristics of the stressful events, the "big picture" (a comprehensive assessment of gross and microscopic findings in the appropriate clinical context) is currently our best tool to understand these processes.

It might be expected that if one might more completely appreciate and more rigorously monitor the complex fetal and placental transition from intrauterine to extrauterine life, changes in fetal well-being relevant to the question of fetal cerebral injury might be discerned. Our own operative hypothesis has been that placental examination can provide clues as to the most likely mechanism and progress of a case culminating in fetal injury, especially by identifying those chronic subclinical insults, antedating birth by weeks to months and occurring without clinically recognized maternal or fetal signs or symptoms, which may set up the fetus to deal poorly with an additional peripartum stress. Support for the latter circumstance is found in studies which associate chronic fetal hypoxia or nutrient deprivation with fetal ischemic white matter injury (20) and which provide evidence for an onset of stress remote from delivery (21). We can consider the following three possibilities in light of placental anatomy and function, and we can generate for each a set of placental lesions which could underlie (1) acute fetal decompensation without chronic fetal stress, (2) acute fetal decompensation with chronic fetal stress, and (3) clinically silent antenatal fetal cerebral injury.

PERTINENT PLACENTAL ANATOMY AND PHYSIOLOGY

Battaglia and Meschia (22) have summarized the factors upon which net *fetal* transfer of nutrients depends: "without attempting to make this subject unnecessarily complex, . . . properties of the placenta, such as maternal and fetal blood flows, the pattern of placental perfusion, the surface, thickness and physicochemical properties of the placental membrane, the metabolic activity of the placenta, the various mechanisms of transfer which are available (e.g., diffusion, carrier mediated transfer, active transfer), and regional differences in placental histology and function." In the most basic physiologic terms, placental function as a nutrient exchanger requires three components: maternal blood flow, fetal–placental blood flow, and placental trophoblast membrane permeability. Any changes reducing maternal or fetal blood flow, or changing surface area or thickness of the vasculosyncytial membrane, will affect placental exchange functions.

Maternal Blood Flow

Maternal uteroplacental flow involves an extensive remodeling of the maternal vasculature, in a process which is well underway by the midtrimester (23). The remodeled maternal vessel has an enormously increased caliber and is not responsive to vasomotor stimuli (Figure 1A). Thus the normally massive increase in blood flow to the pregnant uterus can develop without increased intravascular pressure or resistance. The maternal vasculature terminates in the basal plate. Maternal blood is emptied into a

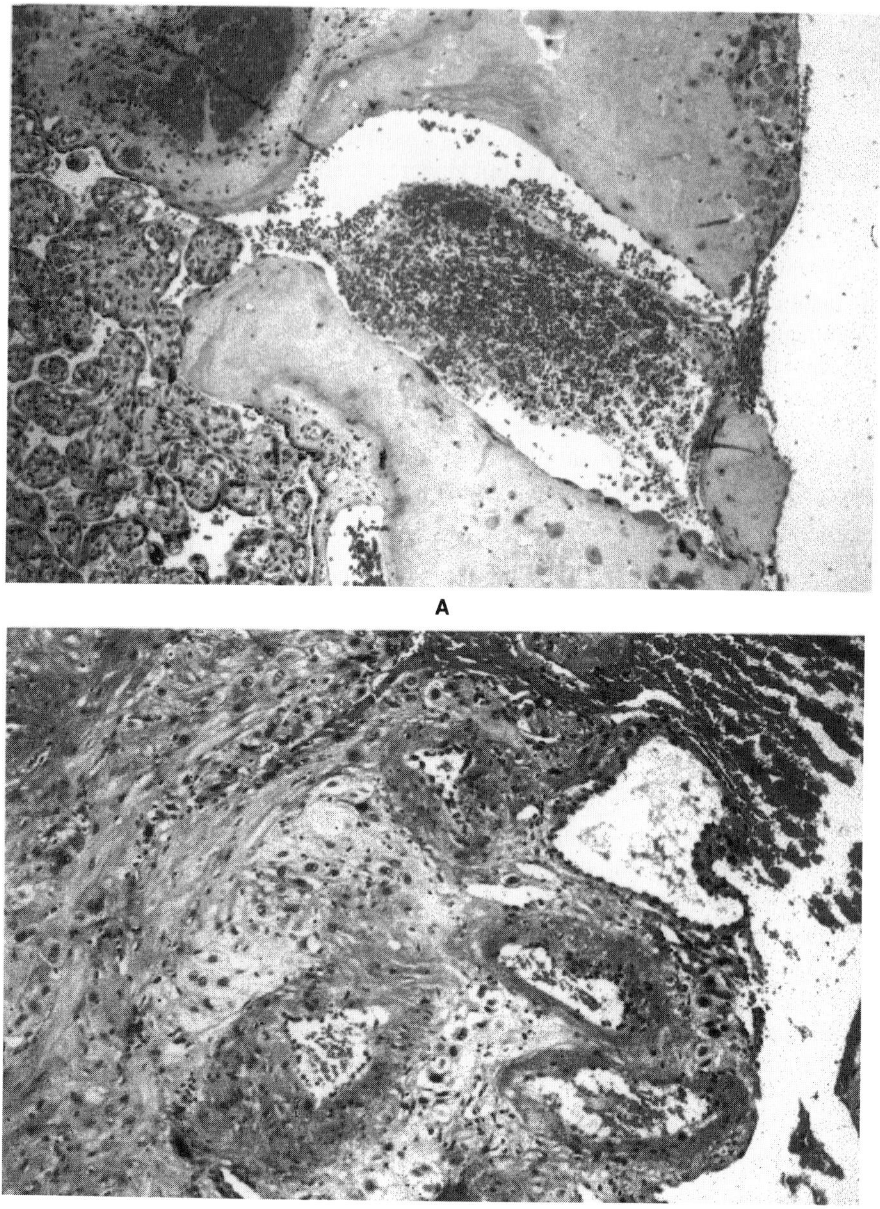

A

B

Figure 1. A: Basal plate, delivered placenta, normal term delivery: converted uteroplacental vessel with trophoblasts embedded within the amorphous fibrinoid wall. The vessel empties into the intervillous blood space. Hematoxylin and eosin, 10× original magnification. (Photomicrograph courtesy of Dr. Edwina J. Popek.) **B:** Basal plate, delivered placenta, late fetal death following paternal leukocyte immunization for recurrent pregnancy loss: multiple loops of spiral arteries with circumferential persistence of a muscular media. There is focal thinning and disorganization of the media, typical of preinvasive (trophoblast-"independent") vascular remodeling. Note numerous interstitial trophoblasts. Hematoxylin and eosin, 10× original magnification.

trophoblast-lined pool, the intervillous space. Due in part to the flow pattern of maternal blood, placental transfer of nutrients into fetal blood appears to be proportional to the concentrations of nutrients in the maternal blood.

Pregnancy compromise has been associated with abnormal conversion of the spiral vasculature in the early months of gestation. In preeclampsia, as well as in idiopathic intrauterine growth retardation in nonhypertensive mothers, histologic evidence of aberrant, incomplete, or failed trophoblast conversion of the vascular bed can be observed both in placental bed biopsies and in uteroplacental vessel segments delivered in the placental basal plate (Figure 1B). Aberrant conversion leads to retention of muscular and elastic elements within the vessels, causing abnormal uterine vascular resistance and capacitance and potentially decreased total uteroplacental vascular flow (and nutrient and oxygen presentation). Flow may also be at a greater pressure and may be more turbulent. Reduced flow or flow at an abnormal pressure may affect the developing placental capillary bed. It is important to recall that fetal effects of preeclampsia (e.g., IUGR) may not manifest for weeks to months after uterine vascular conversion is well underway (approximately 22–24 weeks).

The maternal uteroplacental vasculature can also be compromised by maternal hypercoagulable states and by toxic and environmental factors which may affect vascular function. Maternal hypercoagulable states are associated with pregnancy wastage, which appears to be caused by intrauterine thrombosis and placental infarction (24). Maternal hypercoagulability may be identified in the context of maternal autoimmune diseases such as systemic lupus erythematosus and in otherwise clinically healthy patients. The antibodies associated with maternal hypercoagulable states include the lupus anticoagulant, anti-cardiolipin and/or anti-phospholipid antibodies. They have been variably described to form immune complexes and initiate coagulation, disrupt prostanoid biosynthesis, and/or activate proteins C and S or thrombin; they may also affect placental annexin distributions, thereby disturbing normal placental development, or they may only be epiphenomena reflecting the presence of a second actually deleterious antibody (25,26). The uterine vasculature may be the sole site in which the thrombotic tendency is manifest. The uterine vasculature is unique in that its endothelium is *normally* eroded, and its basement membrane and decidual stromal collagen are *normally* exposed to circulating maternal platelets; this remodeling continues actively into the midtrimester. Fetal death associated with antiphospholipid antibodies typically involves decidual thromboses and placental infarctions, and it typically occurs before the third trimester.

Toxic and environmental factors may also affect maternal vasomotor tone; examples include maternal smoking and maternal cocaine use. Maternal smoking and increased circulating levels of nicotine result in uterine vasoconstriction and reduced uteroplacental flow which may persist for several minutes after cessation of smoking (27). Therefore, while maternal smoking compromises the quality of maternal blood by increasing the concentration of thiocyanate, carboxyhemoglobin, and potential carcinogens, it also intermittently and repetitively reduces the quantity of maternal blood presented to the placenta. Cocaine is an even more powerful vasoconstrictive agent. There is an increased incidence of abruption (28), which is a "decidual vascular accident" in mothers using cocaine. Placental transfer of cocaine may also disturb fetoplacental hemodynamics. Cocaine use may be associated with cerebral damage or dysgenesis (29).

Villous Effects of Abnormal Maternal Blood Flow

When uteroplacental vascular lesions are present, the resultant disturbance in resistance, capacitance, and increased fragility of the vasculature predisposes to "uteroplacental vascular accidents" such as placental infarcts (30) or abruption (31). Marginal separation of the placenta may be related to prematurity (32). In abruption, the placenta is forcibly separated from the uterine wall by retroplacental hemorrhage from abnormal uteroplacental vessels (33). Placental compression by a retroplacental hematoma increases fetal blood volume and may be associated with villous stromal hemorrhage (Figure 2) (34). In some settings, villous stromal hemorrhage may indicate the effects of placental trauma (a "bruise"). Chronic abruption is recognized grossly by retroplacental clot, with villous compression and possibly infarct. Acute abruption may not be grossly recognizable, and it may leave only subtle histologic "footprints." Correlation between clinical and pathologic abruption may be poor, since if the retroplacental blood escapes from behind the placenta to present as clinical vaginal bleeding, nothing is left behind the placenta to generate the typical compressive lesion.

When uteroplacental arteries are occluded, intervillous flow ceases, the intervillous space collapses, and villi become compressed, undergoing ischemic necrosis (an infarct). The gross appearance of placental infarcts varies with the age of the infarct; older lesions, in which blood is more extensively degraded, may appear tan to pink-

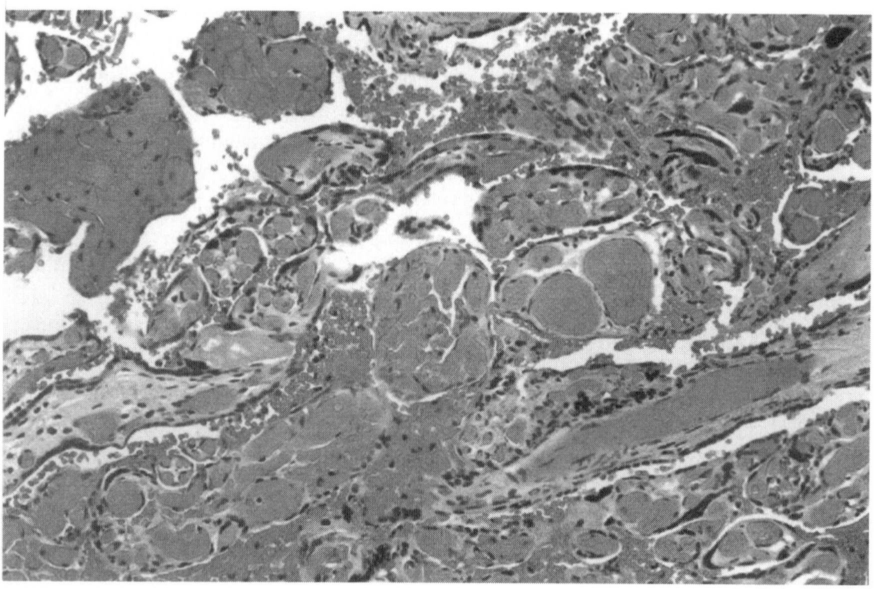

Figure 2. Focus of villous stromal hemorrhage at the margin of a recent placental abruption. Hematoxylin and eosin, 10× original magnification.

tan. More recent lesions may be the same color as the adjacent noninfarcted placenta, but simply have a firm feel—consistent with the collapse of intervillous space. The boundaries of an infarct often can be clearly demarcated by the naked eye (Figure 3). Older lesions are characterized histologically by complete loss of nuclear detail. Central infarcts are believed to be more significant to the fetus, given the greater dependence of the fetus on the central, most healthy area of villous parenchyma. The author personally grossed 500 consecutive placentas from uncomplicated term deliveries in a community hospital; 10% of the placentas had one infarct. Ninety percent of that 10% (9 out of 10 lesions) were located at the placental margin; 90% of that 10% (9 out of 10 lesions) were less than 1 cm^3 in dimension. Therefore we consider placentas with more than one infarct, infarcts located centrally, and infarcts of greater than 1 cm^3 dimension to be outside of the range of normal.

In addition to these larger-scale placental lesions, chronically abnormal uteroplacental vascular perfusion may impair the growth and development of the placenta or, alternatively, lead to diffuse microscopic lesions in a grossly normal parenchyma. The association of small placental size with long-standing poor uteroplacental perfusion has led to the concept that chronic placental nutritional deprivation can impair terminal villous arborization. The clinically relevant distinction among small placentas must be between (1) a primary failure to develop adequate placental mass, or, alternatively,

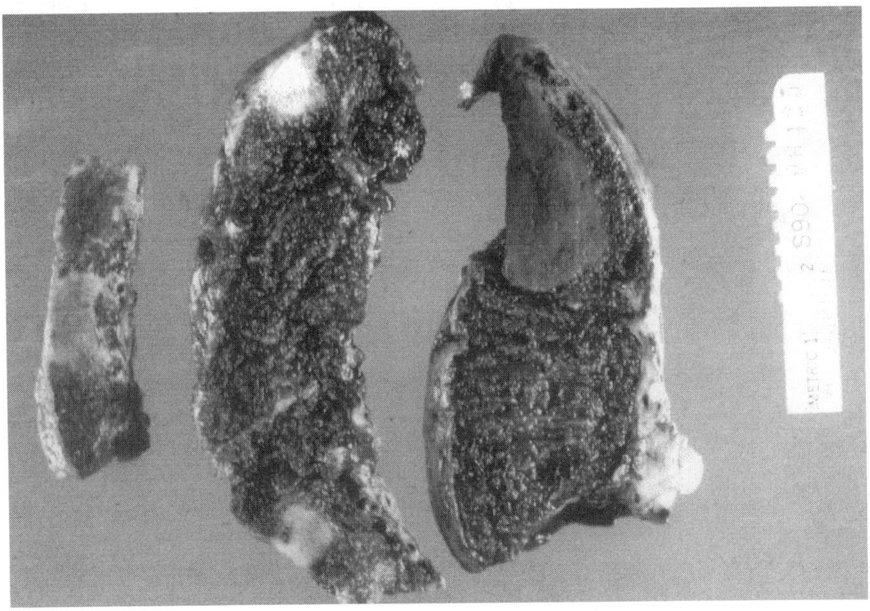

Figure 3. Gross section of a delivered placenta from 28-week stillbirth, born to nonhypertensive mother. Note the varying ages of lesions, reflected in the range of color from tan (second section, extreme right, most blood hemolyzed/degraded) to pink-tan (top section, and second section, extreme left) to dark purple, essentially a condensation of normally blood filled villi (third section, extreme right, at placental margin). Histologically, the placenta showed multifocal lesions of fibrinoid necrosis/atherosis, despite the absence of clinical preeclampsia.

(2) destruction of a normally forming structure by abnormal perfusion patterns, since the latter condition might be expected to be amenable to obstetric intervention. High intervillous pension pressure may affect the growth and development of the terminal capillary net (35,36). Abnormal uteroplacental flow has also been proposed to destroy villous capillaries, which would then yield scarred, shrunken, fibrotic, and hypovascular villi, with reduced number and/or caliber of placental capillaries (Figure 4A–C) (37). Terminal villous capillary injury would result in intraplacental villous stromal bleeding, a potential villous marker of (and intermediate step to) fetomaternal hemorrhage; midtrimester fetomaternal hemorrhage is more frequent in hypertensive pregnancies (38). "Tenney-Parker" changes of the terminal villi, an increase in syncytial nuclear clumping and basophilia, are common in cases of chronic uteroplacental malperfusion. However, it is commonly forgotten that these syncytial histologic features accompany abnormal placental perfusion of either maternal or fetal origin. It is common experience that avascular villi (villi devascularized from intraplacental

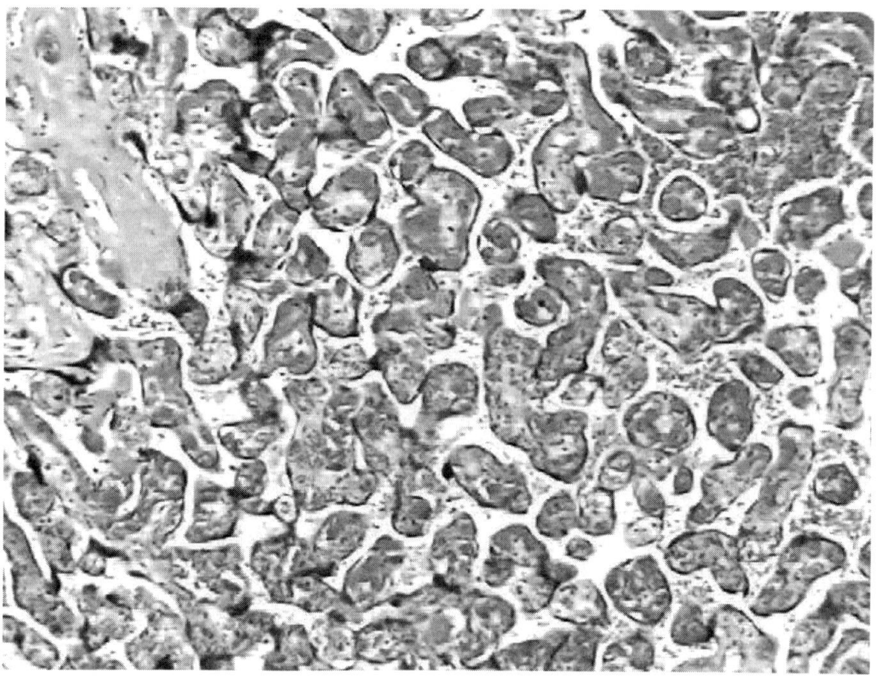

A

Figure 4. **A:** Normal term delivery, villi with numerous vasculosyncytial membranes. Hemotoxylinand eosin, 10× original magnification. **B:** Decreased terminal villous arborization in FGR delivered at 32 weeks with no clinical risk factors. Placenta demonstrated extensive uteroplacental vascular lesions. Hematoxylin and eosin, 4× original magnification. **C:** Same case as 2B. Note the very irregular vascular development, with both poorly vascularized villi and one villus with multiple capillary lumens (*arrow*). Hematoxylin and eosin, 40× original magnification. **D:** Term delivery, history of maternal smoking, AGA infant. Note increased number of capillary lumens, along with their decreased caliber, compared to part A. Hematoxylin and eosin, 40× original magnification.

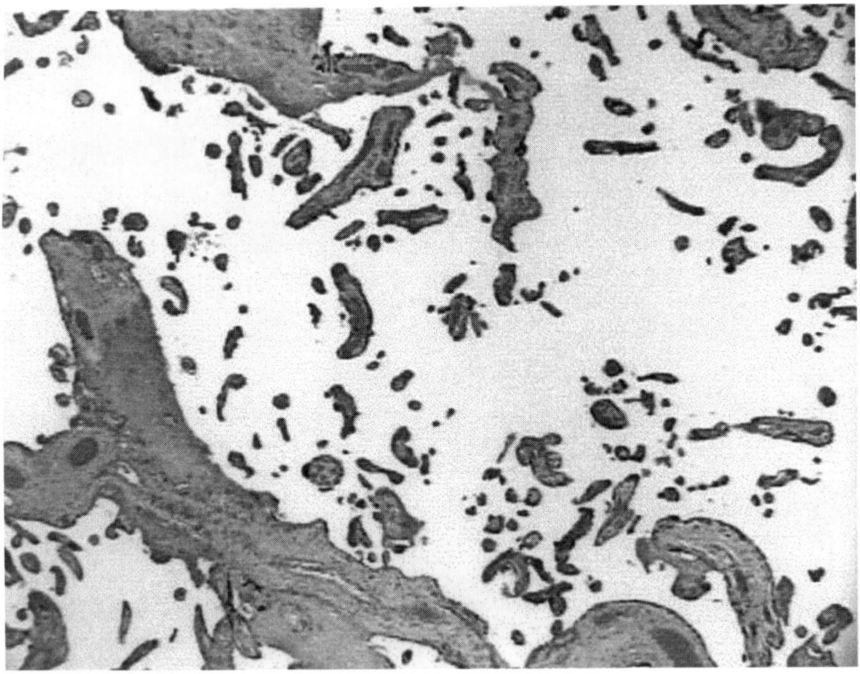

Figure 4. B. *continued*

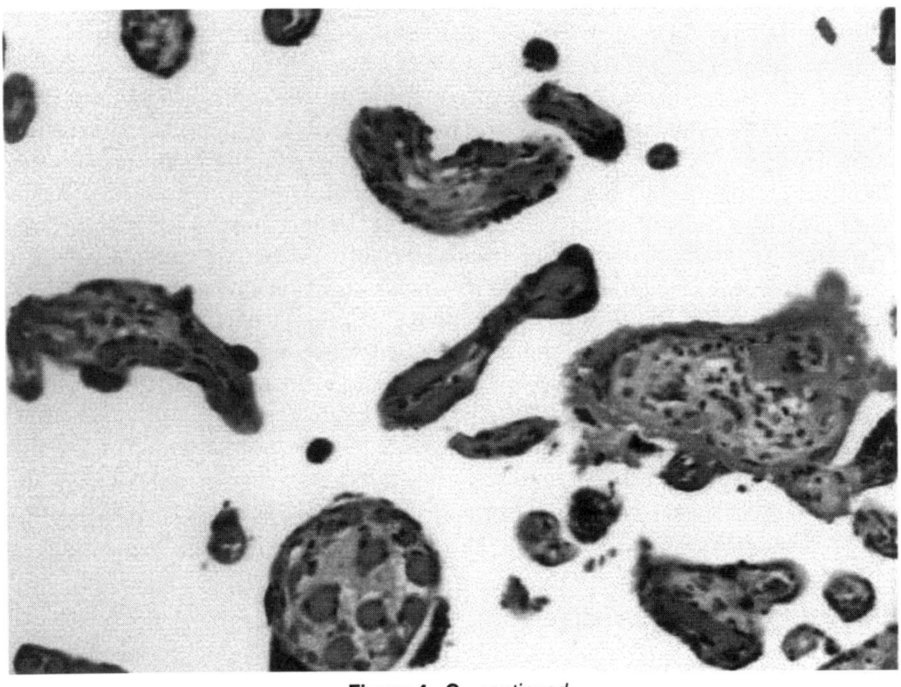

Figure 4. C. *continued*

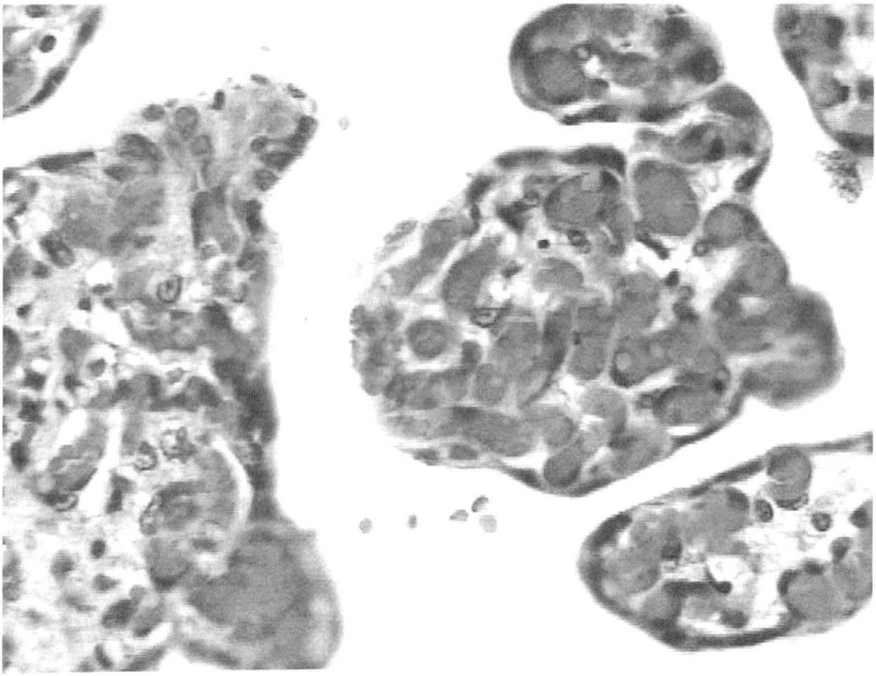

Figure 4. D. *continued*

vascular lesions) will have excess syncytial knotting compared to their normally vascularized neighbors. Experimentally, ligation of a fetal artery in the monkey placenta appeared to result in increased syncytial knotting in the villi rendered avascular (39).

When the total fetoplacental capillary bed is reduced (by whatever cause), the resultant reduction in fetoplacental volume and fetal glomerular filtration rate may lead to oligohydramnios (40) and, hence, to cord entrapment and cord pathology. A reduced capillary bed will have increased resistance, leading to increased fetal cardiac work and myocardial oxygen requirements. Histologic evidence of uteroplacental ischemia has been linked to increased resistance on umbilical artery Doppler velocimetry (41,42). The S/D ratio, an indirect reflection of umbilical–placental resistance, approaches infinity, and end diastolic flow in the umbilical artery may be negative when the placental capillary bed is reduced by more than 50% (37). Perfusion of the placenta at abnormally low oxygen tension is associated with increased basal perfusion pressure, consistent with placental vasoconstriction (43). Chronic vasoconstriction (and increased intraluminal pressure) could lead to vascular lesions via progressive mural hyperplasia (Figure 5A) or via endothelial injury (and lesions of the "hemorrhagic endovasculitis" type; see Figure 6).

Intraplacental Hemodynamics

Placental blood flow may be considered in three different anatomic sites: the umbilical arteries and vein, the chorionic vessels, and the villous capillary bed. The umbilical arteries and vein are the largest volume carriers. With the two arteries wrapped around the vein, low-pressure venous blood is "milked" back through the cord to the fetus courtesy of arterial pulsations. Cases of single umbilical artery are associated with increased likelihood of intrauterine growth retardation (44), possibly related to subtle compromise of normal cord flow.

The placental "macrovasculature" of umbilical and chorionic vessels develops early in gestation. Normal branching of the chorionic vessels may be an important determinant of later placental vascular resistance, since umbilical vascular resistance may be influenced by the number of parallel circulatory units which may develop in relation to the major vascular branches (45).

Factors regulating placental angiogenesis and vasculogenesis are poorly understood. It is believed that, early in pregnancy, villous endothelium is derived from differentiating mesenchymal cells. Not surprisingly, aneuploid placentas commonly

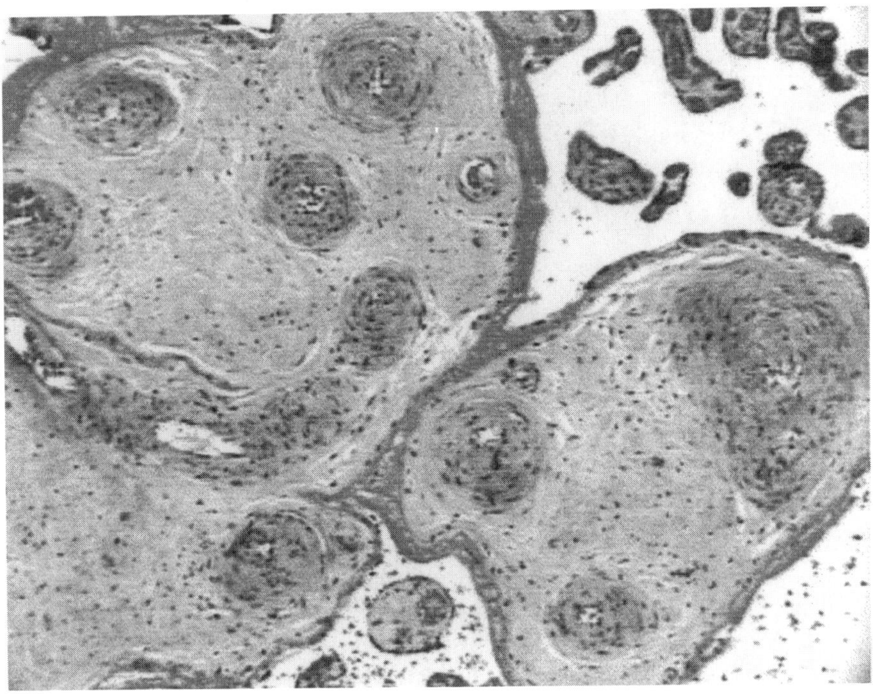

A

Figure 5. A: Clinically, a growth-restricted fetus with absent umbilical arterial end-diastolic flow by Doppler velocimetry, delivered at 34 weeks, no clinical risk factors. Fetal stem villi with uniformly thick-walled vessels with pinpoint lumens. Normally, fetal stem veins have thinner walls than fetal stem arteries, possibly due to the lower intravascular pressure. The histology here suggests that both arteries and veins have undergone medial hyperplasia. Hematoxylin and eosin, 10× original magnification. **B:** Clinically, a growth-restricted fetus with reversed umbilical arterial end-diastolic flow by Doppler velocimetry, delivered at 35 weeks, associated with maternal preeclampsia. Fetal stem villus with both vessels with reduced (*arrow*) to essentially absent media. Since, one fetal stem vessel is obligatorily an artery, we interpret this finding as remodeling of the fetal stem artery so that it resembles a vein. We hypothesize that it is induced by REDF (see text). In this case, the putative vein media (unarrowed vessel) is also markedly reduced. Hematoxylin and eosin, 10× original magnification.

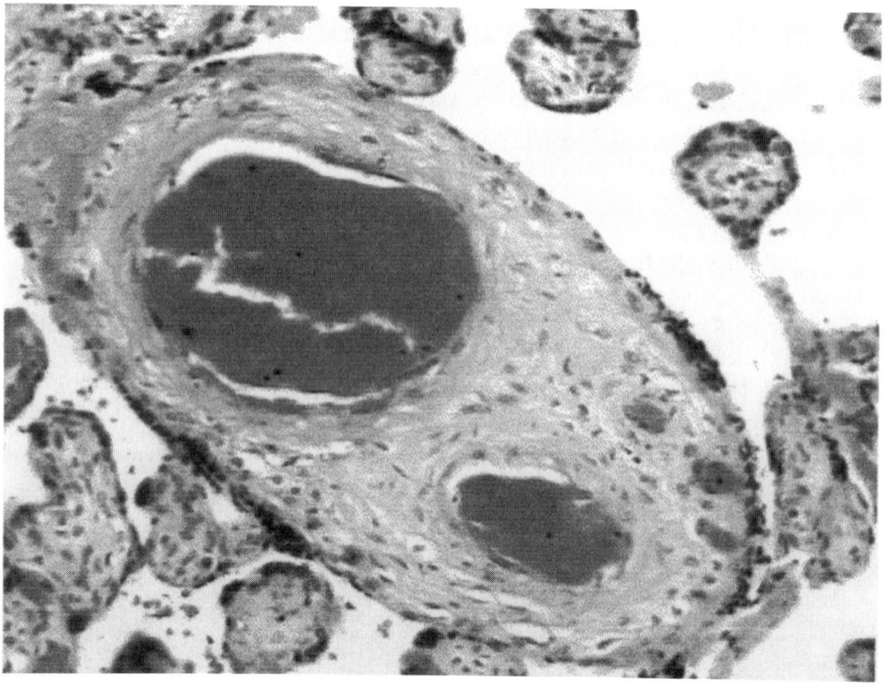

Figure 5. B. *continued*

have aberrant patterns of vascular development (46). Late in pregnancy, vasculogenesis appears to occur by proliferation of existing cells rather than by recruitment of differentiating cells. By the midtrimester, villous elaboration is due in large part to endothelial cell proliferation and capillary growth (47). The placental microvasculature increases in complexity by elongation of the terminal capillary network until about 36 weeks' gestation (48). There appears to be a specific villous proliferative zone within which placental growth is confined by term (49).

Abnormal Fetoplacental Perfusion. Abnormal development of placental vasculature is commonly associated with either restriction of growth by abnormal uteroplacental perfusion (see above) or overstimulation of growth (e.g., maternal diabetes mellitus). Considering first the restriction of normal placental vascular growth, placental vessels can fail to form or they may develop normally, but be removed from function by a variety of processes, such as intraplacental thrombi. The placental vasculature can also be modified by extrinsic forces (related to maternal perfusion) and then be remodeled by aberrant flow patterns within the placenta itself.

Lesions considered to reflect intraplacental vascular pathology include:

1. Mural or occlusive fibrin thrombi in chorionic and fetal stem vessels.
2. Avascular terminal villi, diagnosed when nutrient villi lacked capillaries and had a dense paucicellular eosinophilic stroma.
3. "Hemorrhagic endovasculitis."

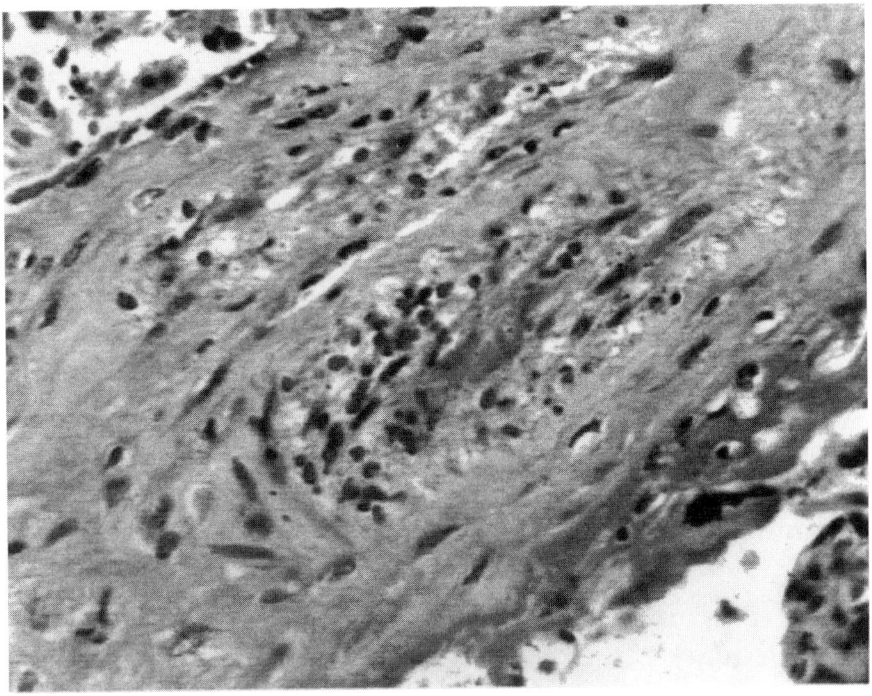

Figure 6. Clinically, delivery at term of well-grown infant with "fetal distress," no known maternal risk factors. Note the obliterated fetal stem vessel lumen, with fragmented erythrocytes in the vicinity. Hematoxylin and eosin, 20× original magnification.

4. Reduction or obliteration of chorionic or fetal stem vessels by mural hyperplasia, identified by a decreased/absent lumen area and increased wall thickness for the level of the fetal vessel (chorionic, large fetal stem artery, small fetal stem artery; see Figure 5A).
5. Mural disorganization, diagnosed when the normal concentric organization of the arterial wall was interrupted over at least 50% of its circumference.
6. Abnormally thin-walled arteries, diagnosed when all vessels in a large or small fetal stem were histologically similar, implying that the obligatory artery in the fetal stem had vein-like characteristics (Figure 5B).

As discussed above, lesions which preclude subsequent placental capillary development or which destroy existing capilary beds would be expected to affect umbilical artery Doppler velocimetry; numerous studies have suggested that this is in fact the case (41–43,50–54). The coincidence of reduced fetal stem artery counts with uteroplacental ischemic pathology (42) support the hypothesis that they are causally related (43,54). However, at least one report (42) identified severe chronic villitis (Figure 7) associated with abnormal umbilical artery Doppler, suggesting that the pathophysiology of abnormal umbilical artery Doppler—and that of the intraplacental vasculature—is more complex. The intraplacental vasculature should be subject to the same range of potential

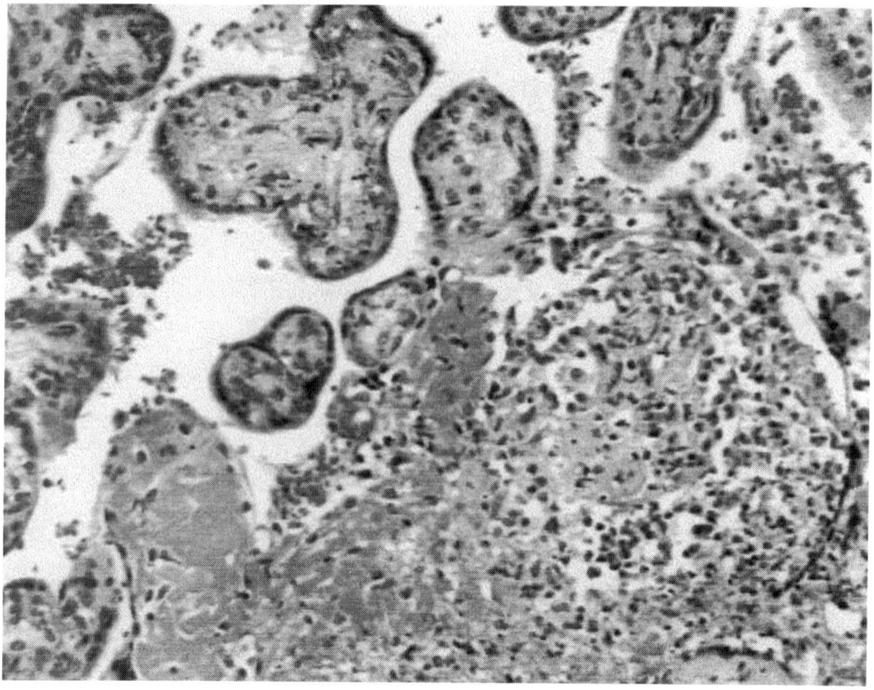

Figure 7. Clinically, explained fetal growth restriction at term, chronic villitis. Hematoxylin and eosin, 20× original magnification.

injuries as any endothelial and vascular structure, including: factors related to intravascular flow (hypoperfusion/reperfusion endothelial injury), hypoxia, cell-mediated or humoral immune mediated endothelial injury, and/or viral infection, as well as features which would modify function (e.g., inflammatory cytokines) of an intact vasculature.

We recently studied the placentas of 52 consecutive, nonanomalous singletons <10th percentile for birthweight (IUGR) admitted to the NICU with umbilical artery Doppler velocimetry obtained within 3 days of delivery between January 1989 and June 1995 (55). We expected that intraplacental vaso-occlusive lesions would be seen in a continuum extending from normal to reversal of end-diastolic umbilical artery Doppler flow. Instead we identified two anatomically distinct subsets of IUGR. The first IUGR subset were cases with intraplacental lesions greater than the mean number of lesions in IUGR placentas with normal umbilical artery Doppler waveforms. In these cases, there were more uteroplacental vascular lesions and lighter placentas, and these features were related to worsening umbilical artery Doppler status. That placentas with intraplacental vaso-occlusive lesions were lighter is consistent with speculations that chronic uteroplacental malperfusion leads to a global reduction or underdevelopment of villous arborization, rather than selective destruction of one vessel type (56–58). This pattern of villous histopathology may not indicate villous hypoxia per se but rather capillary congestion, possibly supporting a primary vasomotor pathology in AEDF.

It would be reasonable to expect that the placental histopathology in cases with absent and reversed end-diastolic flow would have a close resemblance. Although our findings may reflect effects of small sample size, reversed end-diastolic flow cases were striking for the paucity of vaso-occlusive lesions and for a significant increase in structures best described as vein-like fetal stem arteries (Figure 5B). Some cases of reversed end-diastolic flow represent unique vascular maldevelopmental syndromes. Alternatively, in cases of twin-reversed arterial perfusion, a pattern of degenerative and/or dysplastic aortic architecture, reversing the normal differentiation pattern of aortic wall development, has been suggested to parallel the abnormal intraluminal pressure in the reverse-perfused vessel (59). Whether the embryonal vessels forming within primitive chorionic membrane of the placenta will become arteries or veins is believed to be "determined by the direction of flow and its pressure" (60). Our observations suggest that in IUGR with reversed end-diastolic flow, the placental arterial wall structure may be remodeled by the aberrant flow. The development and expansion of the placental vasculature continues throughout the bulk of gestation. Aberrant placental vascular remodeling may exacerbate hemodynamic failure in a compromised fetoplacental unit. In the setting of twin transfusion, maldevelopment of the shared circulation may contribute to the evolution of the intrafetal pathology.

Vascular Proliferative Lesions. Abnormal placental vascular proliferation is commonly related to maternal diseases which are associated with big placentas generally, prime among which is maternal diabetes mellitus, with its potential for abberant fetal serum levels of insulin-like growth factor I and its binding proteins, known to influence placental growth (61). Maternal diabetes mellitus, IUGR, and multiple gestation, conditions in which placental capillary proliferation is common, also share a setting of decreased intrauterine oxygen availability (62): in diabetes, possibly related to increased maternal glycosylated hemoglobin; in IUGR to reduced uteroplacental perfusion; and in multiple gestations, to the dividing up of one uterine blood supply to support multiple siblings, or to the increased lilkelihood of abnormal placentation in multiple gestations. Villous hypervascularity is common in placentas with chronic villitis; we speculate that abnormal macrophage activity may promote abnormal intraplacental vascular proliferation. Capillary proliferation (and hence tortuousity, e.g., Figure 4D) may increase placental microvascular resistance and the diffusion distance of nutrient across the placental membrane, fetoplacental intravascular volume, and fetal cardiac work, but we have repeatedly observed clinically that umbilical S/D ratios generally remain within normal limits even with massive increase in villous capillary number, if other lesions which obliterate the placental vasculature are absent. Chorangioma, a placental vascular tumor or malformation, occurs singly or multifocally and may function as an arteriovenous malformation or vascular shunt. It may present with stillbirth, chronic fetal compromise (e.g., hydrops fetalis and congestive heart failure), or unexplained fetal tachycardia.

Villous Surface Exchange Area

The increase of villous surface exchange area across gestation effectively matches increasing fetal metabolic demands. Placental permeability increases even after the maximal rate of placental growth plateaus. In the human, this increase is achieved probably by the development in the third trimester of vasculosyncytial membranes. Earlier in pregnancy, capilllaries are deep within the villus; by term many capillaries abut the trophoblast basement membrane, with trophoblast nuclei clustering at the side. The vasculosyncytial membrane measures only 0.5–1.0 μm in thickness; the capillary basal lamina and trophoblastic basal lamina may actually fuse, leaving minimal impediment to nutrient diffusion and gas exchange. The microvillous surface increases until about 36 weeks' gestation; however, after this time, the microvillous surface declines until term (63). By term the placental transfer capacity is potentially only limited by rates of maternal and fetal perfusion.

Oxygen and carbon dioxide diffuse across the placenta. The placenta, a very metabolically active tissue, consumes almost 50% of the O_2 delivered to the intrauterine tissues. Fetal arterial pCO_2 can rise due to fetal underperfusion of the placenta (or cord compression). Fetal CO_2 production is approximately equal to pO_2 utilization. Fetal CO_2 diffuses across the placenta rapidly into the maternal blood based on the concentration gradient between fetal and maternal blood. Fetal pCO_2 may drop with maternal hyperventilation and may rise with maternal hypoventilation, impaired placental perfusion, or impaired placental permeability (22).

The fetus has no stores of oxygen. For most other nutrients, including glucose, there is fetal or fetoplacental reserve. The placenta metabolizes much of the glucose obtained from the maternal circulation. The amount of molecular glucose provided to the fetus by the placenta is less than the amount of substrate required to fuel the fetus. Glucose transfer across the placenta is a carrier-mediated event, affected by changes in perfusion (22). A major placental metabolite of glucose is lactate. Throughout gestation, most lactate is provided by the placenta and is a major fetal substrate, since supplied glucose must be reserved for the developing central nervous system. In intrauterine growth retardation, fetal nutrient utilization may decrease (64), leading to underutilization of placental lactate and a lactic acidosis. Under conditions of asphyxia the fetus itself is a net producer of lactate (22). Ketoacids may reduce fetal brain metabolism.

In summary, the placenta transfers molecules into the fetoplacental pool proportionate to their concentrations in the maternal circulation. Features which limit fetal oxygen and nutrient supply, and therefore fetal metabolism, are:

1. Changes in maternal perfusion
2. Changes in fetoplacental blood flow
3. Changes in placental permeability
4. Placental metabolic demands (22)

The principal maternal adaptation favoring fetal oxygenation is a high uterine blood flow. Uniform fetal perfusion of the placenta, production of a fetal hemoglobin with greater oxygen affinity than maternal hemoglobin, and a high fetal cardiac activity and increased fetal tissue perfusion are the main mechanisms by which the fetus optimizes its oxygenation. Normal placental growth and development maximizes placental efficiency while controlling placental metabolic demands (22).

PLACENTAL ANATOMY/PHYSIOLOGY AND CEREBRAL DAMAGE

Anoxia

In terms of our three hypothetical presentations of fetal cerebral injury—namely, acute fetal decompensation without chronic fetal stress, acute fetal decompensation with chronic fetal stress, and clinically silent antenatal fetal cerebral injury—total fetal anoxia could present as acute fetal decompensation due to complete cessation of perfusion in a previously normally functioning fetal–placental unit, as acute fetal decompensation due to complete cessation of perfusion in a previously dysfunctional/damaged fetal–placental unit, or as a clinically silent process culminating in stillbirth.

Complete fetal anoxia would require complete failure of maternal perfusion, complete failure of placental oxygen uptake, or complete failure of oxygen transfer from the placenta to the fetus. Complete failure of maternal perfusion would necessitate maternal circulatory collapse, acute thromboembolism leading to cessation of uterine perfusion, and/or complete abruption. The first two are unlikely to be missed by clinical exam. Maternal circulatory collapse often shows minimal histopathology in the placenta, even when the mother dies. Complete abruption should present with classical clinical symptoms; the placenta in a complete abruption may also be difficult to diagnose, since with a placenta free-floating within the uterine cavity, the typical findings of retroplacental hematoma with villous compression, necrosis, and ischemia will not occur. Villous ischemic changes will only develop if the intervillous perfusion failure lasts long enough to provoke syncytial basophilia and increased syncytial knotting, among the earliest markers of decreased oxygen tension identifiable by routine light microscopy. Villous compression and infarct will only develop if there is sufficient parenchymal compression long enough for histologic changes to be evident. The requirement for parenchymal compression highlights one aspect of the problem of correlating clinical and placental impressions regarding abruption. If retroplacental blood gains access to the cervix (and therefore is clinically evidence as per vaginal bleeding), it is no longer compressing the placenta; unless retroplacental clot remains, the gross and/or histopathology may be equivocal.

Complete failure of placental uptake of oxygen is not recognized; lesions such as "maternal floor infarct" (Figure 8) encase terminal villi in a thick and uniform band of perivillous fibrin/fibrinoid, and they render the bulk of the placenta nonfunctional, but this lesion would more likely lead to fetal hypoxia rather than complete anoxia.

Complete failure of oxygen transfer to the fetus could follow complete occlusion of the umbilical cord (e.g, obstructive cord knots, prolapse or other situations of mechanical cord trauma with cord occlusion, cord rupture). It is our experience that cord

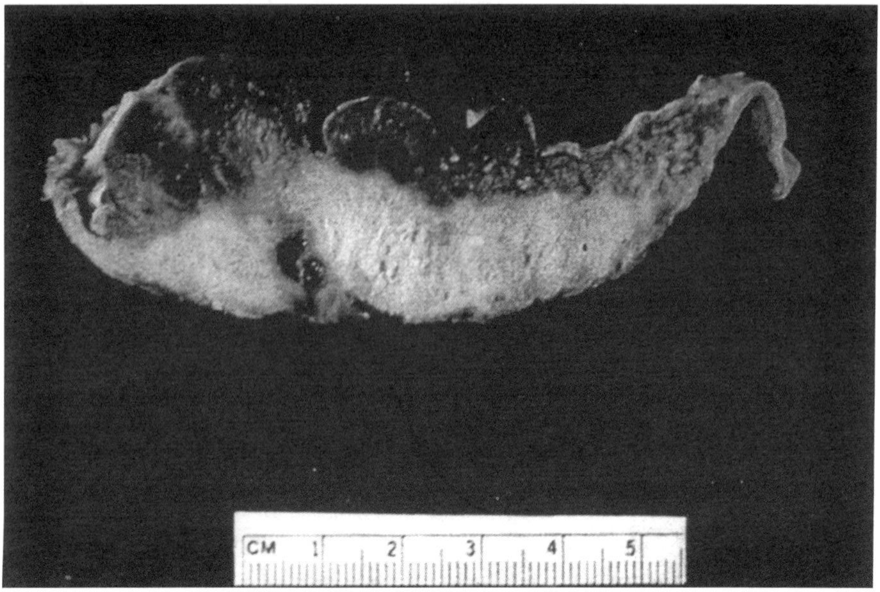

Figure 8. Clinically, late-onset fetal growth restriction and "nonreassuring fetal heart rate tracing" in mother with history of two prior early spontaneous pregnancy losses. Note the large maternal vessel (histologically patent!) in the central basal plate. The lesion is often most extensive centrally (rather than at the placental margins) and may extend to the chorionic plate.

trauma sufficient to cause tissue injury may be associated with acute or even chronic umbilical vasculitis in a nonamniotropic pattern, with occasional histologic evidence of vascular smooth muscle injury. Anecdotally we have observed immunohistochemical patterns which suggest, in cases of cord trauma, that the cells of Wharton's jelly acquire markers of monocyte/macrophage phenotype. The development of an appropriate animal model and/or in vitro manipulation of the Wharton's jelly parenchyma could provide better markers for intrafunicular processes potentially relevant to fetal perfusion. True fetal anoxic insults due to lesions of the chorionic disc and placental villi proper probably do not exist out of the arena of ruptured velamentous vessels with fetal exsanguination—as in vasa previa, or in villous bleeding with fetomaternal transfusion.

Hypoxia

Intrauterine hypoxia could plausibly present as:

1. Acute fetal decompensation without chronic fetal stress
2. Acute fetal decompensation with chronic fetal stress
3. Clinically silent antenatal fetal cerebral injury

The association of placentally mediated hypoxia with fetal asphyxia and cerebral injury is extremely complicated, since it is in this context that the complete range of metabolic intermediary pathways (of systemic acidosis, hypotension, and hypoxemia), the nature of the insult (consistent versus intermittent), and the timing in gestation must be fully considered. Again the simple approach to placental considerations can be used, namely that hypoxia must involve abnormal maternal perfusion, abnormal placental oxygen uptake, or abnormal oxygen transfer from the placenta to the fetus.

Abnormal Maternal Perfusion and Fetoplacental Hypoxia

Uteroplacental Vascular Accidents: Abruption and Infarct. In an abruption, a "uteroplacental vascular accident" causes retroplacental hemorrhage which traumatically detaches the placenta from the uterine lining. This process has both hypoxic and hemodynamic fetal effects. An area of the placenta is acutely rendered incapable of nutrient exchange, acutely decreasing fetal oxygen availability. Placental compression increases fetal placental blood volume and pressure, predisposing to visceral hemorrhage (18). Function of areas distant from the abruption may also suffer from changes in perfusion and resistance of the fetoplacental unit as a whole; it may be difficult to judge the full breadth of abruption-associated placental dysfunction in a poorly sampled placenta, or when only lesional tissue is sampled (as is not uncommonly the case). Villous stromal hemorrhage (bruising) is common in abruption; if fetomaternal bleeding results, the fetus may suffer significant—and often clinically silent—blood loss. This may be relevant in the context of systemic hypotension contributing to fetal decompensation in asphyxia. A chronic fetomaternal hemorrhage following a clinically "stable" abruption may be more common when preformed maternal antibodies to fetal blood are absent (fetomaternal blood group *compatibility*). If an abruption initially increases fetal perfusion and blood volume (hyperperfusion), subsequent placental bleeding may contribute to fetal hypovolemia and hypoperfusion pathology. An abruption may not be a single event. The vasculature in which an abruption occurs is likely to be more generally abnormal, and therefore a second vascular accident (and a second abruption) may be more likely after a first such event. The abruptive process damages the basal plate; this focus of weakened anchorage may extend the abruption given new stresses (e.g., labor).

An infarct is an ischemic (as compared to a hemorrhagic) uteroplacental vascular accident. While infarcts may not be associated with placental disruption which is as extensive as that which may occur in abruption, the infarcted villous tissue is removed from function, which may acutely reduce fetal oxygen availability. Especially at the periphery of infarcts, intraplacental vascular lesions (e.g., fetal stem thrombi) are common, which may potentially cause placental–fetal thromboembolism and direct fetal cerebral injury. The intervillous space at the periphery of infarcts may also demonstrate a prominent acute inflammatory response, possibly recruited in response to the damaged tissue. However, inflammation and cytokines may alter function of adjacent but structurally normal placenta, leading to villous edema or abnormal local perfusion patterns. Since the 40–60 placental functional units are served by 100–150 uteroplacental vessels, a perfusion redundancy (collateral flow) should prevent placental infarct. The presence of even a single, small, but central infarct means that collateral flow is insufficient to maintain placental viability if uteroplacental vessels are compromised. As a corollary, in placentas with central, large, and/or multifocal infarcts, viable villi most commonly show evidence of chronic and diffuse uteroplacental malperfusion; central, large, and/or multifocal infarcts are uncommon in the absence of stigmata of chronic uteroplacental malperfusion. As with abruption, infarcts may be multifocal in both space and time; once the fragility of the uteroplacental circulation has declared itself in an initial lesion, repetitive uteroplacental occlusive events are not uncommon.

Placental Microvascular Lesions and Fetoplacental Hypoxia

Within the villous capillary microcirculation, tissue hypoxia has a potent vasoconstrictive effect on regional placental vasculature (65), shunting blood away from placental regions poorly perfused by maternal blood and directing blood to villi better supplied with oxygen and nutrients. This is analogous to the "ventilation/perfusion matching" of the normal lung. At all levels of the placental circulation, resistance, capacitance, and flow may be acutely modulated by prostanoids and other mediators generated in intraamniotic infection (66,67) as well as by regional placental hypoxia.

Common histologic systems for "grading" severity of placental lesions tend to try to quantitate the volume of frankly lesional tissue, on the assumption that this would best approximate the functional placental compromise. This may not be an accurate assumption; the gross area of histologically lesional tissue may underestimate the degree of altered placental functional capacity. We have identified a subset of IUGR cases admitted to the NICU with severely abnormal umbilical artery Doppler velocimetric studies, but few to no histologic intraplacental vaso-occlusive lesions (see above). Among these cases, the more severe the chronic inflammation, the worse the umbilical artery Doppler status. However, in none of the cases did the estimated volume of lesional tissue exceed 30% of the parenchyma, a level which should preserve placental functional reserve. Placental mass in these cases was not on average 20% greater than age-matched cases with identical umbilical artery Doppler studies and extensive intraplacental vaso-occlusive lesions. These data suggest that chronic-inflammation-associated abnormal umbilical artery Doppler waveforms may be caused by abnormal vascular function—rather than fixed anatomic lesions—due perhaps to local production of cytokines and prostanoids (known to affect placental vasomotor tone) (66). Since malfunction of an anatomically normal placenta may be amenable to in utero therapy (such as transplacental administration of anti-inflammatory agents), it may be clinically relevant to improve in vivo methods of distinguishing between our two possible subtypes of abnormal umbilical artery Doppler waveforms.

A histologic marker of nonspecific placental dysfunction may be villous edema. Villous edema may be more common in cases with acute intrauterine inflammation (68). However, villous edema may be seen in abrupted placentas, cases of maternal diabetes mellitus, and cases with unexplained intrapartum distress. Naeye et al. (68) suggested that increased intravillous pressure may collapse the capillary bed and lead to hypoxia. This is often difficult to appreciate; edematous villi often have normal caliber or even congested vessels. Any process that affects trophoblast epithelial permeability and/or transport, capillary vasomotor tone, or capillary permeability may lead to fluid leakage and villous edema. Therefore, villous edema may be a marker of dysfunction induced by a range of pathology, including the following: endotoxin-induced trophoblast damage, placental macrophage activation and cytokine production, and increased capillary perfusion pressure. One may speculate that the clinical significance of villous edema may vary depending upon its etiology. Villous edema increases the diffusion distance for nutrients across the placenta and thus may impair placental permeability. Other lesions which may affect placental diffusion capacity include thickening of the trophoblast basement membrane or reduced total area of vasculosyncytial membranes.

Placental lesions are significantly related to placental respiratory function. We have reported on umbilical blood gas values in 431 nonanomalous singleton infants born at less than 32 weeks' gestation (69). Placental lesions related to uteroplacental vascular pathology, chronic villitis, and coagulation-related lesions demonstrated general associations with decreased UV and UA pH, decreased UV and UA pO_2, and increased UV and UA pCO_2, while acute infection and villous edema were generally related to increased UV and UA pH, increased UV and UA PO_2, and decreased UV and UA pCO_2. However, this finding was spurious, caused by a relative sparing of severely acutely inflamed placentas of significant uteroplacental vascular, chronic inflammatory, or coagulation related pathology. Stepwise regression isolated four variables with independent predictive value for umbilical cord blood gas values (histologic evidence of abruption, villous infarct, villous hypovascularity, and avascular villi, $R^2 = .10$). When we examined the subset of cases with clinical labor, the data suggested that there is a basic difference in placental functional reserve (or capacity to withstand the stresses of labor) which is best measured by the gestational age of the placenta and which is not marked by histologic lesions. In other words, the more preterm the placenta, the greater may be its relative functional inefficiency and the lesser the ability to withstand stresses including labor. This relative inefficiency is irregardless of pathologic lesions, which may however superimpose compromise on the preterm placenta.

Large Placental Vessel Pathology and Fetoplacental Hypoxia

Cord compression may cause fluctuations in fetal perfusion. Umbilical arterial compression increases placental resistance, fetal cardiac work, and fetal myocardial oxygen requirements; umbilical venous compression may cause hypoxemia (reduced O_2 availability) and ischemia (decreased blood flow). Cord pathology is more common in the crowded intrauterine environment of multiple gestation. In twin gestations, velamentous cord insertion is commonly associated with intrauterine growth retardation of the involved twin (70). From pure mechanics, it is not difficult to understand how a velamentous cord insertion could compromise fetal placental blood flow. Especially following membrane rupture, the umbilical cord would itself be much more susceptible to kinking/obstruction at its insertion. Placental thickness in utero is approximately twice that measured after delivery in the pathology laboratory; active maternal intervillous circulation distends the intervillous space. Therefore, chorionic plate vessels are based on a deformable bed of villi and maternal blood. The vessels which run in the extraplacental membranes are apposed directly to the rigid myometrial wall. Any compression of these vessels will reduce flow, damage their musculature and/or endothelium, and lead to thrombosis, thromboemboli, or chronically—but intermittently—abnormal flow. Thromboemboli originating in damaged sections of the placental arterial tree will lodge in the placental capillary bed, occlude local circulation, and compromise placental function. Equally significant to a fetus may be venous-derived placental thromboemboli with their potential for cerebral embolism. Similar mechanics could reasonably compromise the singleton fetus with a velamentous cord. Furcate umbilical cords (when Wharton's jelly stops above the chorionic insertion and unsupported umbilical vessels traverse to the chorionic plate) are also mechanically vulnerable.

Trauma and other mechanical events are not the only stimuli for generation of thrombi in umbilical and chorionic vessels. Inflammation activates endothelium to promote platelet aggregation and produces local and systemic vasomotor stimuli (generally arachidonic acid derivatives) which can act at different levels within the placental vasculature (66,69). Acute ascending—often bacterial—invasion of the amniotic fluid space leads to intraamniotic accumulation of cytokines and other inflammation-related molecules which diffuse into the placental tissues and vascular structures with the potential for effects on fetoplacental vasomotor tone. Increased umbilical systolic/diastolic ratios have been observed in human fetuses with inflamed umbilical vessels in their delivered placentas (71).

TIMING: GENERAL CONSIDERATIONS

Many of the same events which may cause acute intrapartum damage may, if severe enough, cause antepartum cerebral damage. Insults antedating birth may be (1) acute, temporally limited events and/or (2) chronic disorders which progressively compromise the fetus and which culminate in acute tissue damage prior to birth. Acute and temporally limited processes cause immediate global dysfunction that would resolve with time except in the central nervous system. Examples of time-restricted damage processes include:

1. Maternal abdominal trauma, maternal hypotension, hypovolemia or shock
2. Placental abruption with delayed delivery ("stable" abruption)
3. Umbilical cord compression or vascular compression in membranous cord insertion (see above)
4. Spontaneous fetomaternal or fetofetal transfusion
5. Acute infectious/inflammatory processes that resolve before birth

"Acute time-limited" and "chronic" events may overlap since histological timing of antepartum events in the delivered placenta is imprecise. Since there is often more than one route by which an intrauterine event may affect the fetus and/or placenta, even a "one-shot" event may "ricochet" into a broader range of effects, each with variable time courses. For example, in the ewe, uteroplacental embolization may acutely damage the placenta but also alters placental endocrine function (cortisol and progesterone biosynthesis). Here, an acute event may have result in chronic dysfunction (72). The effects of acute intraamniotic infection may include direct bacterial/toxigenic effects, inflammatory/vasomotor effects, or even abruption, which may be more common in an infected uterus. There may be no single cause for a placental feature such as, for example, circumvallate membrane insertion, which may reflect an acute event (decrease in amniotic fluid pressure) or a chronic process (abnormal depth of placentation) (73). Some "acute" events are the climax of subclinical chronic pathology. A "spontaneous" acute abruption is most commonly the result of maldevelopment of the uterine vasculature since the early weeks of gestation. Obstetricians have come increasingly to appreciate that even normotensive women may demonstrate uterine and placental anatomy histologically to those seen in preeclampsia. Despite the absence of maternal symptoms, the histopathology commonly reflects a pathologic fetoplacental environment, because IUGR is common in such cases (74–76).

Certain processes (e.g., maternal smoking) may primarily have chronic effects. We have observed increased capillary proliferation in many placentas of smoking mothers, and others have described lesions which reasonably should affect placental nutrient exchange efficiency, such as basal lamina thickening (77). Additionally, toxic compounds which circulate in the blood of mothers who smoke may accumulate in the fetus and placenta, with cumulative tissue damage effects (78). There are also direct and chronic effects of maternal smoking on circulation in the umbilical vessels (79), fetal coronary arteries, and aorta (80,81). Maternal smoking is a repetitive act, so neither intermittent types of fetal injury, nor that the uteroplacental circulatory derangement in maternal smoking could culminate in an acute fetoplacental event (e.g., abruption), can be excluded.

Maternal diabetes mellitus may also create a situation of chronic ongoing fetal compromise. In placentas delivered of diabetic mothers, there is often diffusely abnormal villous maturation. Villi are abnormally large and poorly vascularized, with centrally located vessels (rather than vasculosyncytial membranes) and immature-appearing bilayered trophoblast and voluminous stroma. Vasculosyncytial membranes, if present, may be thickened. Because of this abnormal anatomy, these placentas may be more inefficient in nutrient transport. Diabetic placentas are often larger than normal; fetoplacental weight ratios may be decreased, indicating that placental growth may outstrip fetal growth. These disproportionately large organs have disproportionate metabolic demands. The progressive switch of fetal production of hemoglobin F to hemoglobin A may, especially in the presence of high-oxygen affinity hemoglobin A1c in the maternal circulation, reduce fetal capacity to extract oxygen from the maternal circulation and progressively impair fetal oxygen supply with advancing gestational age.

The increasing incidence of multiple gestations (thanks to ART) increases the frequency of concerns for fetal injury. In monozygous twins, there are almost always vascular anastomoses; these vascular communications, often mismatched between artery (high pressure) and venous (low-pressure circulations), may result in both acute and chronic insults. Chronic twin transfusion may lead to (a) chronic hypoxia and relative hypovolemia in the donor and (b) volume overload and congestive heart failure in the recipient. Doppler studies indicate that these anastamoses may be very dynamic, with bidirectional flow in serial evaluations (82). Chronic hypoperfusion/reperfusion injury in both twins may be frequent. Acutely, death of a co-twin may result in variable degrees of exsanguination of the living sibling into the dead baby through the circulatory connections. Acute hypovolemic shock may lead to death of the sibling but homeostasis may also occur with resultant visceral but not cerebral repair. In studies of children in whom antenatal cerebral damage is thought to have occurred, many of them are monochorionic twins (83). Velamentous umbilical cord insertion is common in multiple gestation (84). This mechanically vulnerable cord insertion places the fetal lifeline flush against the rigid and unyielding myometrium, instead of the flexible chorionic plate. In multiple gestation, the "disadvantage" conveyed by a velamentous cord has been linked to chronic donor status or chronic "vascular steal" and to significant fetal morbidity/mortality (70).

Partially treated problem pregnancies pose yet another complication for the diagnostic placental pathologist. Maternal hypercoagulable states are associated with uteroplacental thromboses and placental infarction, which can chronically impair the wellbeing of the fetoplacental unit. Heparin/aspirin therapy is associated with a high rate of subsequent successful pregnancy (85). However, the trophoblast surface (perivillous coagulation) and intraplacental circulation may also be targets of antiphospholipid antibodies (86,87). Despite full anticoagulative therapy, these lesions will persist in frank treatment failures (i.e., those resulting in repeat fetal death) but also in "successes" which result in delivery of preterm IUGR, chronically stressed infants. As therapeutic interventions in poor pregnancy outcome become more prevalent, the pathologist must be able to appreciate the possibility of multiple means of fetoplacental manifestation of a single clinical disease.

Finally, an all-too-common finding in cases of unexplained fetal/neonatal damage is that of chronic villitis. Chronic villitis, chronic inflammation of the placental villi, is believed to indicate a congenital viral infection (88). Recently, chronic villitis has been associated with autoimmune responses of the mother, possibly to the extensive modifications of her tissues by the conceptus and also to allo-immune rejection of the conceptus. Most cases of congenital viral infection are clinically asymptomatic in the mother. Autoimmunity may also be subclinical, with no evidence of maternal systemic disease but only serologic abnormalties. Maternal/fetoplacental allo-immune pathology may also be without any recognized maternal syndrome or specific laboratory abnormality. The actual amount of villi inflamed is often quite small, and it is insufficient to explain fetal compromise on the basis of anatomic placental insufficiency. It is proposed that viral infections are associated with reduced fetal mitosis and decreased cell number. Other effects of chronic inflammation may be changes in placental macrophage activity. Macrophage products may locally affect placental microcirculatory growth, hemodynamics, and trophoblast function. Also, maternal invasion of the conceptus in villitis may lead to intrauterine graft versus host disease and widespread fetal damage.

TIMING AND PLACENTAL PATHOLOGY

Problems

- *Single versus multiple events.* Even those histologic features for which some agreement as to timing exists (e.g., hemosiderin pigment, metabolism of which from hemoglobin requires a minimum 24 hours) (89) cannot distinguish between single or multiple events of intrauterine bleeding.
- *Multiple pathways, with different time frames, can produce a similar lesion.* Interpretation of lesion timing must be made after taking into account the "big picture" of all placental histopathologic features. While trophoblast degenerative knots may develop as quickly as 24 hours after in vitro exposure to lowered oxygen tension (90), trophoblast knots are most common in chronic uterine vascular insufficiency (e.g., preeclampsia). Trophoblast knots which develop as a response to an acute stimulus are associated with normal-appearing villi. Acute events of lowered intervillous oxygen tension, if sufficiently brief, may not be associated with syncytial knotting. Trophoblast knots appearing as part of a more chronic process will have abnormal villous structure, including fibrosis and hypovascularity. Infarctions with loss of nuclear detail will likely be more than 7 days old.
- *Placental responses to insults/stressors may vary with gestational age.* The premature placenta, with its functionally immature macrophages, may be less capable of demonstrating a cellular infiltrate than a term placenta. Small foci of villitis in a preterm placenta may represent a significantly more severe and protracted inflammation than in a term placenta. The possibility that inflammation may present in a different fashion in the very immature placenta should also be considered. Perhaps in the very immature placenta, a cellular infiltrate will not develop. Instead edema, a cardinal sign of inflammation, may be the only histologic evidence of villous inflammation. The gestational age of the placenta at the time of insult and at delivery may affect (a) placental tissue response to intrauterine events and (b) placental–fetal pathophysiology. Similarly, fetal myeloid immaturity may impair the development of fetal vasculitis in intraamniotic infection, "underestimating" the extent of fetal immune activation.

Acute Inflammation

There is relatively little information about the timing of onset and evolution of placental lesions. Even the time course of the evolution of histology related to intraamniotic infection is not well understood. The infiltrate seen histologically in the amnion, chorion-decidua, chorionic plate (composed of maternal neutrophils), and the umbilical cord and chorionic plate vessels (comprised of fetal inflammatory cells) develops along the same principles by which inflammation develops in other tissues, namely, the immune maturity and response capacity of the organism, the immunogenicity of the organism, the size of the organism inoculum, and the duration of exposure to the inflammatory response. It is this author's belief that overall histologic assessment of the density of infiltration and distance traveled, as well as the patterns of acute inflammation in different tissue sites, cannot be related to one of these features (for example, duration of inflammation) independent of the other considerations. The only feature which has the potential to isolate the time course from other considerations may be the lifespan of neutrophils. Aging neutrophils undergo programmed cell death, a process which allows their recognition by macrophages and removal from inflamed sites. In vitro work has shown that >98% of neutrophils maintain viability to 24 hours, and a progressive, time-related increase in macrophage recognition past that time is associated with neutrophil morphology consistent with apoptosis (91). While in other tissues with large population of resident mature macrophages, neutrophil recognition, uptake, and degradation are rapid, in the avascular amnion and chorion, as well as in the parenchyma of the umbilical cord, neutrophil removal might be expected to be slow. The relative proportion of intact to degenerated neutrophils in tissue can provide some crude estimate of the time of onset of neutrophil infiltration in acute intraamniotic infection.

Meconium

Meconium staining has been studied in one in vitro experiment (92). This study suggested that meconium phagocytosis by amniotic macrophages occurred within 1–3 hours, and meconium phagocytosis by chorionic macrophages occurred within 3–6 hours. Staining of the umbilical cord has not been studied critically, since in the cited study the umbilical cord was cut into 1-cm segments and apparently floated in the meconium mixture. The extremely rapid cord staining they described (within 15 min) is in contrast to clinical experience of green membranes commonly accompanied by unstained, creamy white umbilical cords. However, if meconium has access to the cut end of the cord, it would be expected that it would rapidly diffuse into the myxoid, watery Wharton's jelly. Since the experimental design appeared also to allow multidirectional tissue exposure to meconium (membranes were also floated in a meconium mixture), rather than the unidirectional exposure seen in vivo (with meconium-contaminated amniotic fluid as the source of diffusible meconium), additional studies may be required to better understand the timing of meconium tissue effects. Meconium may also confound the interpretation of acute intraamniotic infection; meconium has been shown to enhance bacterial growth in culture systems (93), and enhance deleterious effects of bacteria (94). Whether these are organism-specific or general effects is not known and should be studied. The hypothesis of cerebral-vasospasm-induced cerebral injury deserves careful study by as many investigators as can be recruited to the subject. In a small study of meconium-exposed infants admitted to a Neonatal Intensive Care Nursery (95), fully 55% (18/33) of the infants had meconium histiocytes apposed or intercalated within the chorionic vascular media. These infants had a mean cord arterial pH of 7.24, and mean Apgar score of 8 ± 1.5 (range 3–9) at 5 min; 91% (30/33) required oxygen therapy for less than 72 hours. All were discharged home neurologically intact. Meconium associated with fetal vasculature may not uniformly be associated with fetal injury which manifests as fetal or immediate neonatal significant compromise.

Nucleated Erythrocytes

New insights into intrauterine pathophysiology have complicated the timing issue. For instance, understanding of the mechanisms of release of nucleated erythrocytes by the bone marrow has become more complicated. The traditional pathway of hypoxia inducing erythropoeitin to affect the bone marrow has been invoked to explain the association of excess nucleated erythrocytes in the fetoplacental circulation with increased risk of cerebral compromise (96). However, infection induces both maternal and fetal production of interleukin-6, which has recently been shown to have a direct effect on the bone marrow to stimulate proliferation of immature cells of multiple lineages, including immature (nucleated) erythrocytes (97). In acute intraamniotic infection there are increased fetal circulating levels of interleukin-6. Acute amniotic infection has also been proposed as a risk factor for cerebral damage (98). In the adult, generally a hypoxic stress requires 24–48 hours for detection of circulating nucleated erythrocytes. This time course must vary in the fetus due to the following:

1. Gestational age, with younger ages having greater extramedullary hematopoeisis and facilitated egress of nucleated erythrocytes into the circulation
2. Duration and severity of stress, with protracted duration promoting excessive extramedullary hematopoeisis and a greater bone marrow stress
3. Pressures of additional factors affecting bone marrow "gating" of erythrocytes (such as interleukin-6 in acute infection)

We have demonstrated that acute intraamniotic infection provides a potent stimulus to nRBC release in the preterm fetus (99). Furthermore, working on the hypothesis that hypoxic (and erythropoeitin-mediated) nRBC release and acute inflammatory (cytokine-mediated) nRBC release would differ in the time course of nRBC clearance after delivery, we have identified separate patterns of nRBC clearance: One is related to uteroplacental vascular and placental ischemic lesions, and the other is related to acute inflammatory pathology. Using the cord blood sample and at least one other nRBC value, we extrapolated a time at which nRBC count would approximate zero (the "time to clearance"). The ischemic/hypoxic pattern had a longer time to clearance than the acute inflammatory pattern, consistent with the shorter effect of cytokines as compared to erythropoeitin (100).

Histopathology and Differentiation of Causal Pathways

This is a concern to which perinatal pathologists are frequently asked to respond in courts of law. Placental pathology may be helpful in ruling in—or in ruling out—likely causal pathways for fetal injury. However, it is most common that complicated pregnancies, and especially those which culminate in fetal injury, may demonstrate more than one type of pathological process, almost as if the redundancy and protections built into the human reproductive system require several homeostatic mechanisms to become impaired before any harm can come to the fetus. In these circumstances it is often very difficult to point to a single cause of fetal injury, because the complex gross and microscopic pictures appear to indicate—rather than a single injurious process—a series of pathological straws which, when laid across the camel's back, finally broke it.

In addition to the difficulty of sorting out a single factor from what may be a cumulative pathophysiology, the limitations of human pathophysiology make it likely that somewhere in the pathophysiology, even diverse noxious agents such as acute intraamniotic infection and a cord accident will join in a final common pathway of cell death, within which the pathophysiology set in motion by an acute infection (infectious shock with global failure of the fetal circulation) is indistinguishable from circulatory collapse and failure of tissue perfusion by cord occlusion or by any etiology. Prior to that point, intraamniotic cytokines and other inflammatory mediators may affect fetoplacental vasomotor (including umbilical) function and begin to influence tissue oxygen availability and perfusion. Fetal immune activation may lead to fetal tachycardia (and increased fetal myocardial oxygen requirements) and fetal metabolic responses to infection which increase tissue oxygen utilization more generally. What the pathologist can do is identify what processes are present in the placenta, the relative strengths of those processes, and their possible duration in utero. From that study, the pathologist can describe what are and are not likely significant pathophysiologic processes, and possibly their potential clinical associations. Only from clinicopathologic correlation—the correlation of placental anatomic and histologic findings, with laboratory assessment of mother and baby, and clinical assessment of mother and baby—can the final "big picture" be constructed.

SUMMARY

Given what is understood of placental function, and of pathways which could lead to cerebral damage, specific placental sites and specific pathophysiologic process can be identified in which disturbance of anatomy or changes in functional capacity could contribute to the metabolic and hemodynamic processes that lead to cerebral damage. Lesions may point to clinically silent pathways of fetal damage or may lend support to relevant clinical and biochemical clues. Computer-assisted image analyses (to better quantify and standardize diagnoses of lesions) and immunohistochemistry and in situ hybridization (to more completely describe and better characterize lesions) may become necessary to supplement our present diagnostic capabilities.

REFERENCES

1. Nelson KB, Ellenberg JH. The asymptomatic newborn and risk of cerebral palsy. *Am J Dis Child* 1987;141:1333.
2. Naeye RL. *Disorders of the placenta, fetus, and neonate: diagnosis and clinical significance.* St. Louis: Mosby Year Book, 1992.

3. Low JA, Galbraith JS, Muir DW, Killen HL, Pater EA, Karchmar EJ. Factors associated with motor and cognitive deficits in children after intrapartum fetal hypoxia. *Am J Obstet Gynecol* 1984;148:533.

4. Low JA, Froese AF, Galbraith RS, Sauerbrei EE, McKinven JP, Karchmar EJ. The association of fetal and newborn metabolic acidosis with severe periventricular leukomalacia in the preterm newborn. *Am J Obstet Gynecol* 1990;162:977–982.

5. Low JA, Panagiotopoulos C, Derrick EJ. Newborn complications after intrapartum asphyxia with metabolic acidosis in the term fetus. *Am J Obstet Gynecol* 1994;170: 1081–1087.

6. Low LA, Simpson LL, Tonni G, Chamberlain S. Limitations in the clinical prediction of intrapartum fetal asphyxia.. *Am J Obstet Gynecol* 1995;172(3):805–810.

7. Richardson BS, Rurak G, Patrick JE, et al. Cerebral oxidative metabolism during sustained hypoxemia in fetal sheep. *J Dev Physiol* 1989;11:37–43.

8. Gunn AJ, Parer JT, Mallard EC, et al. Cerebral histologic and electrocorticographic changes after asphyxia in fetal sheep. *Pediatr Res* 1992;31:486–491.

9. Low JA, Froese AB, Galbraith RS, et al. Association between preterm newborn hypotension and hypoxemia and outcome. In Lou HC, Briesen G, Falck Larsen J (eds). *Brain lesions in the newborn.* Alfred Benzon Symposium 37. Copenhagen: Munksgaard, 1994:411–419.

10. Penning DH, Grafe MR, Hammond R, et al. Neuropathology of the near term and midgestation ovine fetal brain after sustained in utero hypoxemia. *Am J Obstet Gynecol* 1994;170:1425–1432.

11. Faro MD, Windle WF. Transeuronal degeneration in brains of monkey asphyxiated at birth. *Exp Neurol* 1969;24:38–53.

12. Ranck JB, Windle WE. Brain damage in the monkey, *Maccaca mulatta,* by asphyxia neonatorum. *Exp Neurol* 1959;1:130–154.

13. Low JA. Relationship of fetal asphyxia to neuropathology and deficits in children. *Clin Invest Med* 1993;16:133–140.

14. Johnston MV, Tresher WH, Taylor GA. Hypoxic and ischemic CNS disorders in infants and children. *Adv Pediatr* 1995;42:1–45.

15. Norman MG. Perinatal brain damage. *Perspect Pediatr Pathol* 1978;4:41–92.

16. Low JA, Simpson LL, Ransey DA. The clinical diagnosis of asphyxia responsible for brain damage in the human fetus. *Am J Obstet Gynecol* 1992;167:11–15.

17. Mallard C, Johnston B, Williams C, et al. *Frequent episodes of brief ischemia sensitize the fetal sheep brain to neuronal loss and induce striatal injury.* Toronto: Society for Gynecologic Investigation, 1993:abstract B8.

18. Wigglesworth JS, Pape K. Haemorrhage, ischemia and the perinatal brain. *Early Hum Dev* 1978;2(2):179–188.

19. Clapp JF III, Peress NS, Wesley M, Mann LI. Brain damage after intermittent partial cord occlusion in the chronically instrumented fetal lamb. *Am J Obstet Gynecol* 1988;159:504–509.

20. Gaffney G, Squier MV, Johnson A. Clinical association of prenatal ischemic white matter injury. *Arch Dis Child* 1994;70:F101–F106.

21. Truwit CL, Barkovitch AJ, Koch TK, Ferriero DM. Cerebral palsy, MR findings in 40 patients. *Am J Neuroradiol* 1992;13:67–78.

22. Battaglia FC, Meschia G (eds). *An introduction to fetal physiology.* London: Academic Press, 1986.
23. Pijnenborg R, Dixon G, Robertson WB, Brosens I. Trophoblastic invasion of human decidua from 8 to 18 weeks of pregnancy. *Placenta* 1980;1:3–19.
24. Feinstein DI. Lupus anticoagulant, thrombosis, and fetal loss. *N Engl J Med* 1985;21:1348.
25. Cowchock S, Smith JB, Gocial B. Antibodies to phospholipids and nuclear antigens in patients with repeated abortions. *Am J Obstet Gynecol* 1986;155:1002–1010.
26. Triplett DA. *Symposia: Pathogenic mechanisms of action: Effects on the coagulation system.* Fifth International Symposium on Antiphospholipid Antibodies, San Antonio, Texas, 1992.
27. Andersen KV, Hermann N. Placenta flow reduction in pregnant smokers. *Acta Obstet Gynecol Scand* 1984;63:707–709.
28. Dombrowski MP, Wolfe HM, Welch RA, Evans MI. Cocaine abuse is associated with abruptio placentae and decreased birth weight, but not shorter labor. *Obstet Gynecol* 1991;77:139–141.
29. Chasnoff IJ, Bussey ME, Savich R, Stack CM. Clinical and laboratory observations: perinatal cerebral infarction and maternal cocaine use. *J Pediatr* 1986;108(3):456–461.
30. Brosens I, Renaer M. On the pathogenesis of placental infarcts in preeclampsia. *J Obstet Gynaecol Br Cwlth* 1972;79:794–799.
31. Dommisse J, Tiltman AJ. Placental bed biopsies in placental abruption. *Br J Obstet Gynaecol* 1992;99:651–654.
32. Harris BA. Peripheral placental separation: a review. *Obstet Gynecol* 1988;43(10):577–581.
33. Wigglesworth S, Singer DB. *Textbook of fetal and perinatal pathology,* Cambridge, MA: Blackwell Scientific Publications, 1991.
34. Mooney EE, al Shunnar A, O'Regan M, et al. Chorionic villous haemorrhage is associated with retroplacental haemorrhage. *Br J Obstet Gynaecol* 1994;101(11):965–991.
35. Karimu AL, Burton GJ. Significance of changes in fetal perfusion pressure to factors controlling angiogenesis in the human term placenta. *J Reprod Fertil* 1994;102(2):447–450.
36. Karimu AL, Burton GJ. The effects of maternal vascular pressure on the dimensions of the placental capillaries. *Br J Obstet Gynecol* 1994;101(1):57–63.
37. Giles WB, Trudinger BJ, Baird PJ. Fetal umbilical artery flow velocity waveforms and placental resistance: pathological correlation. *Br J Obstet Gynecol* 1985;92:31.
38. Los FJ, DeWolf BT, Huisjes HJ. Raised maternal serum-alpha fetoprotein levels and spontaneous fetomaternal transfusion. *Lancet* 1979:1210.
39. Myers RA, Fujikura T. Placental changes after experimental abruptio placentae and fetal vessel ligation of rhesus monkey placenta. *Am J Obstet Gynecol* 1968;100:846–951.
40. Groome LJ, Owen J, Neely CL, et al. Oligohydramnios: antepartum fetal urine production and intrapartum fetal distress. *Am J Obstet Gynecol* 1991;165:1077.
41. Arabin B, Jimenez E, Vogel M, Weitzel HK. Relationship of utero and fetoplacental blood flow velocity wave forms with pathomorphological placental findings. *Fetal Diagn Ther* 1992;7:173–179.
42. Laurini R, Laurin J, Marsal K. Placental histology and fetal blood flow in intrauterine growth retardation. *Acta Obstet Gynecol Scand* 1994;73:529–534.
43. Read MA, Boura ALA, and Walters WAW. Effects of variation in oxygen tension on responses of the human fetoplacental vasculature to vasoactive agents in vitro. *Placenta* 1995;16:667–678.

44. Benirschke K, Kaufmann P. *Pathology of the human placenta,* 2nd ed. New York: Springer-Verlag, 1990:209.

45. Burton GJ; Jauniaux E. Sonographic, stereological and Doppler flow velocimetric assessments of placental maturity. *Br J Obstet Gynecol,* 1995;102(10):818–825.

46. Rochelson B, Kaplan C, Guzman E, Arato M, Hansen K, Trunca C. A quantitative analysis of placental vasculature in the third trimester fetus with autosomal trisomy. *Obstet Gynecol* 1990;75:59–63.

47. Demir R, Kaufmann P, Castelucci M, Erbengi T, Kotowski A. Fetal vasculogenesis and angiogenesis in human placental villi. *Acta Anat* 1989;136:190–203.

48. Teasdae F. Gestational changes in the functional structure of the human placenta in relation to fetal growth: a morphometric study. *Am J Obstet Gynecol* 1980;137:560–568.

49. Kaufmann P, Luckhardt M, Leiser R. Three-dimensional representation of the fetal vessel system in the human placenta. *Troph Res* 1988;3:113–137.

50. McGowan LM, Mullen BM, Ritchie K. Umbilical artery flow velocity waveforms and the placental vascular bed. *Am J Obstet Gynecol* 1987;157:900–902.

51. Fok RY, Pavlova Z, Benirschke K, et al. The correlation of arterial lesions with umbilical artery Doppler velocimetry in placentas of small-for-dates pregnancies. *Obstet Gynecol* 1990;75:578–583.

52. Bracero LA, Beneck D, Kirshenbaum N, et al. Doppler velocimetry and placental disease. *Am J Obstet Gynecol* 1989;161:388–393.

53. Trudinger BJ. Doppler ultrasonography: applications in clinical practice. In Hanson MA, Spencer JAD, Rodeck CH (eds). *The circulation,* vol 1. *Fetus and neonate, physiology and clinical applications.* Cambridge, England: Cambridge University Press, 1993.

54. Rankin JHG, McLaughlin MK. The regulation of placental blood flows. *J Dev Physiol* 1979;1:3–30.

55. Salafia CM, Divon MY, Minior VK, Pezzullo JC. Placental pathology of absent and reversed end-diastolic flow in growth-retarded fetuses. *Obstet Gynecol* 1997;90(5):830–836.

56. Macara L, Kingdom JCP, Kohnen G, et al. Elaboration of stem villous vessels in growth restricted pregnancies with abnormal umbilical artery Doppler waveforms. *Br J Obstet Gynecol* 1995;102:807–812.

57. Hitschold T, Weiss E, Beck T, et al. Low target birth weight or growth retardation? Umbilical Doppler flow velocity waveforms and histometric analysis of the fetoplacental vascular tree. *Am J Obstet Gynecol* 1993;168:1260–1264.

58. Jackson MR, Walsh AJ, Morrow RJ, et al. Reduced placental villous tree elaboration in small-for-gestational age newborn pregnancies: relationship with umbilical artery Doppler waveforms. *Am J Obstet Gynecol* 1995;172:518–525.

59. Park HW, Kapur RP, Shepard TH. Reversed circulation in acardiac fetuses is associated with anatomic inversions in the aortic wall. *Teratology* 1994;49:267–272.

60. Baldwin VJ. Intertwin vascular anastomoses. In *Pathology of multiple pregnancy.* New York: Springer-Verlag, 1994:216.

61. Fant M, Salafia CM, Baxter RC, et al. Circulating levels of IGFs and IGF binding proteins in human cord serum: Relationship to intrauterine growth. *Regul Pept* 1993;48 (1–2):29–39.

62. Altshuler G. Some placental considerations related to neurodevelopmental and other disorders. *J Child Neurol* 1993;8:78.

63. Teasdale F, Jean-Jacques G. Morphometric evaluation of the microvillous surface enlargement factor in the human placenta from mid-gestation to term. *Placenta* 1985;6(5):375–381.

64. Clapp JF, Szeto HH, Larrow R, Hewitt J, Mann LI. Fetal metabolic response to experimental placental vascular damage. *Am J Obstet Gynecol* 1981;140:446–451.

65. Howard RB, Hosokawa T, Maguire MH. Hypoxia induced fetoplacental vasoconstriction in perfused human placental cotyledons. *Am J Obstet Gynecol* 1987;157(5):1261–1266.

66. Mak K K-W, Gude NM, Walters WAW, Boura ALA. Effects of vasoactive autocoids on the human-fetal placental vasculature. *Br J Obstet Gynecol* 1984;91:99–106.

67. Howard RB, Hosokawa T, Maguire MH. Pressor and depressor actions of prostanoids in the intact human fetoplacental vascular bed. *Prostaglandins Leukotrienes Med* 1986;21: 323–330.

68. Naeye R, Maisels J, Lorenz RP, Botti JJ. The clinical significance of placental villous edema. *Pediatrics* 1983;71:588–594.

69. Salafia CM, Minior VK, López-Zeno JA, Whittington SS, Pezzullo JC, Vintzileos AM. Relationship between placental histology and umbilical cord blood gases in preterm gestations. *Am J Obstet Gynecol* 1995;173:1058–1064.

70. Fries MH, Goldstein RB, Kilpatrick SJ, et al. The role of velamentous cord insertion in the etiology of twin-twin transfusion syndrome. *Obstet Gynecol* 1993;81(4):569.

71. Fleming AD, Salafia CM, Vintzileos AM, Rodis JF, Campbell WA, Bantham KF. The relationships amongst umbilical arterial velocimetry, fetal biophysical profile and placental inflammation in preterm premature rupture of the membranes. *Am J Obstet Gynecol* 1991;164:38–41.

72. Clapp JF, Auletta FJ, Farnham J, Larrow RW, Mann LI. The ovine fetoplacental endocrine response to placental damage. *Am J Obstet Gynecol* 1982;144:47–54.

73. Benirschke K, Kaufmann P. *Pathology of the human placenta,* 2nd ed. New York: Springer-Verlag, 1990:386–391.

74. Salafia CM, Ernst L, Pezzullo JC, et al. The very low birth weight infant: maternal complications leading to preterm birth, placental lesions, and intrauterine growth. *Am J Perinatol* 1995;12(2):106–110.

75. Naeye RL. Pregnancy hypertension, placental evidences of low uteroplacental blood flow, and spontaneous Premature delivery. *Hum Pathol* 1989;20:441–444.

76. Arias F, Rodriquez L, Rayne SC, Kraus FT. Maternal placental vasculopathy and infection: Two distinct subgroups among patients with preterm labor and preterm ruptured membranes. *Am J Obstet Gynecol* 1993;168:585–591.

77. Burton GJ, Palmer ME, Dalton EJ. Morphometric differences between the placental vasculature of non-smokers, smokers, and ex-smokers. *Br J Obstet Gynaecol* 1989;96: 907–915.

78. Kuhnert PM, Kuhnert BR, Bottoms SF, Erhard P. Cadmium levels in maternal blood, fetal cord blood, and placental tissues of pregnant women who smoke. *Am J Obstet Gynecol* 1982;142:1021–1025.

79. Busacca M, Balconi G, Pietra A, Vergara-Dauden M, de Gaetano G, Dejana E. Maternal smoking and prostacyclin production by cultured endothelial cells from umbilical arteries. *Am J Obstet Gynecol* 1984;148:1127–1129.

80. Lehtovirta P, Pesonen E, Sarna S. Effect of smoking on the fetal coronary arteries. *Acta Path Microbiol Immunol Scan Sect A* 1984;92:189–193.

81. Eriksen PS, Marsal K. Circulatory changes in the fetal aorta after maternal smoking. *Br J Obstet Gynecol* 1987;94:301–305.

82. Pretorius DH, Manchester D, Barkin S, Parker S, Nelson TR. Doppler ultrasound of twin transfusion syndrome. *J Ultrasound Med* 1988;7:117–124.

83. Bejar R, Vigliocco G, Gramajo H, Solana C, Benirschke K, Berry C, Coen R, Resnik R. Antenatal origin of neurologic damage in newborn infants. *Am J Obstet Gynecol* 1990;162:1230–1236.

84. Benirschke K. Multiple pregnancy. In Benirschke K and Kaufmann P (eds). *Pathology of the human placenta,* 3rd ed. New York: Springer-Verlag, 1995:739.

85. Cowchock FS. Prevention of fetal death in the antiphospholipid antibody syndrome. *Lupus* 1996;5(5):467–472.

86. Salafia CM, Parke AL, Starzyk KA, Ernst LM, Lopez-Zeno JA. Obstetric complications in the APL syndrome. In Ascherson R (ed). *The APL syndrome.* Boca Raton, FL: CRC Press, 1996.

87. Salafia CM, Cowchock FS. Placental pathology and antiphospholipid antibodies: a descriptive study. *Am J Perinatol* 1997;14(8):435–441.

88. Altshuler G, Russell P. The human placental villitides: a review of chronic intrauterine infection. In Grundmann E and Kirsten WH (eds). *Current topics in pathology.* Heidelberg: Springer-Verlag, 1975:64–112.

89. Muir R, Niven JSF. The local formation of blood pigments. *J Pathol* 1935;41:183–197.

90. Tominaga T, Page EW. Accomodation of the human placenta to hypoxia. *Am J Obstet Gynecol* 1966;94:679–691.

91. Savill JS, Wyllie AH, Henson JE, et al. Macrophage phagocytosis of aging neutrophils in inflammation: programmed cell death in the neutrophil leads to its recognition by macrophages. J *Clin Invest* 1989;83:865–875.

92. Miller PW, Coen RW, Benirschke K. Dating the time interval from meconium passage to birth. *Obstet Gynecol* 1985;66(4):459–462.

93. Florman AL, Teubner D. Enhancement of bacterial growth in amniotic fluid by meconium. *J Pediatr* 1969;74(1):111–114.

94. Bryan CS. Enhancement of bacterial infection by meconium. *John Hopkins Med J* 1967;121:9.

95. Salafia CM, Holzman I. Meconium aspiration syndrome: placental pathology and respiratory disease. Society of Perinatal Obstetricians 1997 Annual Meeting Abstract #112. *Am J Obstet Gynecol* 1997;176(1, Part 2):S42.

96. Altshuler G, Herman AA. Placenta within the medicolegal imperative. *Arch Pathol Lab Med* 1991;115:688–695.

97. Heinrich PC, Castell JV, Andus T. Review article: Interleukin-6 and the acute phase response. *Biochem J* 1990;265:621–636.

98. Naeye RL. Amniotic fluid infections, neonatal hyperbilirubinemia, and psychomotor impairment. *Pediatrics* 1978;62:497–503.

99. Salafia CM, Starzyk KA, Pezzullo JC, Ghidini A, Rosenkrantz TS. Early neonatal nucleated erythrocyte counts in preterm deliveries: clinical and pathological correlations. *J Soc Gynecol Invest* 1997;4(3):138–143.

100. Salafia CM, Pezzullo JC, Ghidini A, Rosenkrantz TS. Patterns of change in early neonatal nucleated erythrocyte counts in preterm deliveries. *J Soc Gynecol Invest* 1997;4: 178–182.

6

EXCITOTOXICITY AND PATTERNS OF BRAIN INJURY FROM FETAL OR PERINATAL ASPHYXIA

Michael V. Johnston, M.D. and Alexander H. Hoon, Jr., M.D., M.P.H.
Kennedy Krieger Institute and Johns Hopkins University, School of Medicine, Baltimore, Maryland

Modern brain imaging techniques, especially cranial ultrasound and magnetic resonance imaging (MRI), can provide information about the selective patterns of injury produced by asphyxia in the developing brain, and these patterns often provide information about its timing during gestation (1–4). For example, cranial ultrasound imaging is quite sensitive for detecting intracranial hemorrhage and damage to the immature white matter from periventricular leukomalacia (PVL) or hemorrhagic infarction (4–6). Both intracranial hemorrhage and white matter injury are most likely to occur in fetuses or premature infants born at less than 34 weeks' gestation. PVL is most common at 28 weeks' gestation and rarely occurs after 32 weeks. Routine clinical head ultrasound imaging in premature and other sick infants demonstrates a close relationship between injury to the periventricular white matter and the type of cerebral palsy known as *spastic diplegia,* where spasticity in the legs is worse than in the arms. Ischemia and infection are the most common causes of PVL with some contribution

Asphyxia and Fetal Brain Damage, Edited by Dev Maulik, M.D., Ph.D.
ISBN 0-471-18427-6

from metabolic and endocrine disorders (7,8). In contrast, as the fetus matures in the third trimester and the neonatal period, the focus of injury from asphyxia or infection shifts from the midline germinal matrix and white matter structures to the neuron-rich gray matter structures, especially the motor cerebral cortex and basal ganglia (9,10). These patterns of selective regional vulnerability in the developing brain are determined by age-dependent changes in cerebral circulation as well as by changes in cellular metabolism and neuronal connectivity.

PVL AND OTHER INJURIES TO DEVELOPING WHITE MATTER

The developing cerebral white matter is the most vulnerable region of the fetal brain prior to 32 weeks' gestation. Figure 1 shows a cranial ultrasound image of symmetric cystic periventricular white matter injury in a premature infant along with a magnetic resonance image of the same infant, both obtained at 5 weeks postnatal age. Despite the immaturity of myelin at this age, the MRI image shows severe damage at the edges of each lateral ventricle suggesting that an ischemic injury has destroyed tissue in the watershed regions between major arterial supplies in the immature brain. Recent evaluation of cerebral blood flow using the experimental technique of near infrared spectroscopy suggests that loss of autoregulation of cerebral vasculature may play a role in some cases (11). Clinically, there is a direct quantitative relationship between the size of cysts in the periventricular white matter as visualized on ultrasound and the incidence of disabling cerebral palsy (12,13). This picture of extensive cyst formation is virtually always associated with severe disability. These images show an injury at the severe end of the spectrum with clearly defined cavities that appear like "Swiss cheese" at postmortem examination. However, in some infants, smaller cysts can collapse over time, often leaving ventriculomegaly as the only sign of white matter injury (14,15). Figure 2 demonstrates another visual pattern of PVL seen on an MRI image after a delay of several months. In this case the T_2-weighted image demonstrates bright signal extending within the white matter along each lateral ventricle. This appearance is probably produced by extensive gliosis in the damaged white matter, and the changes may persist for many years.

Although fluctuations in cerebral perfusion pressure in combination with immaturity of cerebral blood vessels serving the periventricular white matter can predispose this region to ischemia, the age-dependent vulnerability of the fetal white matter is also related to the special sensitivity of the immature oligodendroglia, the cells that synthesize myelin. The periventricular zone in the premature infant is composed primarily of sparsely covered axons surrounded by immature oligodendroglia. In vitro experiments indicate that immature oligodendroglial precursor cells are vulnerable to oxidative stress from oxygen free radicals (16). One effect of the oxygen free radicals is to trigger genetic programs for apoptosis or programmed cell death. In part, this sensitivity may be related to a high concentration of oligodendroglial iron that is available to react with oxygen radicals to form hydroxyl ions through the Fenton reaction. Release of the neurotransmitter glutamate during ischemia may also contribute to free radical stress in premature infants by competing with the uptake of the

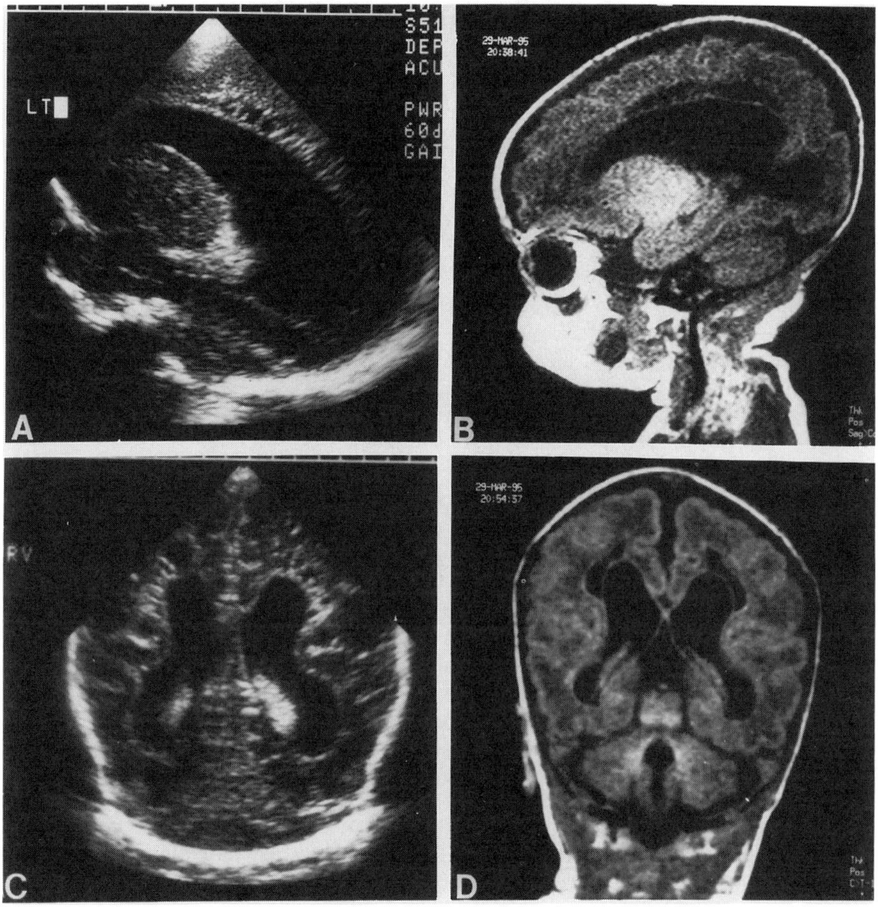

Figure 1. Cranial ultrasound and MRI images of severe periventricular leukomalacia (PVL) in a 5 week old female infant born at 29 weeks gestation. Panels A and B show parasagittal ultrasound and MRI images obtained on the same day. Panels C and D show coronal views. Note the prominent, symmetrical cysts at the lateral edge of each ventricle, and extending along the ventricles in the sagittal orientation.

amino acid cysteine which is needed to synthesize the antioxidant glutathione. Cytokines stimulated by infections in the mother and/or fetus can also contribute to oxidative stress for oligodendroglia, possibly by activating cascades that produce the free radical gas nitric oxide or the cyclooxygenase cascade (17). These results of in vitro basic science studies of developing oligodendroglia suggest that as term approaches, the oligodendroglia develop metabolic defenses against the higher oxygen environment that will be encountered when the fetus makes the transition from intrauterine to extrauterine life. The maturational studies fit well with clinical observations that the white matter becomes remarkably less vulnerable to injury as the end of gestation approaches.

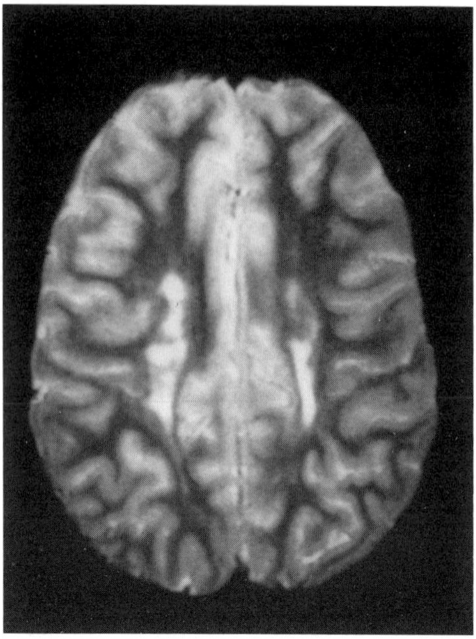

Figure 2. An axial T_2 weighted MRI image of a teenage boy with spastic diplegia resulting from a prenatal injury. Note the white, high signal extending rostral caudally in the periventricular white matter, which should be black at this age in normal myelin. At this stage in PVL, any cysts have collapsed and a gliotic scar remains with enlargement of the ventricles reflecting the loss of white matter. There was no scarring in the basal ganglia in this patient.

Severe intraventricular hemorrhage (IVH) can also cause damage to the developing white matter, but the pattern is usually unilateral or very asymmetric (Figure 3). In preterm infants, IVH encompasses a spectrum of hemorrhagic disorders, from Grade 1 germinal matrix hemorrhage to intraventricular hemorrhage, with or without ventricular dilatation. Periventricular hemorrhagic infarction (PHI), which was previously termed Grade 4 IVH, is now recognized as a complication of IVH resulting from venous infarction and asymmetric hemorrhagic necrosis in periventricular white matter (18). The common motor sequelae of PHI include hemiplegia or asymmetric quadriplegia. Lower-grade hemorrhage is not associated with a substantial increase in neurologic disability. In contrast, ventriculomegaly in premature infants is associated with a high rate of cerebral palsy, probably because it reflects loss of periventricular white matter (15).

HYPOXIC-ISCHEMIC ENCEPHALOPATHY IN TERM INFANTS

As the vulnerability of the white matter diminishes in the last trimester, neurons become more vulnerable to asphyxia that is severe enough to cause hypoxia-ischemia encephalopathy. The major developmental change that correlates with the increasing

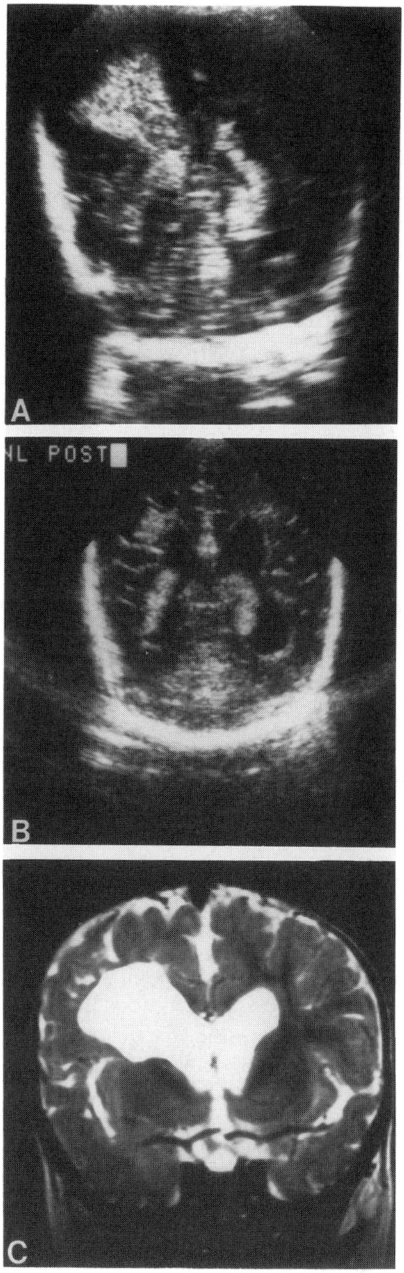

Figure 3. Periventricular hemorrhagic infarction (PHI) in an infant born at 28 weeks gestation. Panel A shows a grade IV intraventricular hemorrhage at 5 days of age on coronal cranial ultrasound. Panel B shows resolution of the intraventricular clot with early formation of a porencephalic cyst at 6 weeks of age. Panel C shows a coronal T_2 weighted MRI at 18 months of age showing ventriculomegaly and a porencephalic cyst.

vulnerability of neurons to asphyxia appears to be the elaboration of neuronal synaptic connections that use the excitatory neurotransmitter glutamate. Glutamate is the most prominent excitatory neurotransmitter in the brain, playing important roles in motor and sensory functions (3). During severe hypoxia-ischemia, neuronal depolarization and calcium entry into presynaptic nerve terminals leads to release of large amounts of glutamate into the extracellular space where it can stimulate multiple subtypes of glutamate receptors. The *N*-methyl-D-aspartate (NMDA) type glutamate receptor is the most important subtype in the "excitotoxic cascade" that is triggered in the immature brain, and strategies that inhibit this receptor's action are strongly neuroprotective against ischemic brain injury in immature animal models (Table 1) (19–22). NMDA channel opening is enhanced by a reduction in the neuron's transmembrane electrical potential, a feature referred to as "voltage dependence." In the presence of elevated concentrations of glutamate and glycine, coagonists for the NMDA receptor, reductions in neuronal energy metabolism associated with asphyxia can lead to membrane depolarization that facilitates the opening of the NMDA ion channel, allowing toxic levels of calcium to flood into the neuron. Therefore, NMDA channel opening can be triggered by a mismatch between neuronal energy demands and limited supplies of oxygen and metabolic substrates including glucose, fatty acids, and ketone bodies. Development of interneuronal synaptic connections enhances neuronal energy requirements because of the expensive demands of membrane ion pumps associated with synaptic activity.

Despite the fact that neurons in the developing brain become more vulnerable to hypoxic-ischemic injury as the fetus approaches term, it is important to note that the infant's brain is far less vulnerable to damage than that of an older child or an adult. The overall synaptic activity and energy needs of the normal neonate are minuscule com-

Table 1. The excitotoxic cascade that mediates brain injury from severe asphyxia

Ischemia stimulates calcium entry into nerve terminals and neuronal depolarization; glutamate uptake pumps reverse.
Glutamate accumulating extracellularly, combined with membrane depolarization, leads to opening of NMDA receptor channels.
Calcium floods through NMDA channels, raising intraneuronal calcium.
Calcium triggers several potentially toxic events including:
Stimulates nitric oxide synthase (NOS) to produce nitric oxide
Activates catalytic enzymes, lipases, proteases, and nucleases
Overstimulation of non-NMDA receptors synergistically raises intracellular calcium, depolarizes membranes
Calcium overload in mitochondria enhances production of oxygen free radicals from electron transport chain
Delayed induction of enzymes including neuronal NOS and cyclooxygenase following reperfusion leads to a vicious cycle of production of oxygen free radicals including superoxide and nitric oxide.
Oxygen free radicals, including combination of superoxide with nitric oxide to form peroxynitrite, lead to mitochondrial disruption, apoptotic neuronal death, and membrane disruption with necrosis.

pared to the adult (23,24). Most full-term infants can withstand a hypoxic episode severe enough to produce metabolic acidosis lowering the arterial pH to 7.0 with no brain injury. Infants are far more tolerant of periods of hypothermic circulatory arrest used as a support technique for cardiac surgery than older children or adults. However, if a critical threshold of hypoxia-ischemia is exceeded, the infant is vulnerable to NMDA-receptor-mediated excitotoxic neuronal injury because this receptor is present in a biochemical form that is "turned on" compared to the adult. The glutamate receptor subunits coded for in the immature brain build a channel that is less easily blocked by antagonists, including magnesium, and is more easily opened than the adult form (20,25). This state of affairs is suited to the major roles that NMDA receptors play in activity-dependent changes in normal brain development. Therefore, while the term neonate's brain is relatively protected, if a critical threshold for severe asphyxia is exceeded, the excitotoxic cascade is triggered in areas of rapidly developing neuronal circuitry.

The basal ganglia, especially the putamen and lateral aspects of the thalamus, and sections of the cerebral cortex, especially the motor strip anterior to the Rolandic fissure, are selectively vulnerable to hypoxic-ischemic brain injury in the term fetus as shown in Figure 4. MRI scans performed months to years after an acute severe episode of asphyxia severe enough to cause encephalopathy and multiorgan dysfunction at term typically show this very selective pattern of scarring (9). Clinically, this pattern is

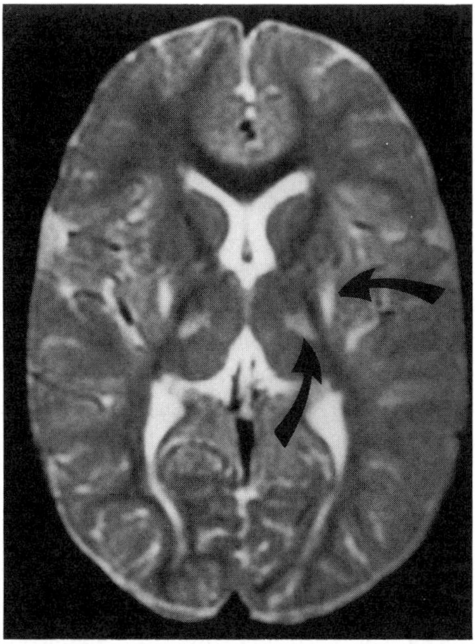

Figure 4. An axial T_2 weighted MRI image of a toddler with extrapyramidal cerebral palsy and scarring in the posterior ventral putamen and lateral thalamus following perinatal asphyxia and hypoxic-ischemic encephalopathy at near term in gestation. Additional views showed normal white matter.

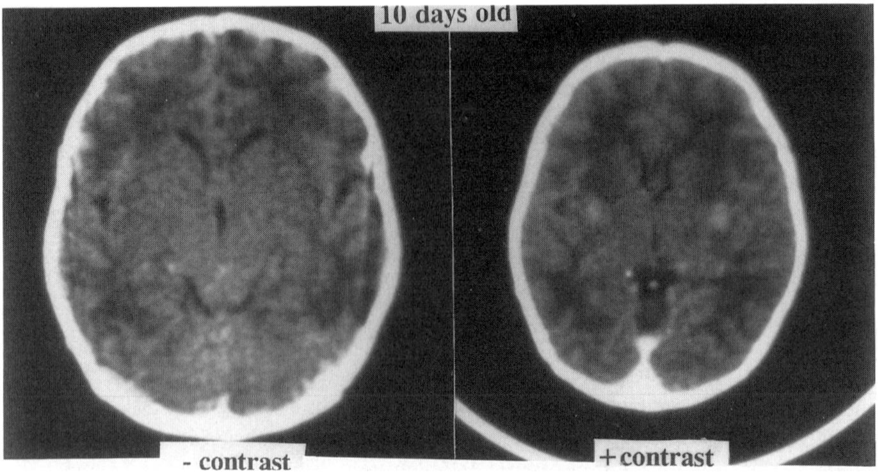

Figure 5. Panel A shows an unenhanced CT scan in a ten day old infant born at term who was asphyxiated and had hypoxic-ischemic encephalopathy at birth. Panel B shows the same infant after injection of contrast material. Very localized contrast enhancement is seen bilaterally in the region of the basal ganglia, probably in the putamen. The contrast enhances areas with breakdown of the blood brain barrier related to asphyxial injury. The focal enhancement is in the same region as the areas of scarring seen on MRI imaging (Figure 4) in older children with extrapyramidal cerebral palsy from asphyxia with HIE in the third trimester.

associated with a pattern of extrapyramidal cerebral palsy that produces rigidity, dystonia, diminished fine motor ability in the hands greater than in the legs, and muteness or dysarthric or dystonic speech (10). In contrast to similar insults prior to 32 weeks' gestation, this selective injury to basal ganglia and/or motor cortex is not accompanied by injury to the periventricular white matter. However, it is noteworthy that hypoxia-ischemia at term selects for injury neurons that participate in motor programs, similar to the myelinating motor pathways targeted for injury in the preterm fetus earlier in gestation. These patterns of selective vulnerability in the developing brain are the neurobiological basis for the syndrome of congenital motor dysfunction referred to as cerebral palsy. Several epidemiologic studies of cerebral palsy, including the NINDS Perinatal Collaborative Project, have also demonstrated that the developing motor system is far more vulnerable than cognitive function to asphyxial brain injury (26).

Figure 5 shows a computerized tomographic (CT) image of a 10-day-old full-term infant asphyxiated at birth who sustained injury to the putamen bilaterally and later manifested signs of extrapyramidal cerebral palsy. In these images, injection of contrast material produced enhancement selectively in the basal ganglia bilaterally. The precise cellular explanation for the selective vulnerability of the putamen and thalamus in acute severe asphyxia is unclear. However, it is noteworthy that positron emission tomographic (PET) scans of glucose metabolism in asphyxiated infants demonstrate focally enhanced glucose metabolism in the basal ganglia within a few hours, suggesting that oxidative metabolism is disrupted (27). PET scanning in normal infants showed that the glucose metabolic rate in term neonates is highest in the basal ganglia (28). The immature human basal ganglia also have large numbers of glutamate receptors in the neonatal period; and in regions such as the globus pallidus, the number is higher in infants than in the adult nervous system. Therefore the vulnerability of the basal ganglia to asphyxia in term infants may reflect the coincidence of relatively high metabolic demands and a high concentration of activated excitatory amino acid receptors in neuronal circuits serving motor functions that are developing exponentially at birth.

DELAYED NEURONAL DAMAGE AND HYPOXIC-ISCHEMIC ENCEPHALOPATHY

Clinical experience and experimental work indicate that the expression and evolution of hypoxic-ischemic injury is delayed for hours to days following an asphyxial insult severe enough to cause damage. Evolution of delayed injury is manifested by the clinical syndrome of hypoxic-ischemic encephalopathy (HIE) that includes coma, seizures, severe hypotonia, and severe electroencephalographic abnormalities (29,30). Assessment of energy metabolism in asphyxiated human infants using nuclear magnetic spectroscopy indicates that following resuscitation, energy metabolism returns to normal for 8–12 hours or longer (31). This latent interval is followed by a delayed energy failure associated with clinical signs of HIE. Results from the Perinatal Collaborative Study indicated that there is a strong correlation between the incidence of seizures in the neonatal period following very low Apgar scores at 5 minutes and later cerebral palsy (32). Studies of intrauterine asphyxia in sheep demonstrate that asphyxia severe enough to damage the brain produces seizures that are delayed by 8 hours or more following an acute insult (33). In a model of carotid ligation/hypoxemia injury in infant rats, mild hypothermia induced for only 2 hours following the acute insult can extend the latent interval by as much as a week (34). These results suggest that the insult triggers delayed events that eventually lead to brain damage, and that these events are modifiable with mild hypothermia. Other recent data from our laboratory indicate that delayed induction of neuronal NOS enzyme activity can play an important role in delayed reperfusion injury. Inhibition of neuronal NOS activity significantly reduces neuronal injury, especially the component related to programmed cell death or apoptosis (35). The events responsible for delayed injury following asphyxia are of great interest for developing effective neuroprotective therapeutic strategies. NMDA receptor blockade appears to be of limited value if delayed even a few hours after an acute hypoxic-ischemic insult (21). However, interventions such as hypothermia, aimed at the delayed events, may extend the "therapeutic window" for glutamate antagonists and other drugs.

OTHER PATTERNS OF ASPHYXIAL INJURY

Several other patterns of brain injury are recognized in near-term infants including parasagittal cortical infarction, multicystic encephalopathy, and cortical porencephalic cysts (18). The syndrome of parasagittal cortical infarction is related to watershed infarction of cortical tissue in the territory between the middle cerebral and anterior cerebral artery, typically reflected as a linear area of injury running from frontal cortex backward to parietal cortex. Infants with this pattern of injury usually have significant hypotension or shock as part of their hypoxic-ischemic injury. From a clinical standpoint, these infants often have weakness in the shoulder girdle, the area that is represented in the watershed area of infarction in the cortex. Cortical porencephalic cysts, often associated with hemiparetic cerebral palsy, usually result from infarctions in one cortical territory such as the middle cerebral artery. Many porencephalic cysts occur in fetal life, and they appear relatively larger than later occurring cysts. The etiology of these arterial infarctions is often unclear, but clotting disorders related to infection or to genetic disorders contribute to the incidence of this disorder. It is important to distinguish vascular-based porencephaly from the congenital malformation called *schizencephaly* that has a developmental or genetic basis (36) (Figure 6). Unlike porencephalic cysts which are typically encompassed by a membrane of brain tissue, schizencephaly is usually open and the wall of the malformation is

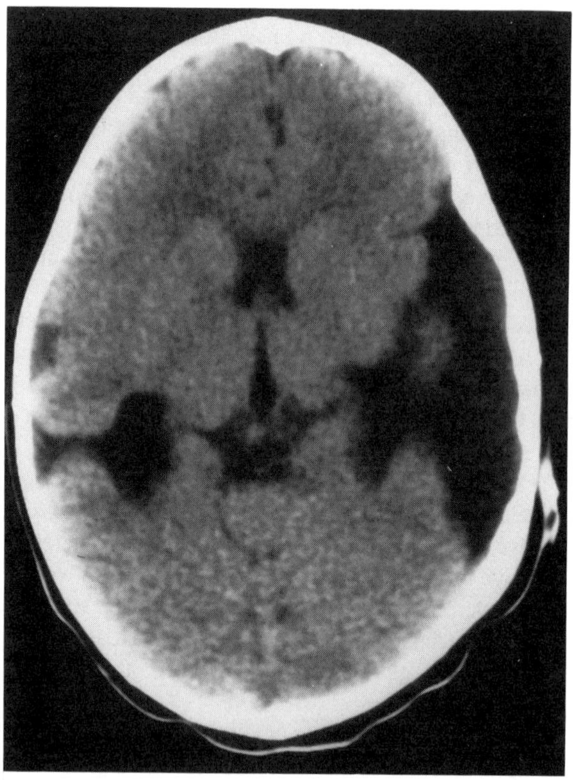

Figure 6. CT image of a child with cerebral palsy of mixed spastic and extrapyramidal type. Unexpectedly, the child had schizencephaly, a developmental brain malformation originating early in gestation. Unlike porencephaly, the clefts in the hemispheres are open to the cerebrospinal fluid space and the cavity is covered by a layer of cerebral cortex. In some families schizencephaly is linked to specific genetic mutations.

often covered by a layer of cortex (2). Multicystic encephalomalacia is a devastating disorder involving much of the cerebral cortex in certain infants. It is a relatively unique disorder and its etiology is not well understood. In some cases congenital infection, probably associated with involvement of cortical blood vessels, has been shown to play a role. Although infants with this disorder often have low Apgar scores, seizures, other signs of encephalopathy and associated medical disorders such as meconium aspiration, a cause and effect with asphyxia has not been well documented. More information about this disorder is needed.

CONCLUSION

Modern neuroimaging along with a growing body of clinical and experimental science is providing a clearer picture of the relationships between the timing of asphyxial insults to the brain and the patterns of injury. Both human and experimental data indicate that different parts of the brain display striking selectivity in their vulnerability to injury at different ages. A major distinction can be made between the early window of vulnerability of the cerebral white matter to injury prior to 32–34 weeks' gestation and the emerging vulnerability of the neurons in the basal ganglia and cerebral cortex in the third trimester and neonatal period. In the case of white matter injury or PVL, the window of vulnerability appears to be created in part by the inadequacy of antioxidant protective mechanisms against free radicals in the immature oligodendroglia that are destined to form the periventricular myelin. In the term infant, it is the developing interneuronal synaptic connections that create vulnerability to excitotoxic injury from asphyxia. Patterns of selective vulnerability seen on neuroimaging can often provide information about the timing of injury, but it is important to note that the precise cause of injury may still remain uncertain based on imaging alone. For example, PVL white matter injury can look very similar whether produced by infection or asphyxia because both etiologies can trigger the same final common pathways to injury. A better understanding of the pathogenesis of these disorders and their appearance on neuroimaging is providing more accurate diagnosis and timing of injury as well as the prospect of intervention in the future.

ACKNOWLEDGMENT

This work was supported, in part, by United Cerebral Palsy Research and Education grant R-706-96.

REFERENCES

1. Barkovich AJ. MR and CT evaluation of profound neonatal and infantile asphyxia. *J Neuroradiol* 1992;13:959–972.
2. Barkovich AJ, Chuang SH, Norman D. MR of neuronal migration anomalies. *Am J Neuroradiol* 1987;8:1009–1017.

3. Johnston MV, Ishiwa S. Ischemia and excitotoxins in development. *Ment Retard Dev Disabil* 1995;1:193–200.
4. Volpe JJ. Current concepts of brain injury in the premature infant. *Am J Roentgenol* 1989;153:472–477.
5. Babcock DS. Sonography of the brain in infants: role in evaluating neurologic abnormalities. *Am J Radiol* 1995;165:417–423.
6. Gould SJ, Howard S, Hope PL. Periventricular intraparenchymal cerebral hemorrhage in preterm infants: the role of venous infarction. *J Pathol* 1987;151:197–202.
7. Kuban KCK, Leviton A. Cerebral palsy. *N Engl J Med* 1994;330:188–195.
8. Perlman JM, Risser R, Broyles RS. Bilateral cystic periventricular leukomalacia in the premature infant. *Pediatrics* 1996;97:822–827.
9. Menkes JH, Curran J. Clinical and MR correlates in children with extrapyramidal cerebral palsy. *AJNR* 1994;15:451–457.
10. Hoon AH, Reinhardt EM, Kelley RI, Brieter SN, Morton DH, Naidu S, Johnston MV. Brain MR Imaging in suspected extrapyramidal cerebral palsy: observations in distinguishing genetic–metabolic from acquired etiologies. *J Pediatr* 1997;131:240–245.
11. du Plessis AJ, Newburger J, Jonas RA, Hickey P, Naruse H, Tsuji M, Walsh A, Walter G, Wypij D, Volpe JJ. Cerebral oxygen supply and utilization during infant cardiac surgery. *Ann Neurol* 1995;37:488–497.
12. Pinto-Martin JA, Riolo S, Cnaan A, Holzman C, Susser MW, Paneth N. Cranial ultrasound prediction of disabling and nondisabling cerebral palsy at age two in a low birth weight population. *Pediatrics* 1995;95:249–254.
13. Rogers B, Msall M, Owens T, Guernsey K, Brody A, Buck G, Hudak M. Cystic periventricular leukomalacia and type of cerebral palsy in preterm infants. *J Pediatr* 1994;125: 51–58.
14. Dubowitz LMS, Bydder GM, Mushin J. Developmental sequence of periventricular leukomalacia. *Arch Dis Child* 1985;60:349–355.
15. Paneth N, Rudelli R, Kazam E, Monte W. *Brain damage in the preterm infant.* London: MacKeith Press, 1994:209pp.
16. Oka A, Belliveau MJ, Rosenberg PA, Volpe JJ. Vulnerability of oligodendroglia to glutamate: pharmacology, mechanisms and prevention. *J Neurosci* 1993:1441–1453.
17. Leviton A. Preterm birth and cerebral palsy: is tumor necrosis factor the missing link? *Dev Med Child Neurol* 1993;35:549–558.
18. Volpe JJ. *Neurology of the newborn,* 3rd ed. Philadelphia: WB Saunders, 1995.
19. McDonald JW, Silverstein FS, Johnston MV. MK-801 protects the neonatal brain from hypoxic-ischemic damage. *Eur J Pharmacol* 1987;140:359–361.
20. McDonald JW, Johnston MV. Physiological and pathophysiological roles of excitatory amino acids during central nervous system development. *Brain Res Rev* 1990;15:41–70.
21. Hagberg H, Gilland E, Diemer, NH, Andine P. Hypoxia-ischemia in the neonatal rat brain: histopathology after post-treatment with NMDA and non-NMDA receptor antagonists. *Biol Neonate* 1994;66:205–213.
22. Ikonomidou C, Mosinger JL, Shahid Salles K. Sensitivity of the developing rat brain to hypobaric/ischemic damage parallels sensitivity to NMDA neurotoxicity. *J Neurosci* 1989;9:2809–2828.
23. Vannucci RC. Experimental biology of cerebral hypoxia-ischemia: relation to perinatal brain damage. *Pediatr Res* 1990;27:317–326.

24. Altman DI, Perlman JM, Volpe JJ, Powers WJ. Cerebral oxygen metabolism in newborns. *Pediatrics* 1993;92:99–104.
25. Burgard EC, Hablitz JJ. Developmental changes in NMDA and non-NMDA receptor mediated synaptic potentials in rat neocortex. *J Neurophysiol* 1993;69:230–240.
26. Paneth N, Stark RI. Cerebral palsy and mental retardation in relation to indicators of perinatal asphyxia. *Am J Obstet Gynecol* 1983;147:960–966.
27. Blennow M, Ingvar M, Lagercrantz H, Stone-Elander S, Eriksson L, Forssberg H, Ericson K, Flodmark O. Early [18F]FDG positron emission tomography in infants with hypoxic-ischemic encephalopathy shows hypermetabolism during the postasphyctic period. *Acta Paediatr* 1995;84:1–7.
28. Chugani HT, Phelps ME. Maturational changes in cerebral function in infants determined by 18FDG positron emission tomography. *Science* 1986;231:840–843.
29. Johnston MV, Trescher WH, Taylor GA. Hypoxic and ischemic central nervous system disorders in infants and children. *Adv Pediatr* 1995;42:1–45.
30. Levene MI, Grindulis H, Sands C, Moore JR. Comparison of two methods of predicting outcome in perinatal asphyxia. *Lancet* 1986;I:67–68.
31. Azzopardi D, Wyatt JS, Cady EB, Delpy DT, Baudin J, Stewart AL, Hope PL, Hamilton PA, Reynolds EOR. Prognosis for newborn infants with hypoxic ischemia brain injury assessed by phosphorus magnetic resonance spectroscopy. *Pediatr Res* 1989;25:445–451.
32. Nelson KB, Ellenberg JK. Apgar scores as predictors of chronic neurologic disability. *Pediatrics* 1981;68:36–44.
33. Williams CE, Gunn AJ, Mallard C, Gluckman PD. Outcome after ischemia in the developing sheep brain: an electroencephalographic and histological study. *Ann Neurol* 1992;31:14–21.
34. Trescher WH, Ishiwa S, Johnston MV. Brief post-hypoxic-ischemic hypothermia markedly delays neonatal brain injury. *Brain Dev* 1997;19:326–338.
35. Tseng EE, Brock MV, Lange MS, Blue ME, Troncoso JC, Lowenstein CJ, Johnston MV, Baumgartner WA. Neuronal nitric oxide synthase inhibition reduces neuronal apoptosis following hypothermic circulatory arrest. *Ann Thorac Surg* 1997;64:1637–1647.
36. Brunelli S, Faiella A, Capra V, Nigro V, Simeone A, Cama A, Boncinelli E. Germline mutations in the homeobox gene EMX2 in patients with severe schizencephaly. *Nature Genetics* 1996;12:94–96.

7

MANAGEMENT STRATEGIES FOR PERINATAL HYPOXIC-ISCHEMIC ENCEPHALOPATHY

Robert C. Vannucci, M.D.
Department of Pediatrics, The Pennsylvania State University College of Medicine, The Milton S. Hershey Medical Center, Hershey, Pennsylvania

INTRODUCTION

Perinatal cerebral hypoxia-ischemia remains a frequent cause of the chronic handicapping conditions of cerebral palsy, mental retardation, learning disability, and epilepsy (1). Estimates suggest that between 2 and 4 out of every 1000 full-term newborn infants suffer asphyxia at or shortly prior to birth, and this incidence approaches 60% in small preterm infants. Depending upon gestational age, between 10% and 60% of asphyxiated infants who exhibit hypoxic-ischemic encephalopathy actually expire during the newborn period; and of the survivors, 25% will exhibit permanent neuropsychologic deficits. Given these incidence figures, physicians have searched

Asphyxia and Fetal Brain Damage, Edited by Dev Maulik, M.D., Ph.D.
ISBN 0-471-18427-6

for strategies to prevent or minimize the long-term consequences of perinatal cerebral hypoxia-ischemia.

In the past, therapeutic interventions for perinatal hypoxic-ischemic encephalopathy consisted of those drugs which reduced the severity of cerebral edema arising from hypoxia-ischemia (2). Such agents included osmotic diuretics (mannitol, furosemide), glucocorticosteroids, and barbiturates. One by one, these drugs and other manipulations to treat brain swelling have been discarded, such that presently no agent has been proven useful to ameliorate perinatal hypoxic-ischemic brain damage in the clinical setting. Accordingly, there is no uniform standard of care in the brain-oriented therapy of newborn infants sustaining cerebral hypoxia-ischemia, and it remains for future research to uncover new and effective strategies for the neurologically compromised infant.

PHARMACOLOGIC AGENTS UNDER EXPERIMENTAL INVESTIGATION

Given the absence of an effective management program for perinatal hypoxic-ischemic encephalopathy, it is important that physicians and scientists seek new approaches to the treatment of fetuses and newborn infants suffering cerebral hypoxia-ischemia. Drugs currently under intense investigation, especially in experimental animals, include inhibitors of oxygen free-radical generation and free-radical scavengers, antagonists of excitatory amino acids, calcium channel blockers, and nitric oxide synthase inhibitors.

Oxygen Free Radical Inhibitors and Scavengers

A free radical is an atom or molecule that contains an uneven number of electrons in its outer most orbital. A free radical, such as $\bullet O_2^-$ or $\bullet OH_2^-$ can combine sequentially with nonradicals, the result of which are new free radicals. This characteristic enables free radicals to initiate and perpetuate chain reactions, the peroxidation of unsaturated fatty acids being a prominent example. In this regard, it is assumed that the manner in which oxygen free radicals cause or contribute to brain damage relates to their ability to attack the fatty acid moiety of plasma and subcellular membranes (3–5). Polyunsaturated fatty acids seem especially prone to peroxidative attack by free radicals, which initiate and perpetuate chain reactions within the hydrophobic core of the lipid bilayer, leading ultimately to membrane fragmentation. The brain is especially rich in polyunsaturated phosopholipids and, accordingly, is susceptible to free radical attack. Free iron (Fe) (iron not bound to protein) and nitric oxide (see below) are important contributors to oxidative injury, because they transform mildly reactive oxygen species to more toxic free radicals (5,6). Prevention of the formation of these reactive products can be achieved by elimination of hydrogen peroxide, superoxide, or the catalyst of the reaction, specifically Fe.

Oxygen free radicals are generated during and following hypoxia-ischemia in several ways. First, free radicals are produced within mitochondria when cytochrome oxidase is not fully saturated with oxygen, thereby liberating free radicals at more proximal steps. These oxygen free radicals cannot be consumed further and "leak" out into the cytoplasm. Other sources of oxygen free radicals during hypoxia-ischemia and especially during the reperfusion interval of recovery are as byproducts in the synthesis of prostaglandins from arachidonic acid (7–9) and the conversion of hypoxanthine to xanthine and uric acid (4,10,11). Therefore, drugs that inhibit the formation of oxygen free radicals or that rapidly destroy free radicals, once formed, might be efficacious in reducing the severity of hypoxic-ischemic brain damage.

Drugs potentially efficacious in favorably influencing the outcome of hypoxic-ischemic brain damage include those agents which inhibit specific reactions in the production of prostaglandins and of xanthine, the formation of which involves the generation of oxygen free radicals (see above). Both allopurinol and oxypurinol, which are xanthine oxidase inhibitors/scavengers, protect immature rats from hypoxic-ischemic brain damage even when the drugs are administered early during the recovery phase following resuscitation (12–14). Indomethacin, a cyclo-oxygenase and phospholipase inhibitor, also has been shown to ameliorate ischemic brain damage, at least in adult animals (15), and substantially reduces free radical generation during reperfusion from hypoxia-ischemia in newborn pigs (16). Finally, members of a class of compounds called 21-amino steroids (lazeroids) have been shown to be neuroprotective in both adult and immature animal models of cerebral hypoxia-ischemia (17,18). The compounds apparently prevent Fe-dependent lipid peroxidation by scavenging peroxyl radicals, and their site of action is predominantly within cerebral blood vessels, thereby reducing reperfusion injury (Table 1).

Excitatory Amino Acid Antagonists

Several lines of research in experimental animals have implicated a role for the excitatory amino acid, glutamate, in the production of hypoxic-ischemic brain damage in the immature and adult brain. First, glutamate is directly toxic to mature neurons in culture (19). Second, neurons in culture and hippocampal slices die upon exposure to anoxia, but their death can be prevented by the presence of magnesium (Mg^{2+}), which blocks glutamate receptors within the calcium (Ca^{2+}) ion channel, or by specific glutamate anatgonists (20–22). Third, direct injection of glutamate or glutamate agonists into specific regions of brain in vivo produces neuronal injury iden-

Table 1. Oxygen free radical inhibitors/scavengers

Antioxidant enzymes
Polyethylene glycol superoxide dismutase (PEG-SOD)
Polyethylene glycol catalase (PEG-catalase)
Free radical inhibitors
Allopurinol/oxypurinol
Indomethacin
Elimination of free iron
Deferoxamine
Free radical scavengers
Alpha-tocopherol (vitamin E)
21-Amino steroids (lazeroids)

tical to that seen after hypoxia-ischemia (23–25). Fourth, deafferentation of the glutaminergic excitatory input into the hippocampus reduces the damage produced by hypoxia-ischemia (26). These studies provide convincing evidence that excessive exposure of neurons to glutamate, as occurs during hypoxia-ischemia, leads to morphologic alterations characteristic of ischemic neuronal necrosis.

Given the premise that excessive stimulation of neuronal surface receptors by glutamate promotes cellular death and that glutamate release from the axon terminal into the synaptic cleft occurs during hypoxia-ischemia (19,27–29), it has been rational to search for pharmacologic agents which would either inhibit glutamate release or block its postsynaptic action. Inhibitors of glutamate release from the nerve terminal (e.g., baclofen) have not been investigated as potential neuroprotective drugs, whereas antagonists of glutaminergic cell surface receptors have undergone extensive study in experimental animals (30,31). Of the several available antagonists, those which affect the NMDA and AMPA/QA receptors or the ion channels they subserve have received the most attention. Available compounds include phencyclidine, dextromethrophan, ketamine, MK-801, and NBQX, among others. These compounds have been found efficacious in reducing the extent of hypoxic-ischemic brain damage in adult animals even if administered up to 24 hours after the metabolic insult (32). Experimental studies in immature animals have shown that, as in adult animals, glutamate receptor antagonists are capable of reducing the severity of hypoxic-ischemic brain damage. First, systemically administered MK-801 prevents the tissue necrosis produced by the direct injection of the glutamate agonist, NMDA, into the striatum of 7-day postnatal rats (33). Second, MK-801 protects against hypoxic-ischemic brain damage in immature rats even if the drug is administered during the course of or up to 1 hour after the metabolic insult (33–36). Pretreatment of the animals entirely prevents tissue injury from occurring (36). The protective effect of MK-801 or MBQX, which exceeds by far the effect of other glutamate receptor antagonists, appears greater in immature rats compared to their adult counterparts (37,38). The age-related difference in the efficacies of the glutamate receptor antagonists favoring the immature brain appears to reside in the sensitivity of the developing brain to excitatory neurotransmitter toxicity, which, in turn, arises from developmental alterations in the density and distribution of glutamate receptor subtypes (39–41), in glutamate binding to its receptors, or in transmembrane biochemical events initiated by receptor activity. Indeed, it has been suggested that the NMDA and AMPA receptor antagonists presently are the most potent drugs available to ameliorate the potentially devastating effect of cerebral hypoxia-ischemia (31).

As mentioned previously, the divalent cation, Mg^{2+}, acts as a glutamate receptor antagonist to the extent that it blocks the neuronal influx of Ca^{2+} within the ion channel. In this regard, magnesium sulfate has been shown to reduce the severity of hypoxic-ischemic brain damage in immature rats (42–44). However, the solution does not improve neuropathologic outcome when administered prior to and during the course of asphyxia produced by umbilical cord occlusion in near-term fetal lambs (45). In this model, magnesium caused no greater alterations in systemic blood pressure, heart rate, or cerebral blood flow than that seen in nontreated fetuses subjected to asphyxia. In the clinical setting, a retrospective study has suggested that premature fetuses whose mothers received magnesium sulfate for the treatment of preeclampsia or as a tocolytic agent are less likely to develop cerebral palsy compared to a gestational-age-matched group of fetuses not exposed to the drug (46). Based on the investigation, the authors speculated that magnesium sulfate might provide a protective effect against brain damage in immature fetuses and newborn infants. Indeed, Levene et al. (47) currently are conducting a controlled, randomized trial to ascertain the protective effect of magnesium sulfate in asphyxiated full-term infants.

Calcium Channel Blockers

Owing to its multiple functions, calcium (Ca^{2+}) is often considered an intracellular second messenger. The divalent cation is intimately involved as a cofactor in numerous biochemical reactions, thereby acting as a regulator of cellular metabolic homeostasis. Accordingly, a disruption of intracellular free Ca^{2+} concentrations has wide-ranging deleterious effects on neuronal function (3,27).

The mechanisms by which alterations in Ca^{2+} balance which occur during cerebral hypoxia-ischemia contributes to brain damage relates to disturbances in those biochemical reactions subserved by the cation (48). Ca^{2+} activates numerous intracellular reactions, the continued stimulation of which by elevated concentrations of free Ca^{2+} compromises the viability of the neurons. These reactions include the activation of several lipases, proteases, and endonucleases, all of which attack the structural integrity of the cell. Ca^{2+} also activates phospholipase C, which promotes a progressive breakdown in the phospholipid components of the plasma and subcellular membranes. Ca^{2+} also contributes to the formation of oxygen free radicals via the formation of xanthine and prostaglandins (see above). Finally, increased concentrations of intracellular Ca^{2+} lead to an uncoupling of oxidative phosphorylation within mitochondria, because the energy formed during recovery from hypoxia-ischemia is immediately consumed in an attempt to reverse and then maintain the electrochemical (ion) gradient across the mitochondrial membrane. This "futile" cycling of ions restricts the production and transfer of ATP into the cytosol to be used for structural repair and reestablishment of ion gradients across the plasma membrane. Taken together, the toxic effects of excessive free Ca^{2+} accumulation are adequate to cause membrane disintegration and death of the neuron (27,48).

Given the potential neurotoxicity of Ca^{2+} when free intracellular concentrations increase to dangerous levels, drugs have been developed which inhibit Ca^{2+} influx into neurons. Of the numerous calcium channel blockers currently available for experimental and clinical research, flunarizine and nimodipine appear most efficacious in reducing the extent of hypoxic-ischemic brain damage, at least in adult animals (49–51). Furthermore, several investigators independently have shown an amelioration of neuropathologic alterations in immature rats subjected to hypoxia-ischemia and pretreated with the Ca^{2+} channel blocker, flunarizine (52–54). However, the neuroprotective effect of calcium channel blockers is not nearly as great as that of the excitatory amino acid antagonists in the experimental setting, and any efficacy of the calcium channel blockers in the clinical setting has been marginal at best (31). Also in the clinical setting, Levene et al. (55) administered the calcium channel blocker, nicardipine, to four severely asphyxiated newborn infants. Heart rate increased in all four infants, while mean arterial blood pressure decreased in three. Two infants had a sudden and dramatic fall in systemic blood pressure. As a result of their findings, the investigators cautioned against the use of these drugs in asphyxiated infants.

Inhibitors of Nitric Oxide Production

Recent experiments suggest that the free radical gas, nitric oxide (NO), is involved in the cascade of metabolic events which causes or contributes to the occurrence of hypoxic-ischemic brain damage (56–58). NO is produced in selective neurons of the brain, and the pathway for its synthesis involves the direct conversion of L-arginine to citrulline by the catalytic, cytosolic enzyme NO synthase. NO production is linked to the activation of glutamate cell surface receptors, especially NMDA receptors, which activation leads to Ca^{2+} influx into neurons and its binding to calmodulin (see above). Once formed, NO influences numerous metabolic events, primarily through an activation of the second messenger enzyme, guanylate cyclase, with the formation of cyclic GMP. In excessive concentrations, NO can act as a neurotoxic agent and might constitute a final common pathway for amino acid excitotoxicity in brain, as has also been proposed for Ca^{2+} (3). Experiments in adult animals suggest that NO mediates neuronal death following cerebral ischemia (59,60) and that the severity of neuronal loss can be reduced by the prior administration of inhibitors of NO synthase activity (61–63). A similar protective effect also has been observed in the immature rat subjected to cerebral hypoxia-ischemia (64,65), but NO synthase inhibition appears to accentuate neuronal injury in fetal sheep (66).

SUMMARY

The pathophysiologic mechanisms for the production of perinatal hypoxic-ischemic brain damage described above provide multiple avenues of therapeutic intervention for the prevention of brain tissue injury. These pharmacologic interventions are summarized in Table 2. In addition, there is a hierarchy of neuroprotection, to the extent

Table 2. Therapeutic interventions

Free radical inhibitors/scavengers
Allopurinol/oxypurinol
Indomethacin
PEG-SOD
Excitatory amino acid antagonists
MK-801 and analogues; NBQX
Calcium channel blockers
Flunarizine, nimodipine
Nitric oxide synthase inhibitors
N-nitro-L-arginine
Miscellaneous
Monosialogangliosides
Growth factors

Table 3. Hierarchy of neuroprotection

1. Glutamate receptor antagonists
2. Free radical inhibitors/scavengers
3. Nitric oxide synthase inhibitors
4. Calcium channel blockers
5. Others

that at least presently glutamate receptor antagonists appear the most efficacious in reducing or preventing the occurrence of perinatal hypoxic-ischemic brain damage (Table 3). It is anticipated that other neuroprotective agents will be developed in the experimental animal, which ultimately might prove beneficial in the clinical setting.

NONPHARMACOLOGIC INTERVENTIONS

In addition to the potentially new pharmacologic strategies to protect the perinatal brain from hypoxic-ischemic brain damage, nonpharmacologic approaches have proved beneficial. These interventions include hyperglycemia, hypercapnia, and systemic hypothermia.

Hyperglycemia

Several investigations have indicated that hyperglycemia superimposed upon cerebral hypoxia-ischemia or isolated ischemia accentuates brain damage in adult experimental animals and humans (67–70). Such is not the case in perinatal animals, at least in the immature rat. In this regard, Vannucci and Mujsce (71) demonstrated that hyperglycemia to blood glucose concentrations in the range of 600 mg/dl entirely prevents the occurrence of brain damage in an immature rat model of cerebral hypoxia-ischemia. Hyperglycemia with blood glucose concentrations ranging from 300 to 400 mg/dl has no beneficial effect, nor is it deleterious to the brain subjected to hypoxia-ischemia (72). Further investigations have shown that hyperglycemia superimposed on cerebral hypoxia-ischemia results in an enhanced anaerobic glycolytic flux compared to normoglycemic controls (73). The enhanced glycolysis, in turn, leads to better preservation of cerebral high-energy reserves in the hyperglycemic animals, thus accounting for the greater resistance of these animals to hypoxic-ischemic brain damage. However, hyperglycemia has been shown to increase hypoxic-ischemic brain damage in newborn pigs (74), in contrast to the findings in immature rats. In addition, glucose supplementation during recovery following resuscitation from cerebral hypoxia-ischemia appears to accentuate brain damage in immature rats (75).

Carbon Dioxide

Recent clinical investigations suggest that premature infants who require mechanical ventilation to prevent or minimize hypoxemia arising from respiratory distress syndrome are at increased risk for the development of periventricular leukomalacia if hypocapnia occurs during the course of respiratory management (76–78). A causal relationship between low pCO_2 and hypoxic-ischemic brain damage was not established in any of the studies; but given the multiple effects of carbon dioxide (CO_2) on hemodynamics and cerebral metabolism, a cause-and-effect relationship is certainly plausible. The question remained as to the contribution of hypocapnia to hypoxic-ischemic brain damage and whether or not hypercapnia is neuroprotective.

To resolve the issue, Vannucci et al. (79) subjected immature rats to cerebral hypoxia-ischemia with or without CO_2 added to the hypoxic gas mixture to which the animals were exposed. The results showed that normocapnic (pCO_2 = 39 mmHg) cerebral hypoxia-ischemia is associated with less severe brain damage than in hypocapnic (pCO_2 = 26 mmHg) hypoxia-ischemia and that mild hypercapnia (pCO_2 = 54 mmHg) is more protective than normocapnia. Further studies were conducted which ascertained that mild hypercapnia is associated with greater preservations of cerebral blood flow, glucose utilization, and high-energy phosphate reserves than seen during either hypocapnic or normocapnic cerebral hypoxia-ischemia (80). From their findings, the investigators recommended further corroboration in other animal models as well as a clinical reappraisal of the ventilatory management strategies of sick newborn human infants, especially as regards the prevention of hypocapnia and the occurrence of permissive mild hypercapnia.

Hypothermia

Systemic cooling of the brain by as little as 3–6°C has been shown to reduce the extent of tissue injury that follows several cerebral insults in adult experimental animals, including stroke, trauma, and hypoglycemia (81–83). Hypothermia also protects the perinatal brain from hypoxic-ischemic damage. In this regard, Yager et al. (84) demonstrated in immature rats that a reduction in systemic temperature by 3°C during cerebral hypoxia-ischemia provides partial benefit, and a 6°C decrease completely protects the brain from injury (see also reference 85). Presumably, hypothermia reduces cerebral energy demands, such that during hypoxia-ischemia high-energy phosphate reserves are maintained relatively at normal levels (86). Systemic hypothermia during the first 3 hours of reperfusion following hypoxia-ischemia also protects the immature rat brain from damage (87), although this observation has not been universal (84). Similar findings have been observed in newborn pigs (88,89).

CONCLUSIONS

Since the original article on management strategies for perinatal hypoxic-ischemic encephalopathy which appeared in *Pediatrics* in 1990 (2), much progress has been made toward elucidating those pharmacologic and nonpharmacologic interventions which might protect the fetus or newborn human infant from hypoxic-ischemic brain damage. Clinical trials have or are currently being conducted and hopefully will provide information regarding which interventions will protect the immature brain from neuronal injury. Further controlled, prospective studies are warranted, which hopefully will be designed and conducted within the next few years.

ACKNOWLEDGMENT

The author's research is presently supported by Grant #P01 HD30704 from The National Institute of Child Health and Human Development.

REFERENCES

1. Vannucci RC. Hypoxic-ischemic encephalopathy: clinical aspects. In Fanaroff AA, Martin RJ (eds) *Neonatal–perinatal medicine IV.* Philadelphia: Mosby-Yearbook, 1997: 877–891.
2. Vannucci RC. Current and potentially new management strategies for perinatal hypoxic-ischemic encephalopathy. *Pediatrics* 1990;85:961–968.
3. Siesjö BK. Cell damage in the brain: a speculative synthesis. *J Cereb Blood Flow Metab* 1981;1:155–185.
4. McCord JM. Oxygen-derived free radicals in postischemic tissue injury. *N Engl J Med* 1985;312:159–163.
5. Nelson CW, Wei EP, Povlishock IT, Kantos HA, Moskowitz MA. Oxygen radicals in cerebral ischemia. *Am J Physiol* 1992;263:H1356–H1362.
6. Beckman JS, Beckman TW, Chen J, Marshal PA, Freeman BA. Apparent hydroxyl radical production by peroxynitrite: implications for endothelial injury from nitric oxide and superoxide. *Proc NatlAcad Sci* 1990;87:1620–1624.
7. Majewska M, Strosznajder J, Lazarewicz J. Effect of ischemic anoxia and barbiturate anesthesia on free radical oxidation of mitochondrial phospholipids. *Brain Res* 1978;158: 423–434.
8. Rehncroná S, Westerberg E, Akesson B, Siesjö BK. Brain cortical fatty acids and phospholipids during and following complete and severe incomplete ischemia. *Stroke* 1978;9:327–335.
9. Bhakoo KK, Crockard HA, Lascelles PT. Regional studies of changes in brain fatty acids following experimental ischaemia and reperfusion in the gerbil. *J Neurochem* 1984;43: 1025–1031.
10. de Haan HH, Van Reempts JLH, Vles JSH, de Haan J, Hasaart THM. Effects of asphyxia on the fetal lamb brain. *Am J Obstet Gynecol* 1993;169:1493–1501.
11. Saugstad OD. Role of xanthine oxidase and its inhibitor in hypoxia: reoxygenation injury. *Pediatrics* 1996;98:103–107.
12. Palmer C, Vannucci RC, Towfighi J. Reduction of perinatal hypoxic-ischemic brain damage with allopurinol. *Pediatr Res* 1990;27:332–336.
13. Palmer C, Roberts RL. Reduction of perinatal brain damage with oxypurinol treatment after hypoxic-ischemic injury. *Pediatr Res* 1991;29:362 [Abstract].
14. Palmer C, Towfighi J, Roberts RL, Heitjan DF. Allopurinol administered after inducing hypoxia-ischemia reduces brain injury in 7-day-old rats. *Pediatrics* 1993;33:405–411.

15. Sasaki T, Nakagomi T, Kirino T, et al. Indomethacin ameliorates ischemic neuronal damage in the gerbil hippocampal CA1 sector. *Stroke* 1988;19:1399–1403.
16. Pourcyrous N, Leffler CW, Bada HS, Korones SB, Busija DW. Brain supeoxide anion generation in asphyxiated piglets and the effect of indomethacin at therapeutic dose. *Pediatr Res* 1993;34:366–369.
17. Beck T, Bielenberg GW. The effects of 21-aminosteroids on overt infarct size 48 hours after middle cerebral artery occlusion in the rat. *Brain Res* 1991;560:159–162.
18. Bågenholm R, Andiné P, Hagberg H. Effects of 21-amino steroid tirilazad mesylate (U74006F) on brain damage and edema after perinatal hypoxia-ischemia in the rat. *Pediatr Res* 1966;40:399–403.
19. Rothman SM, Olney JW. Glutamate and the pathophysiology of hypoxic-ischemic brain damage. *Ann Neurol* 1986;19:105–111.
20. Kass IS, Lipton P. Mechanisms involved in irreversible anoxic damage to the *in vitro* rat hippocampal slice. *J Physiol* 1982;332:459–472.
21. Rothman SM. Synaptic activity mediates death of hypoxic neurons. *Science* 1983;220: 536–527.
22. Novelli A, Reilly JA, Lysko PG, Henneberry RC. Glutamate becomes neurotoxic via the *N*-methyl-D-aspartate receptor when intracellular energy levels are reduced. *Brain Res* 1988;451:205–212.
23. Coyle JT, Bird SJ, Evans RH, Gulley RL, Nadler JV, Nicklas WJ, Olney JW. Excitatory amino acid neurotoxins: selectivity, specificity and mechanism of action. *Neurosci Res Prog Bull* 1981;19:329–427.
24. McBean GJ, Roberts PJ. Chronic infusion of L-glutamate causes neurotoxicity in rat striatum. *Brain Res* 1984;290:372–375.
25. Steiner HX, McBean GJ, Kohier C, Roberts PJ, Schwarcz R. Ibotenate-induced neuronal degeneration in immature rat brain. *Brain Res* 1984;307:117–124.
26. Pulsinelli WA. De-afferentation of the hippocampus protects CA1 pyramidal neurons against ischemic damage. *Stroke* 1985;16:144.
27. Siesjö BK, Bengtsson F. Calcium fluxes, calcium antagonists, and calcium-related pathology in brain ischemia, hypoglycemia, and spreading depression: a unifying hypothesis. *J Cereb Blood Flow Metab* 1989;9:127–140.
28. Andiné P, Sandberg M, Bågenholm R, Lehmann A, Hagberg H. Intra- and extracellular changes of amino acids in the cerebral cortex of the neonatal rat during hypoxia-ischemia. *Develop Brain Res* 1991;64:115–120.
29. Silverstein FS, Naik B, Simpson J. Hypoxia-ischemia stimulates hippocampal glutamate efflux in perinatal rat brain: an in vivo microdialysis study. *Pediatr Res* 1991;30: 587–590.
30. Albers G, Goldberg MP, Choi DW. *N*-methyl-D-aspartate antagonists: ready for clinical trial in brain ischemia? *Ann Neurol* 1989;25:398–403.
31. McCulloch J. Amelioration of ischemic and hemorrhagic injury by pharmacological intervention. In Lou HC, Greisen G, Larsen JF (eds), *Brain Lesions in the Newborn: Hypoxic and Haemodynamic Pathogenesis*. Copenhagen: Munksgaard, 1994:485–499.
32. Sheardown MJ, Suzdak PD, Nordholm L. AMPA, but not NMDA, receptor antagonism is neuroprotective in gerbil global ischemia, even when delayed 24 hours. *Eur J Pharmacol* 1993;236:347–353.
33. McDonald JW, Silverstein FS, Johnston MW. Neuroprotective effects of MK-801, TCP, PCP, and CPP against *N*-methyl-D-aspartate induced neurotoxicity in an in vivo perinatal rat model. *Brain Res* 1989;490:33–40.

34. McDonald JW, Silverstein FS, Johnston MV. MK-801 protects the neonatal brain from hypoxic-ischemic damage. *Eur J Pharmacol* 1987;140:359–361.

35. Ford LM, Sanberg PR, Norman AB. Mk-801 prevents hippocampal neurodegeneration in neonatal hypoxic-ischemic rats. *Arch Neurol* 1989;46:1090–1096.

36. Hattori H, Morin AM, Schwartz PH, Fujikawa DG, Wasterlain CG. Posthypoxic treatment with MK-801 reduces hypoxic-ischemic damage in the neonatal rat. *Neurology* 1989;39: 713–718.

37. McDonald JW, Trescher WH, Johnston MV. Susceptibility of brain to AMPA induced excitotoxicity transiently peaks during early postnatal development. *Brain Res* 1992;583: 54–70.

38. Hagberg H, Gilland E, Diemer N-H, Andiné P. Hypoxia-ischemia in the neonatal rat brain: histopathology after post-treatment with NMDA and non-NMDA receptor antagonists. *Biol Neonate* 1994;66:205–213.

39. Greenamyre JT, Olson JMM, Penney JB, Young AB. Autoradiographic characterization of *N*-methyl-D-aspartate-, quisqualate- and kainate-sensitive glutamate binding sites. *J Pharmacol Exp Ther* 1985;233:254–263.

40. Greeyamyre JT, Penney JB, Young AB, Hudson C, Silverstein F, Johnston MV. Evidence for transient perinatal glutamatergic innervation of globus pallidus. *J Neurosci* 1987;7: 1022–1030.

41. McDonald JW, Johnston MV. Physiological and pathophysiological roles of excitatory amino acids during central nervous system development. *Brain Res Rev* 1990;15:41–70.

42. McDonald JW, Silverstein FS, Johnston MV. Magnesium reduces *N*-methyl-D-aspartate (NMDA)-mediated brain injury in perinatal rats. *Neurosci Lett* 1990;109:234–238.

43. Thordstein M, Bagenholm R, Thiringer K, Kjellmer I. Scavengers of free oxygen radicals in combination with magnesium ameliorate perinatal hypoxic-ischemic brain damage in the rat. *Pediatr Res* 1993;34:23–26.

44. Marret S, Gressens P, Gadissiux J-F, Evrard P. Prevention by magnesium of excitotoxic neuronal death in the developing brain. An animal model for clinical intervention studies. *Dev Med Child Neurol* 1995;37:473–484.

45. De Haan HH, Gunn AJ, Williams CE, Heymann MA, Gluckman PD. Magnesium sulfate therapy during asphyxia in near-term fetal lambs does not compromise the fetus but does not reduce cerebral injury. *Am J Obstet Gynecol* 1997;176:18–27.

46. Nelson KB, Grether JK. Can magnesium sulfate reduce the risk of cerebral palsy in very low birth weight infants? *Pediatrics* 1995;95:263–269.

47. Levene M, Blennow M, Whitelaw A, Hankø E, Fellman V, Hartley R. Acute effects of two different doses of magnesium sulphate in infants with birth asphyxia. *Arch Dis Child* 1995;73:F174–F177.

48. Vannucci RC. Experimental biology of cerebral hypoxia-ischemia: relation to perinatal brain damage. *Pediatr Res* 1990;27:317–326.

49. Deshpande JK, Wieloch T. Flunarizine, a calcium entry blocker, ameliorates ischemic brain damage in the rat. *Anesthesiology* 1986;64:215–224.

50. Alps BJ, Haas WK. The potential beneficial effect of nicardipine in a rat model of transient forebrain ischemia. *Neurology* 1987;37:809–814.

51. Germano IM, Bartkowski HM, Cassel ME, Pitts LH. The therapeutic value of nimodipine in experimental focal cerebral ischemia. *J Neurosurg* 1987;67:81–87.

52. Silverstein FS, Buchanan K, Hudson C, Johnston MV. Flunarizine limits hypoxia-ischemia induced morphologic injury in immature rat brain. *Stroke* 1986;17:477–482.

53. Gunn AJ, Mydlar T, Bennet L, Faull RLM, Gorter S, Cook C, Johnston BM, Gluckman PD. The neuroprotective actions of a calcium channel antagonist, flunarizine, in the infant rat. *Pediatr Res* 1989;25:573–576.

54. Gunn AJ, Williams CE, Mallard EC, Tan WKM, Gluckman PD. Flunarizine, a calcium channel antagonist, is partially prophylactically neuroprotective in hypoxic-ischemic encephalopathy in the fetal sheep. *Pediatr Res* 1994;35:657–663.

55. Levene MI, Gibson NA, Fenton AC, Papathoma E, Barnett D. The use of a calcium-channel blocker, nicardipine, for severely asphyxiated newborn infants. *Dev Med Child Neurol* 1990;32:567–574.

56. Johns RA. EDRF/nitric oxide. *Anesthesiology* 1991;75:927–931.

57. Dawson TM, Dawson DL, Snyder SH. A novel neuronal molecular message in brain: the free radical, nitric oxide. *Ann Neurol* 1992;32:297–311.

58. Szabó C. Physiological and pathophysiological roles of nitric oxide in the central nervous system. *Brain Res Bull* 1996;41:131–141.

59. Nowicki JP, Duval D, Poignet H, Scatton B. Nitric oxide mediates neuronal death after focal cerebral ischemia in the mouse. *Eur J Pharmacol* 1991;204:339–340.

60. Maiese K, Wagner J, Boccone L. Nitric oxide: a downstream mediator of calcium toxicity in the ischemic cascade. *Neurosci Lett* 1994;166:43–47.

61. Ashwal S, Cole DJ, Osborne T, Pearce WJ. Low dose L-NAME reduces infarct volume in the rat MCAO/reperfusion model. *J Neurosurg Anesthesiol* 1993;5:241–249.

62. Kuluz JW, Prado RJ, Dietrich WD, Schieien CL, Watson BD. The effect of nitric oxide synthase inhibition on infarct volume after reversible focal cerebral ischemia in conscious rats. *Stroke* 1993;24:2023–2029.

63. Nishikawa T, Kirsch JR, Koehier RC, Bredt DS, Snyder SH, Traystman RJ. Effect of nitric oxide synthase inhibition on cerebral blood flow and injury volume during focal ischemia in cats. *Stroke* 1993;24:1717–1724.

64. Trifiletti RR. Neuroprotective effect of N^G-nitro-L-arginine in focal stroke in the 7-day old rat. *Eur J Pharmacol* 1992;218:197–198.

65. Hamada Y, Hayakawa T, Hattori H, Mikawa H. Inhibitor of nitric oxide synthesis reduces hypoxic-ischemic brain damage in the neonatal rat. *Pediatr Res* 1994;35:10–14.

66. Marks KA, Mallard CE, Roberts I, Williams CE, Gluckman PD, Edwards AD. Nitric oxide synthase inhibition attenuates delayed vasodilation and increases injury after cerebral ischemia in fetal sheep. *Pediatr Res* 1996;40:185–191.

67. Myers RE, Yamaguchi S. Nervous system effects of cardiac arrest in monkeys. Preservation of vision. *Arch Neurol* 1977;34:65–74.

68. Kalimo H, Rehncrona S, Sderfeldt B, Olsson Y, Siesjö BK. Brain lactic acidosis and ischemic cell damage: 2. Histopathology. *J Cereb Blood Flow Metab* 1981;1:313–327.

69. Pulsinelli WA, Waldman S, Rawlinson D, Plum F. Hyperglycemia converts neuronal damage into brain infarction. *Neurology* 1982;32:1239–1246.

70. Pulsinelli WA, Levy DE, Sigsbee B, Scherer P, Plum F. Increased damage after ischemic stroke in patients with hyperglycemia with or without diabetes mellitus. *Am J Med* 1983;74:540–544.

71. Vannucci RC, Mujsce DJ. The effect of glucose on perinatal hypoxic-ischemic brain damage. *Biol Neonate* 1992;62:215–224.

72. Voorhies TM, Rawlinson D, Vannucci RC. Glucose and perinatal hypoxic-ischemic brain damage in the rat. *Neurology* 1986;36:1115–1118.

73. Vannucci RC, Brucklacher RM, Vannucci SJ. The effect of hyperglycemia on cerebral metabolism during hypoxia-ischemia in the immature rat. *J Cereb Blood Flow Metab* 1996;16:1026–1033.
74. LeBlanc MH, Huang M, Vig V, Patel D, Smith EE. Glucose affects the severity of hypoxic-ischemic brain injury in newborn pigs. *Stroke* 1993;24:1055–1062.
75. Sheldon RA, Partridge JC, Ferriero DM. Postischemic hyperglycemia is not protective to the neonatal rat brain. *Pediatr Res* 1992;32:489–493.
76. Greisen G, Munck H, Lou H. Severe hypocarbia in preterm infants and neurodevelopmental deficit. *Acta Pediatr Scand* 1987;76:401–404.
77. Graziani L, Spitzer AR, Mitchell DG, et al. Mechanical ventilation in preterm infants: neurosonographic and developmental studies. *Pediatrics* 1992;90:515–522.
78. Ikonen RS, Ianas MO, Koidikko MJ, Laippala P, Kuusinen EJ. Hyperbilirubinemia, hypocarbia and periventricular leukomalacia in preterm infants: relationship to cerebral palsy. *Acta Pediatr Scand* 1992;81:802–807.
79. Vannucci RC, Towfighi J, Heitjan DF, Brucklacher RM. Carbon dioxide protects the perinatal brain from hypoxic-ischemic damage. An experimental study in the immature rat. *Pediatrics* 1995;95:868–874.
80. Vannucci RC, Brucklacher RM, Vannucci SJ. Effect of carbon dioxide on cerebral metabolism during hypoxia-ischemia in the immature rat. *Pediatr Res* 1997;42:24–29.
81. Busto R, Dietrich WD, Globus MY-T, Valdes I, Schenberg P, Ginsberg MD. Small differences in intraischemic brain temperature critically determine the extent of ischemic neuronal injury. *J Cereb Blood Flow Metab* 1987;7:729–738.
82. Clifton GL, Jiang JY, Lyeth BG, Jenkins LW, Hamm RJ, Hayes RL. Marked protection by moderate hypothermia after experimental traumatic brain injury. *J Cereb Blood Flow Metab* 1991;11:114–121.
83. Agardh CD, Smith ML, Siesjö BK. The influence of hypothermia on hypoglycemia-induced brain damage in the rat. *Acta Neuropathol* 1992;83:379–385.
84. Yager J, Towfighi J, Vannucci RC. Influence of mild hypothermia on hypoxic-ischemic brain damage in the immature rat. *Pediatr Res* 1993;34:525–529.
85. Young RSK, Olenginski TP, Yagel SK, Towfighi J. The effect of graded hypothermia on hypoxic-ischemic brain damage: a neuropathologic study in the neonatal rat. *Stroke* 1983;14:929–934.
86. Yager JY, Asselin J. Effect of mild hypothermia on cerebral energy metabolism during the evolution of hypoxic-ischemic brain damage in the immature rat. *Stroke* 1996;27:919–926.
87. Thoresen M, Bågenholm R, Løberg EM, Apricena F, Kjellmer I. Posthypoxic cooling of neonatal rats provides protection against brain injury. *Arch Dis Child* 1996;74:F3–F9.
88. Laptook AR, Corbett RJT, Sterett R, Burns DK, Tollefsbol G, Garcia D. Modest hypothermia provides partial neuroprotection for ischemic neonatal brain. *Pediatr Res* 1994;35:436–442.
89. Thoresen M, Penrice J, Lorek A, Cady EB, Wylezinska M, Kirkbride V, Cooper CE, Brown GC, Edwards AD, Wyatt JS, Reynolds EOR. Mild hypothermia after severe transient hypoxia-ischemia ameliorates delayed cerebral energy failure in the newborn piglet. *Pediatr Res* 1995;37:667–670.

8

POSTNATAL NEUROIMAGING TO TIME HYPOXIC-ISCHEMIC CEREBRAL INJURY

Jeffrey M. Perlman, M.B.

Department of Pediatrics, University of Texas Southwestern Medical Center, Dallas, Texas

Advances in neuroimaging techniques over the past two decades have provided the clinician with the opportunity to study the impact of fetal asphyxia on the developing brain. The ability to identify and time acute brain injury in the postnatal period has both medical and legal implications. In this chapter I will discuss the neuropathologic subtypes attributed to hypoxic ischemic cerebral injury in the developing brain, the clinical setting for such injury, and the role of specific neuroimaging techniques to identify and time such injury.

NEUROPATHOLOGY

The neuropathology of hypoxic ischemic cerebral injury, resulting in motor and cognitive deficits often characterized as cerebral palsy (CP), may be considered in the context of five basic subtypes: (1) parasagittal brain injury, (2) periventricular

Asphyxia and Fetal Brain Damage, Edited by Dev Maulik, M.D., Ph.D.
ISBN 0-471-18427-6

leukomalacia, (3) focal/multifocal ischemic injury, (4) status mamoratus, and (5) selective neuronal necrosis (1). Although these lesions frequently overlap in a particular infant, the nature of the insult, the maturation of the brain, and the vascular development of the brain usually result in one dominant lesion; each is briefly reviewed below:

1. *Parasagittal Cerebral Injury.* Parasagittal cerebral injury, the principal ischemic lesion of the term infant, refers to bilateral cortical and adjacent subcortical white matter necrosis involving the superior medial and, particularly, the posterior aspects of the cerebral convexities. The necrosis occurs within border zones also referred to as "watershed areas" between the end branches of the major cerebral vessels, regions which are extremely vulnerable to decreases in cerebral perfusion pressure (1). Injury to this region involves the motor cortex that subserves proximal extremity function, with the upper extremities more severely affected than the lower extremities (1). The most frequent long-term consequence of injury to this region is spastic quadriplegia.

2. *Periventricular Leukomalacia.* Periventricular leukomalacia, the principal ischemic lesion of the preterm infant, refers to bilateral white matter necrosis adjacent to the external angles of the lateral ventricles involving the centrum semiovale and the optic and acoustic radiations. The periventricular white matter resides within border zones between the penetrating branches of the major cerebral vessels. These border zones corresponding to the parasagittal areas of the term infant are also exquisitely sensitive to decreases in cerebral perfusion (1). This region of cerebral white matter is traversed by descending fibers from the motor cortex. The fibers subserving function of lower extremities are more likely to be affected by moderate lesions, and because of extension laterally into the centrum semiovale and corona radiata with more severe lesions, upper extremity involvement occurs as well (1). The long-term manifestations include spastic diplegia and spastic quadriplegia, with visual and cognitive deficits with more severe injury (1).

3. *Focal/Multifocal Ischemic Brain Necrosis.* Focal/multifocal ischemic brain necrosis is characterized by injury to all cellular elements caused by an infarction within a vascular distribution. The middle cerebral artery is the most common vascular territory affected, with the left side twice as commonly involved as the right side (2,3). Experimental data in monkeys support the importance of ischemia in the genesis of this lesion (4). Neuropathologic sequelae includes (a) porencephaly, (b) multicystic encephalomalacia, and (c) hydranencephaly. The long-term neurologic manifestations will reflect the location and extent of the primary lesion and include spastic hemiplegia, spastic quadriplegia, and/or seizures (1).

4. *Status Mamoratus.* Status mamoratus used to be regarded as the rarest lesion associated with perinatal hypoxia ischemia; however, recent data would suggest it occurs more frequently. The lesion is characterized by neuronal injury within the basal ganglia—that is, within the thalamus, the caudate nucleus, the globus pallidus, and the putamen (1). The condition rarely occurs in isolation and invariably is associated with one of the other neuropathologic manifestation subtypes described above. In its isolated form, the long-term neurologic manifestation is choreoathetosis.

5. *Selective Neuronal Necrosis.* Selective neuronal necrosis (SNN) is commonly observed in hypoxic ischemic encephalopathy and invariably coexists with one or more of the lesions listed above. Specific neurons are vulnerable including CA1 region (Sommers sector) and subiculum of the hippocampus; caudate nucleus, putamen, and globus pallidus of the basal ganglia; and the fifth and seventh cranial motor nuclei nerves within the pons and the dorsal vagal nuclei. The pathogenesis of SNN appears to be related to oxygen deprivation, although recent evidence points to the potential of excitotoxic amino acids (1).

Brain Development and Its Relevance to Neuropathology

The maturation of the developing brain is an important determinant of a specific lesion. Moreover, this characteristic may be an extremely useful adjunct in the timing of a specific lesion. For example, a neuronal migrational disturbance must be sustained during the peak time for migrational events to occur within the cortex (i.e., 12–20 weeks). The brain response to tissue injury which also appears to be developmentally regulated can be used to time an insult. For example, the immature brain has a limited ability to react to tissue injury; and characteristically, the damaged tissue undergoes liquefaction necrosis and resorption. By contrast, in the more mature brain, there is an *astroglial response* in response to tissue injury. It has been suggested that this response is encountered in the middle to late second trimester (5).

A second major factor contributing to the specificity of brain injury relates to vascular development (see above). Thus, in the preterm infant, the periventricular white matter resides within border zones of the end branches of the middle, anterior, and posterior cerebral arteries (6). Cerebral microangiography has shown that active development of the periventricular vasculature is most prominent from approximately 28 to 36 weeks, which is the most vulnerable time for injury to this region (7). By contrast, in the term infant, it is the parasagittal region which resides within border zones between the penetrating branches of the major cerebral arteries that is most vulnerable to reductions in cerebral blood flow. Once again the distribution of a specific lesion may help to time the cerebral insult.

Brain Imaging Techniques Used to Diagnose Hypoxic-Ischemic Brain Injury

The diagnosis in the liveborn of the five lesions described above has been based primarily on brain imaging techniques that include cranial ultrasonography, computerized tomography, and magnetic resonance imaging. Each of these imaging modalities has advantages and disadvantages, and they may complement each other when used to evaluate hypoxic-ischemic brain injury. *Ultrasound,* because of its portability and ease of performing serial evaluations, has become the most common imaging method used for this purpose (8,9). However, resolution is limited to lesions greater than 5–8 mm, and the peripheral field of view is limited. *Computed tomography* likewise has limited ability to detect lesions less than 5 mm and to differentiate gray-white interface, especially in the preterm infant. Imaging of the posterior fossa also is limited with tomography because of beam-hardening interface. *Magnetic resonance imaging* has far superior resolution, particularly with high-field machines (1.5 tesla), and currently it is being used more frequently to assess brain structure (10,11).

SPECIFIC LESIONS AND NEUROIMAGING TECHNIQUES

Parasagittal Cerebral Injury

Parasagittal brain injury previously has been identified most readily by radionuclide brain scanning (12). Recent data suggest that the lesion now may be best identified by magnetic resonance imaging, which has superior localization compared with radionuclide scanning.

Periventricular Leukomalacia

Periventricular leukomalacia is identified in the neonatal period most readily by cranial ultrasound (13–15). The ultrasonic evolution of this lesion is characterized by the appearance of bilateral periventricular echogenicity, especially in the peritrigonal regions, which, after an interval of time ranging from 1 to 3 weeks, become echolucent with cyst formation. Ventriculomegaly, often with disappearance of cysts, is the usual sonographic outcome. The respective neuropathological correlates of these findings are necrosis accompanied by vascular congestion or hemorrhage or both; cyst formation; decreased myelination; and gliosis with eventual collapse of cysts. Magnetic resonance imaging is extremely useful in the identification of periventricular white matter injury, particularly in subsequent months or years (see below).

Focal and Multifocal Ischemic Brain Injury

Focal and multifocal brain injury can be identified by using ultrasound, computed tomography, or magnetic resonance imaging (10,16,17). These lesions often cannot be readily visualized in the first days after the insult. However, increased echogenicity on cranial ultrasound scan may provide initial evidence for this lesion. Smaller or more peripherally placed lesions, for example, posterior parietal lesions, may be missed when using cranial ultrasound imaging.

Status Marmoratus

Injury to basal ganglia is best detected by magnetic resonance imaging (8). Cranial ultrasonography also is useful in detecting this lesion.

Selective Neuronal Necrosis

In our experience, brain imaging modalities have not been particularly useful during the neonatal period for identification of cortical neuronal injury. Experience with magnetic resonance imaging in this setting is limited. The sequelae of selective neuronal necrosis (e.g., cortical atrophy) can be detected readily by magnetic resonance or computed tomographic imaging at long-term follow-up (following hospital discharge). Selective neuronal necrosis is more commonly assessed by neurophysiological techniques, the most frequent being the electroencephalogram (EEG), which shows patterns such as burst suppression indicative of profound neuronal necrosis (1). Brain stem auditory evoked responses and visual evoked responses are of some use in identifying cortical neuronal injury.

Comparison of Neuroimaging Techniques

Keeney et al. (10) compared three imaging techniques to evaluate a variety of neuropathological subtypes following hypoxic-ischemic injury. As shown in Table 1, cranial ultrasonography is useful in the diagnosis of periventricular leukomalacia and basal ganglia injury, but less so with focal ischemic injury. Computerized tomography is extremely limited in the diagnosis of all three basic lesions. These data would indicate that ultrasonography is an excellent screening method for the initial assessment of brain structure. As shown in Table 2, for more specific resolution of peripheral lesions, magnetic resonance imaging appears to be the most sensitive and specific modality.

Table 1. Comparison of magnetic resonance imaging with computed tomography and ultrasonography in the diagnosis of hypoxic-ischemic[a] brain injury

	Percent Verified	
Lesion Identified by MRI (No.)	HUS	CT
Periventricular leukomalacia (12)	83	25
Basal ganglia hemorrhage (5)	80	33
Focal parenchymal hemorrhage (15)	63	45

[a]Adapted from reference 10, with permission. MRI denotes magnetic resonance imaging; HUS, head ultrasonography; CT, computed tomography.

Table 2. Neuroimaging techniques in the evaluation of acute neonatal brain injury

Pathological Substrate	HUS	CT	MRI
Selective neuronal necrosis[a]	–	–	–
Parasagittal cerebral injury	–	–	?
Periventricular leukomalacia	+	–	+
Status marmoratus	+	±	+
Focal and multifocal brain injury	+	+	+

[a]Best diagnosed by neurophysiological techniques (e.g., electroencephalogram). The minus sign "–" denotes "not useful"; the plus sign "+" denotes "useful." HUS denotes head ultrasonography; CT, computed tomography; MRI, magnetic resonance imaging.

Timing of Hypoxic-Ischemic Cerebral Injury

Hypoxic-ischemic cerebral injury can develop in the antenatal, perinatal, or postnatal period.

Antenatal Injury. In most cases (60–70%), the genesis of hypoxic-ischemic cerebral injury that results in cerebral palsy occurs prior to labor and delivery; that is, it is antenatal in origin (18–20). The time of onset of an antenatal ischemic insult is critical to the evolution of a specific lesion. Thus, cerebral ischemia prior to the 20th week of gestation results in a neuromigrational defect (e.g., schizencephaly; see Figure 1); ischemia occurring between the 28th and the 34th week of gestation usually results in periventricular leukomalacia (Figure 2); and when ischemia occurs between the 34th week and 40th week of gestation, focal/multifactorial cerebral injury may develop (21). Factors that have been associated with antenatal hypoxic-ischemic cerebral injury include multiple pregnancy, maternal bleeding in the third trimester, and maternal drug use (e.g., cocaine); however, in most cases, the etiology is idiopathic (22–25). The latter becomes an extremely relevant point with regard to the timing of a cerebral insult, particularly when there are associated perinatal difficulties. To expand upon this further, infants with antepartum hypoxic ischemic brain injury may present in one of four ways: (1) There may be no problems either antepartum, during labor, or in the neonatal period. (2) There may be no antepartum problems; however, intrapartum problems may be encountered (e.g., meconium-stained amniotic fluid; fetal heart rate abnormalities followed by a normal neonatal course). (3) There may be no antepartum problems; however, there may be signs of intrapartum distress (e.g., meconium-stained amniotic fluid) or difficulties in the delivery room (i.e., the need for intensive resuscitation, prolonged low Apgar scores, etc.), and the infant may exhibit clinical signs of HIE, including seizures as well as

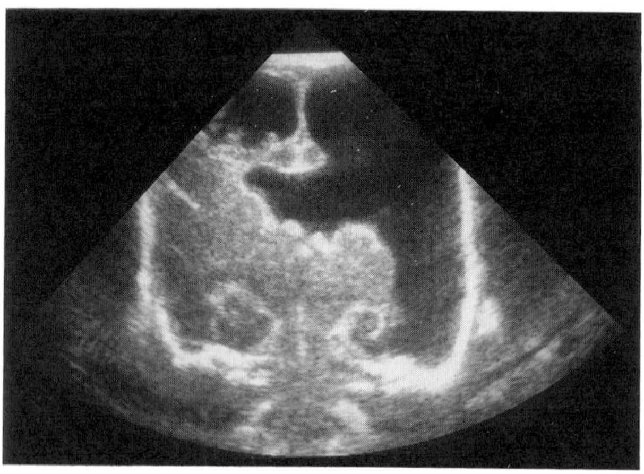

Figure 1. Coronal section of brain. Note the large cystic lesion on the left communicating with the frontal horn of the lateral ventricle. Also note the cystic area in right frontal cortex. The appearance is typical of a schizencephalic defect.

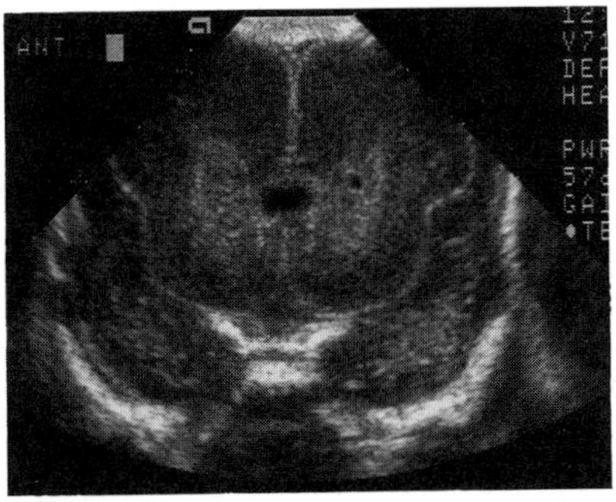

Figure 2. Coronal section of brain obtained on the first day of life from a 1300-g premature infant. Note the cystic lesion in left periventricular white matter (see Case 1 in the text).

systemic organ injury in the early neonatal period; these findings are consistent with intrapartum hypoxic ischemic cerebral injury. (4) All three scenarios may be preceded by known events associated with antenatal brain injury (10).

Intrapartum Injury. Currently available data indicate that perinatal hypoxic ischemic brain injury accounts for approximately 10–20% of all the cases that subsequently evolve to cerebral palsy. Several clinical characteristics usually in combination provide evidence for an intrapartum insult. These include fetal heart rate abnormalities (i.e., fetal bradycardia), meconium in amniotic fluid, an extended low Apgar score, acidosis in cord arterial blood sample (i.e., cord arterial pH $\leq$7.00, base deficit $\geq$14 mEq/liter), and evolution to a syndrome of hypoxic-ischemic encephalopathy including seizures and clinical signs of systemic organ injury (e.g., renal injury) (21). Since antenatal injury may superimpose on a perinatal insult, neuroimaging is critical as an adjunct to potentially time a hypoxic-ischemic insult. Specifically, neuroimaging may provide evidence for antenatal brain injury or identify the postnatal evolution of brain injury. The value of postnatal neuroimaging to time a hypoxic-ischemic cerebral insult is indicated in the following series of case illustrations.

Case 1. Baby A was a 1300-g, 28-week, AGA, to a mother whose pregnancy was uncomplicated until the onset of preterm labor. The labor was complicated by fetal heart rate abnormalities—that is, variable decelerations resulting in delivery via cesarean section. At birth, the infant was noted to be flaccid with a heart rate of 80 beats per minute. Resuscitation included intubation and positive pressure ventilation. The Apgar scores were 2 at 1 min and 6 at 5 min. The umbilical arterial blood gas revealed a cord pH 7.07, pCO_2 of 74 mmHg, and base deficit −11.8 mEq/liter. The infant remained intubated for 5 days secondary to persistent apnea.

A cranial ultrasound scan (HUS) on the first postnatal day revealed a cystic lesion adjacent to the left lateral ventricles within periventricular white matter (Figure 2). The lesion persisted on two subsequent HUS scans. A final scan prior to discharge revealed resolution of the cyst, with moderate left lateral ventriculomegaly. The infant's subsequent clinical was remarkable only for recurrent apnea and bradycardia which resolved by the 34th week of postconceptual age. At early follow-up the infant has developmental motor delay.

INTERPRETATION OF THE CASE. The documentation of a cystic lesion within white matter by cranial ultrasonography on the first postnatal day is consistent with injury prior to the delivery process. The evolution to cyst formation occurs at approximately 5–7 days following a known insult with an initial appearance of hyperechogenicity prior to the cyst formation. In the preterm infant, failure to obtain a cranial sonogram at birth would have rendered timing of the lesion more difficult.

Case 2. BW was a 2945-g, 42-week, appropriate-for-gestational-age female, born to a 36-year-old G_1,P_0 mother. The pregnancy was uncomplicated; however, labor was complicated by late decelerations resulting in a cesarean section delivery. Resuscitation in the delivery room included brief bag and mask ventilation. The Apgar scores were 7 at 1 min and 9 at 5 min. The umbilical arterial blood gas determination revealed a pH of 7.21, pCO_2 of 62 mmHg, base deficit of –5.2 mEq/liter. The infant's subsequent clinical course was considered within normal limits for age. A cranial ultrasound scan was performed because of a small but unexplained decrease in hematocrit from 60% to 50% over the first three days of life. The scan revealed an area of increased echogenicity within the left temporo-occipital distribution of the middle cerebral artery (Figure 3a). A magnetic resonance imaging scan confirmed the ultrasound abnormalities and defined the lesion as a large focal cerebral infarction within the distribution of the middle and posterior cerebral arteries (Figure 3b). A CT scan

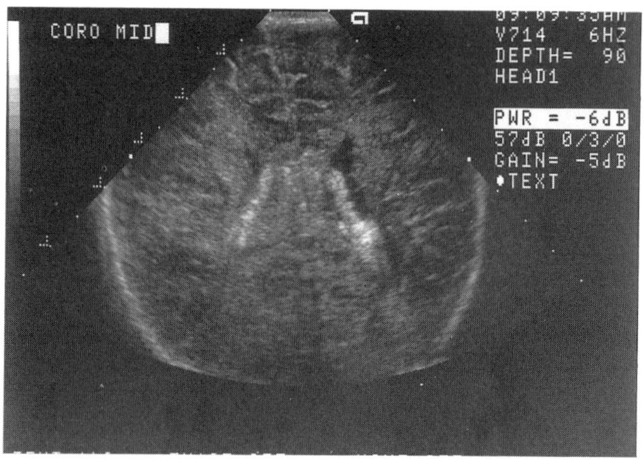

a

Figure 3. (a) Coronal ultrasound scan obtained in the first week of life. Note the increased echogenicity on the right in the distribution of the right middle cerebral artery. **(b)** MRI from the same infant one day later. T_2-weighted axial image. Note the increased signal intensity in the distribution of the right middle and posterior cerebral arteries. **(c)** CT scan from the same patient at 3 months of age. Note the evolution to a porencephalic cyst in the distribution of the previously noted infarction.

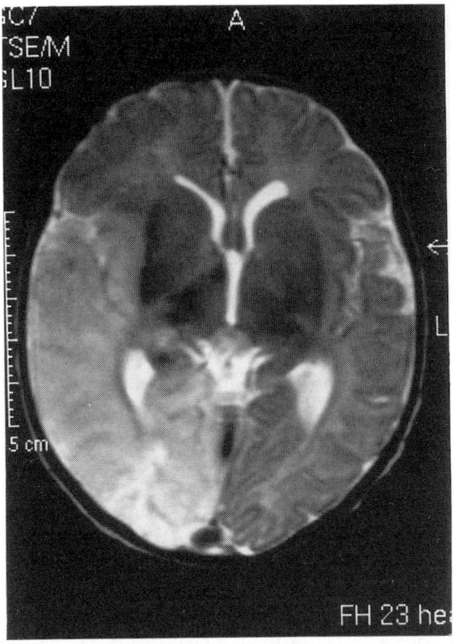

Figure 3. b. *continued*

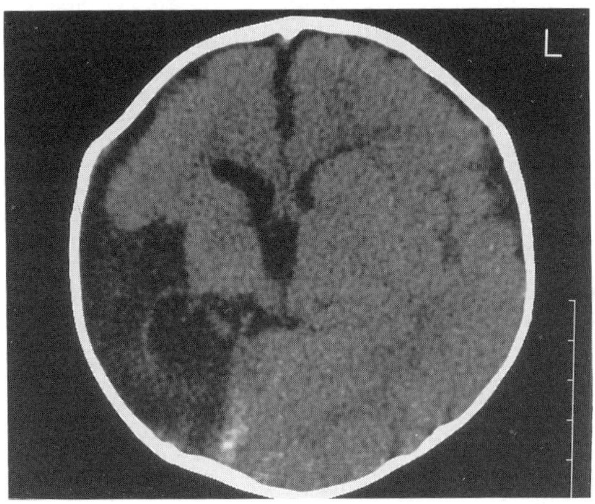

Figure 3. c. *continued*

obtained two months later revealed a porencephalic cyst in the distribution of the previous noted lesion (Figure 3c).

INTERPRETATION OF THE CASE. This infant delivered after an uncomplicated pregnancy, had evidence of fetal decelerations but no other problems. The postnatal course was benign. On a neuroimaging screening evaluation, a diagnosis of a neonatal stroke was made. Since the postnatal clinical course was unremarkable, the findings suggests an onset either prior to or during labor. We have previously demonstrated that the majority of cases of neonatal stroke occur in the absence of overt signs of perinatal distress and/or asphyxia (15). If no imaging had been performed in the immediate neonatal period, it would have been very difficult to time the development of the porencephalic cyst noted on the CT scan at 2 months of age.

Postnatal Injury. Postnatal injury resulting in brain injury is more commonly observed in the premature infant and less so in the term infant. In the premature infant, the most striking example is periventricular–intraventricular hemorrhage where the lesion develops between the second and fifth postnatal day and is often preceded by a known provocative event. Similarly, in the term infant, the development of a hemorrhagic/ischemic lesion beyond the immediate neonatal period is often precipitated by a major clinical event—for example, postcannulation of the major cerebral vessels for extra corporeal membrane oxygenation therapy.

Delayed Neuroimaging to Time a Hypoxic-Ischemic Insult

In several recent studies, neuroradiologic imaging techniques, specifically computed tomography and magnetic resonance imaging, have been performed later in childhood to define the neuropathology of cerebral palsy in vivo (26,27). In some of the first studies, Wiklund et al. (26) used tomography to study 28 preterm infants and 83 term infants with hemiplegic cerebral palsy between 5 and 16 years of age. Half of the preterm infants had evidence of periventricular leukomalacia, 20% had neural maldevelopment indicative of early fetal brain injury, and in 25%, tomographic findings were normal. As shown in Table 3, in term infants the tomographic findings suggested prenatal injury in over half of cases—that is, periventricular leukomalacia in 37% and maldevelopment in 17%. By contrast, about 20% had cortical and subcortical injuries suggestive of a perinatal injury, and findings were considered normal in 27%.

In another study, shown in Table 4, 11 preterm and 29 term infants were evaluated with magnetic resonance imaging (27). The predominant finding in the preterm infants was evidence for periventricular white matter damage in over 80%. This was indicative of hypoxic ischemic brain injury. As noted previously, it is difficult to distinguish the exact chronology of onset of these lesions. By contrast, 50% of the term infants' magnetic resonance imaging findings were consistent with antenatal brain damage (i.e., gyral abnormalities such as *polymicrogyri* consistent with mid-

Table 3. Computed tomographic findings in 83 term infants with hemispheric cerebral palsy

Type of Lesion	Percent of Total
Maldevelopment	17
Periventricular atrophy	37
Cortical or subcortical atrophy	19
Normal	27

Table 4. Magnetic resonance imaging findings in term infants with cerebral palsy

Type of Lesion	Percent of Total
Migration abnormalities	31
Periventricular leukomalacia	21
Hydrencephaly	3
Cortical or subcortical injury	17
Others	28

second-trimester injury) and isolated periventricular leukomalacia (Table 4). In approximately one-fourth of these, the magnetic resonance findings, coupled with clinical events, were suggestive of intrapartum hypoxic ischemic injury. This figure is similar to that obtained in several large-scale epidemiological studies of infants with cerebral palsy noted previously (18–20,28).

CONCLUSION

It cannot be assumed with any degree of medical certainty that brain injury manifesting as cerebral palsy in a given child is due to perinatal asphyxia. Thus, whenever neurological abnormalities develop in the newborn, an accurate diagnosis should be pursued vigorously, using both clinical and neuroimaging modalities.

REFERENCES

1. Volpe JJ. *Neurology of the newborn,* 2nd ed. Philadelphia: WB Saunders, 1995.
2. Barmada M, Modssy J, Shuman RM. Cerebral infarcts with arterial occlusion in neonates. *Ann Neurol* 1979;6:495–502.
3. Perlman JM, Rollins NK, Evans D. Neonatal stroke: clinical characteristics and cerebral blood flow velocity measurements. *Pediatr Neurol* 1994; 11:281–284.
4. Myers RE. Cerebral ischemia in the developing primate fetus. *Biomed Biochim Acta* 1989;48:S137–S142.
5. Gilles FH. Neuropathologic indicators of abnormal development. In Freeman J, (ed). *Prenatal and perinatal factors associated with brain disorders.* Bethesda, MD: National Institutes of Health, 1985;85:1149.
6. DeReuck J. The human periventricular arterial blood supply and the anatomy of cerebral infarctions. *Eur Neurol* 1973;5:321.
7. Takashima S, Tanaka K. Development of cerebrovascular architecture and its relationship to periventricular leukomalacia. *Arch Neurol* 1978;35:11.
8. Babcock DS, Ball W Jr. Post asphyxial encephalopathy in full term infants. Ultrasound diagnosis. *Radiology* 1983;148:417–423.

9. Siegel MJ, Shackelford GD, Perlman JM, et al. Hypoxic ischemic cerebral injury in term infants. Diagnosis and prognosis by ultrasound. *Radiology* 1984;152:395–399.

10. Keeney SE, Adcock EW, McArdle CB. Prospective observations of 100 high-risk neonates by high-field (1.5 tesla) magnetic resonance imaging of the central nervous system. II. Lesions associated with hypoxic-ischemic encephalopathy. *Pediatrics* 1991;87:431.

11. Barkovich AJ, Westmark K, Partridge C, Sola A, Ferriero D. Perinatal asphyxia: MR findings in the first 10 days. *Am J Neuroradiol* 1995;16:427–438.

12. O'Brien MJ, Ash JM, Gilday DL. Radionuclide brain scanning in perinatal hypoxia ischemia. *Dev Med Child Neurol* 1979;21:161–1 73.

13. Fawer CL, Calame A, Perentes E et al. Periventricular leukomalacia. A correlation study between real-time ultrasound and autopsy findings. Periventricular leukomalacia in the neonate. *Neuroradiology* 1985;27:292–300.

14. Chow PP, Horgan JG, Taylor KJ. Neonatal periventricular leukomalacia: real-time sonographic diagnosis with CT correlation. *Am J Roentgenol* 1985;145:155–160.

15. Dubowitz LM, Bydder GM, Mushin J. Developmental sequence of periventricular leukomalacia: correlation of ultrasound, clinical and nuclear magnetic resonance findings. *Arch Dis Child* 1985;60:349–355.

16. Fujimoto S, Yokochi K, Togari H, et al. Neonatal cerebral infarction. CT findings and prognosis. *Brain Dev* 1992;14:48–52.

17. Rollins NC, Morriss M, Evans D, Perlman JM. The role of early MR in the evaluation of the term infants with seizures. *Am J Neuroradiol* 1994;15:239–248.

18. Stanley F, Alberman E (eds). *The epidemiology of the cerebral palsy.* Philadelphia: JB Lippincott, 1984.

19. Blair E, Stanley FJ. Intrapartum asphyxia—a rare cause of cerebral palsy. *J Pediatr* 1988;112:515–519.

20. Torfs CP, Van der berg BJ, Oeschali FW. Prenatal and perinatal factors in the etiology of cerebral palsy. *J Pediatr* 1990;116:615–619.

21. Perlman JM. Intrapartum hypoxic ischemic cerebral injury—Medicolegal issues. *Pediatrics* 1997;99:851–857.

22. Nelson KB, Ellenberg JH. Antecedents of cerebral palsy multivariate analysis of risk. *N Engl J Med* 1986;315:81–86.

23. Larroche JC. Fetal encephalopathies of circulatory origin. *Biol Neonate* 1986;50:61–74.

24. Bejar R, Gustavo V, Gramajo H, et al. Antenatal origin of neurologic damage in newborn infants. II. Multiple gestations. *Am J Obstet Gynecol* 159:357–363.

25. Scher MS, Belfar H, Martin J, Painter MJ. Destructive brain lesion of presumed fetal onset: antepartum causes of cerebral palsy. *Pediatrics* 1991;88:898–906.

26. Wiklund LM, Uvebrant P, Flodmark O. Computed tomography as an adjunct in etiological analysis of hemiplegic cerebral palsy. II. Children born at term. *Neuropediatrics* 1991;22:121–125.

27. Truwit CL, Barkovich AJ, Koch TK, Ferriero DM. Cerebral palsy: MR findings in 40 patients. *Am J Neuroradiol* 1992;13:67–75.

28. Perlman JM, Cunningham FG. Fetal and neonatal hypoxic ischemic cerebral injury. Supplement to *Williams Obstetrics,* No. 21. (Cunningham, McDonald, Gant, eds), December 1993.

9

HOW TO TIME WHEN HYPOXIC-ISCHEMIC FETAL BRAIN DAMAGE TOOK PLACE

Richard L. Naeye, M.D.

Department of Pathology, Milton S. Hershey Medical Center, The Pennsylvania State University College of Medicine, Hershey, Pennsylvania

INTRODUCTION

It has long been widely assumed that abnormal fetal heart rates, low Apgar scores, metabolic acidosis at birth, and neonatal seizures are indications that cerebral palsy had a hypoxic-ischemic origin during labor and delivery. All of these findings can also be present when the brain damage took place before labor began (1–5). As a result, it is not known what portion of the hypoxic-ischemic cerebral palsy in the general population originated pre-labor and what portion was the result of damage during labor and delivery. If a substantial portion originated before labor began, there is a pressing need to document this fact, determine its cause, learn how to recognize its antecedents, and discover how the resulting risks might be managed. The first step in reaching these goals is to find a reliable way to accurately determine the time when

Asphyxia and Fetal Brain Damage, Edited by Dev Maulik, M.D., Ph.D.
ISBN 0-471-18427-6

damaging hypoxemia began in individual children with hypoxic-ischemic cerebral palsy. This chapter describes a simple method that might often meet this need.

We obtained the first clue to how this time might be determined from a paper by Siri et al. (6), who found that lymphocyte numbers and erythropoietin levels increased in the blood of an adult made hypoxemic in a high-altitude chamber. This finding led us to analyze lymphocyte and normoblast counts in the blood of neonates who had developed quadriplegic cerebral palsy as the result of damaging antenatal hypoxia-ischemia. First, we established the time of the hypoxic-ischemic injury by one of the following markers: (a) the sudden, unexpected appearance of severe, sustained fetal bradycardia, (b) the mother's unsolicited report that fetal movements markedly decreased or ceased at a specific time prior to the start of labor, and (c) the sudden onset in one gravida of severe abdominal pain accompanied by massive vaginal bleeding due to a complete placental abruption (1). Eleven of the children had placental abruptions as the cause of their cerebral palsy, two had umbilical cord compressions, two had large feto-maternal hemorrhages, and one had a thrombotic occlusion of the umbilical vein. Lymphocyte counts in the blood of these children were consistently greater than 10,000/mm^3 within an hour after their hypoxemia-ischemia began and routinely decreased to far less than 10,000/mm^3 at the end of 24 hours (1). The mean value of lymphocyte counts in 84 normal neonates used as controls was 4430 ± 1418/mm^3 (1).

The next challenge was to determine if the aforementioned lymphocyte cycle is reliable enough in its timing and specific enough for hypoxia-ischemia to be clinically valid in establishing when hypoxic-ischemic brain damage took place. To make these determinations a number of questions need to be asked and answered. Are the aforementioned lymphocyte findings present in larger populations of children who have hypoxic-ischemic cerebral palsy? Do various types of nonhypoxic fetal stress produce a similar lymphocyte response? How soon after severe hypoxia-ischemia begins do large numbers of lymphocytes enter the fetal blood? Can this lymphocyte response take place at levels of hypoxemia and ischemia less severe than those that produce brain damage?

To answer the first question we searched our 1988–1995 medical center records and consultation files to locate 25 children whose hypoxic-ischemic cerebral palsy had been documented by MRI or CT scan brain images. The previously mentioned clinical indicators were then employed to establish when their damaging hypoxemia had begun. Their blood lymphocyte counts exceeded 10,000/mm^3 after the hypoxemia began and consistently decreased to normal or subnormal levels 24 hours later (Figure 1).

Do various types of fetal stress that are not acute hypoxic-ischemic in nature produce a similar lymphocyte response? One-minute Apgar scores of 0–3 in neonates were used as the indicator of such stress. We located 35 children born in our hospital during 1993 who fell into this category. Fourteen were born with severe bacterial pneumonia as the cause of their low Apgar scores. Eleven had major congenital malformations and 10 had been subjected to very severe, chronic low uteroplacental blood flow before birth. The placentas of these last 10 were markedly growth-retarded and had multiple infarcts and abnormally small villi with excessive numbers of syn-

Fig. 1

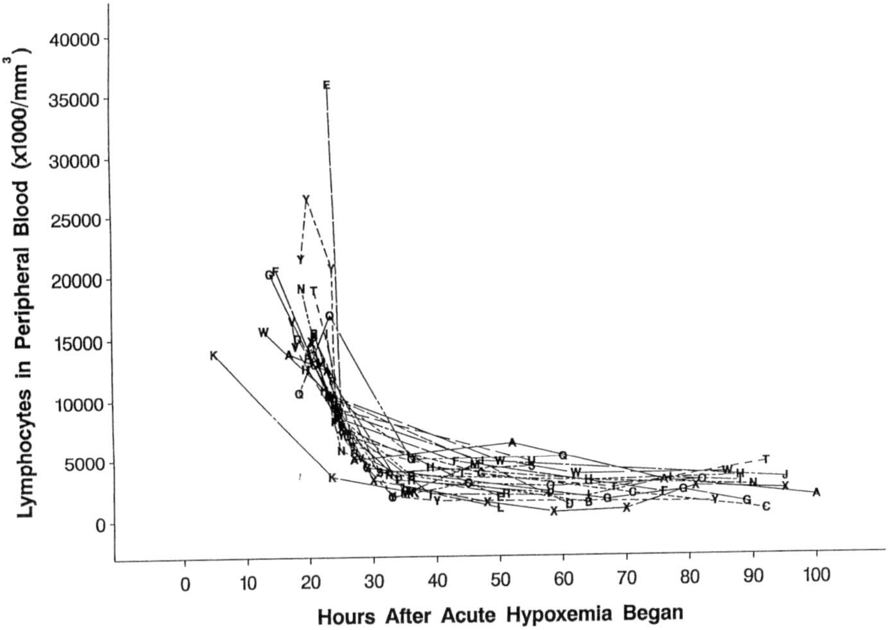

Figure 1. Lymphocyte counts (×1000/mm^3) in the blood of neonates following the start of severe, acute antenatal hypoxemia. The letters A–Y represent the 25 children who now have hypoxic-ischemic cerebral palsy.

cytial knots. These placental findings are well-known consequences of chronic low uteroplacental blood flow (7). None of the children in the three groups had blood lymphocyte counts that exceeded 10,000/mm^3 during the 24 hours following their births (1). These lymphocyte counts ranged from 1830/mm^3 to 7700/mm^3 (1).

How soon after severe hypoxia-ischemia begins do large numbers of lymphocytes enter the fetal blood? We have pursued several lines of investigation to try to answer this question. First we located four children who had experienced an interval of 10–15 min between the onset of severe hypoxemia-ischemia and death (2). The first of these children was stillborn 15 min after the start of severe bradycardia caused by a complete placental abruption. The other three were victims of the sudden infant death syndrome (SIDS). Their lymphocyte counts were evaluated because the hearts of some SIDS victims have continued to beat after they quit breathing. Such intervals presumably do not last longer than 15 minutes before the heart stops. The stillborn child had a blood lymphocyte count of 15,490/mm^3 and all three SIDS victims had lymphocyte counts greater than 10,000/mm^3. Thus large numbers of lymphocytes may be able to enter the blood of fetuses and young infants within 15 minutes after severe hypoxemia begins. Other studies suggest the interval is close to 25 minutes (8).

There is always the possibility that some nonhypoxemic process initiated the lymphocytosis in the just-described four children, so blood counts of neonates born with large diaphragmatic hernias were also analyzed to determine the following: How soon after hypoxemia begins can large numbers of lymphocytes enter the blood (8)? Hypoxemia is absent in these children before birth but often starts within minutes after they are born. At our institution these children have usually had arterial blood pH, pO2, and base excess values determined just after birth and at short intervals thereafter. We studied 12 such children who had been markedly cyanotic for 0.5 to 1.4 hours before their blood was drawn for leukocyte counts. Their lymphocyte counts ranged from $9768/mm^3$ to $19,767/mm^3$. These counts reinforce the likelihood that lymphocytes can enter the blood in large numbers within a half hour after the start of severe hypoxemia.

Can the cycle of lymphocyte numbers that increase and later decrease take place at levels of hypoxemia that do not produce brain damage? To answer this question, blood counts need to be analyzed from a large number of neonates whose time when hypoxemia began is known and its severity documented. Forty-two children who were born with diaphragmatic hernias met this requirement (8). As previously mentioned these children usually experience hypoxemia within an hour after they are born. In our cases, varying degrees of this hypoxemia then continued until their hernias were surgically repaired. All 42 had multiple recorded arterial blood pH and base excess values along with simultaneously measured blood lymphocyte counts measured within 5 hours of their births. pH values just below 7.00 and base excess values of –14 or –15 were the thresholds at which their blood lymphocyte counts exceeded $10,000/mm^3$. Brain damage most often occurs with arterial blood pH values less than 7.0 and base excess values more negative than –20, so the threshold at which large numbers of lymphocytes can enter the blood appears to be close to that at which brain damage can take place.

How might blood lymphocyte counts be used in routine clinical practice to identify when severe hypoxia-ischemia began before birth? These counts should be routinely obtained in neonates whose clinical findings raise the possibility of severe antecedent hypoxia-ischemia. The first should be made within an hour of birth. If it is greater than $10,000/mm^3$, subsequent counts should be made at 2- to 3-hour intervals until the counts fall below $10,000/mm^3$. A line should then be drawn between the counts to identify the time that the counts decreased to below $10,000/mm^3$. This latter time after birth in hours is then subtracted from 24 to indicate the number of hours before birth when severe ischemia and hypoxemia began. For example, if a child had a lymphocyte count of $13,000/mm^3$ 2 hours after birth and $9000/mm^3$ 4 hours later, plotting these two numbers against the times the blood was drawn (2 and 6 hours after birth) show that the lymphocyte count decreased below $10,000/mm^3$ at about 5 hours after birth. Subtracting 5 from 24 placed the start of severe hypoxemia at 19 hours before birth. We have recently found that brain damage is usually complete within 2 hours after severe hypoxia-ischemia begins.

We next attempted to determine if normoblast counts in neonates' blood could be used to identify the time before birth that hypoxia-ischemia damaged their brains. Normoblast counts are an obvious candidate for this purpose because it has long been known that normoblasts are present in the blood of many fetuses and neonates who are hypoxemic (1,9,10). To determine if such counts could be used as timers, it must first be determined if they have a time predictable cycle of entry and exit from the blood. If such a cycle exists, all of the questions asked about the lymphocyte cycle need to be asked and answered for normoblasts. In a preliminary study we found that normoblast numbers routinely increased many-fold in the blood of fetuses after hypoxemia started and then decreased in number 24 hours later (1). However, unlike lymphocytes, normoblasts sometimes remained in the blood in large numbers beyond 24 hours (1). The normoblast counts that remained elevated beyond 24 hours were in neonates whose hypoxemia continued after birth (1,2). In this latter situation, normoblast counts cannot be used to indicate when hypoxemia began.

The answers to other important questions about the normoblast cycle point up additional limitations that must be considered in its interpretation as previously mentioned. The hypoxic-acidotic threshold at which lymphocytes enter the blood is close to the threshold at which large numbers of brain damage takes place (1). This is only partially true for normoblasts. The arterial blood pH threshold value at which normoblasts enter the blood is about 7.0, which is the same as the value for lymphocytes. However, normoblasts enter the blood in large numbers at a base excess value of –11 mEq/ml, which is not as close to the level at which brain damage can occur as the –15 value at which large numbers of lymphocytes enter the blood.

Is the time at which large numbers of normoblasts enter the blood predictable after hypoxia-ischemia begins? In our studies, normoblasts in large numbers began to enter the blood of neonates about 20 min after the start of hypoxemia, which is earlier than the time that large numbers of lymphocytes enter the blood following the start of severe hypoxemia. This conclusion was based on the following. Several children whose large diaphragmatic hernias led to severe hypoxemia soon after birth had large numbers of normoblasts in their blood at 20 min after birth. This suggests that large numbers of normoblasts can enter the blood about 20 min after severe hypoxemia begins. When a large number of normoblasts but not lymphocytes are present in a child's blood, the possibility that severe hypoxemia began more than 24 hours earlier needs to be considered.

Do nonhypoxemic stresses lead large numbers of normoblasts to enter the blood? The answer so far is no. Normoblast counts were consistently less than 500/mm^3 within an hour of birth in the previously mentioned children who had 1-min Apgar scores of 0–3 due to causes other than acute hypoxemia (1).

CONCLUSIONS

Findings of our studies indicate that undertaking serial lymphocyte counts in the blood of neonates, starting at birth and continuing for at least 24 hours thereafter, can sometimes establish when brain-damaging hypoxia-ischemia started before birth. Lymphocyte counts increased to greater than 10,000/mm^{3}within 15–25 min after the start of severe hypoxia-ischemia and reliably returned to normal or subnormal levels 24 hours later. Such counts are easy to obtain, inexpensive, and available at most facilities where babies are born in the industrial nations. Blood normoblast numbers have a similar (but not as time-reliable) cycle of increase and decrease after hypoxemia begins. The level of metabolic acidosis initiated by hypoxemia must be more severe for large numbers of lymphocytes than for normoblasts to enter the blood.

REFERENCES

1. Naeye RL, Localio AR. Determining the time before death when ischemia and hypoxemia initiated cerebral palsy. *Obstet Gynecol* 1995;86:713–719.
2. Naeye RL. Can meconium in the amniotic fluid injure the fetal brain? *Obstet Gynecol* 1995;86:720–724.
3. Volpe JJ. *Neurobiology of the newborn.* Philadelphia: WB Saunders 1985: Chapter 9.
4. Nelson KB, Dambrosia JM ,Ting TY, Grether JK. Uncertain value of electronic fetal monitoring in predicting cerebral palsy. *N Engl J Med* 1996;334:613–618.
5. MacDonald D. Cerebral palsy and intrapartum fetal heart rate monitoring. *N Engl J Med* 1996;334:659–660.
6. Siri WE, VanDyke DC, Winchell HS, Pollycove M, Parker HG, Cleveland AS. Early erythropoietin, blood and physiological responses to severe hypoxia in man. *J Appl Physiol* 1966;21:73–80.
7. Naeye RL. *Disorders of the placenta and fetus and neonate: diagnosis and clinical significance.* New York: Mosby-Yearbook, 1992:138.
8. Naeye RL, Localio AR. Lymphocytosis in neonates, a consequence of severe hypoxemia. Submitted for publication.
9. Fox H. The incidence and significance of nucleated erythrocytes in the foetal vessels of the mature human placenta. *J Obstet Gynaecol Br Cwlth* 1967;74:40–43.
10. Phelan JP, Ahn MO, Korst LM, Martin GI. Nucleated red blood cells: a marker for fetal asphyxia? *Am J Obstet Gynecol* 1995;173:1380–1384.

10

HEMATOLOGIC MARKERS TO DATE FETAL NEUROLOGIC INJURY

Lisa M. Korst, M.D. and Jeffrey P. Phelan, M.D.

Department of Obstetrics and Gynecology, Cedars-Sinai Medical Center, Los Angeles, California (LMK); and Department of Obstetrics and Gynecology, Pomona Valley Hospital Medical Center, Pasadena, California (JPP)

INTRODUCTION

Cerebral palsy occurs in approximately 1–2 cases per 1000 live births (1,2). But cerebral palsy due to fetal asphyxia is even rarer, with a reported incidence of 1–2 cases per 10,000 live births (3). Because of the lasting emotional and financial impact on families and our society, physicians and researchers have attempted to prevent cerebral palsy by determining what causes fetal asphyxial brain injury (4). To date, their success has been limited, and effective preventive measures continue to remain elusive.

For each asphyxiated newborn, two questions immediately arise: When did the hypoxic episode occur, and what caused it? The answer to these questions requires an understanding of what is currently known about fetal asphyxial brain injury. In regard to timing of the episode, historically it has been believed that most cases of fetal asphyxial injury occur intrapartum. Catastrophic events occurring during labor, such as a cord prolapse or placental abruption, have long been known to lead to prolonged

Asphyxia and Fetal Brain Damage, Edited by Dev Maulik, M.D., Ph.D.
ISBN 0-471-18427-6

fetal heart rate (FHR) decelerations, fetal asphyxia, and permanent brain injury. In some cases, acute prolonged FHR decelerations can occur without any identifiable cause or warning and can lead to an asphyxiated fetus. However, a growing body of evidence has now developed that suggests that fetuses may undergo asphyxial events throughout gestation and not necessarily just during labor. Studies in primate colonies (5,6), animal (7), brain pathology (8,9), brain imaging (10,11), and dental enamel (12,13) provide evidence of prelabor asphyxial events associated with permanent brain injury. Although these data have established that prelabor asphyxial events can and do occur, the rarity and lack of predictability of these events have precluded population-based studies and the determination of the proportion of cerebral palsy cases due to intrapartum or prelabor asphyxia.

How do these asphyxial events occur? Through the use of animal models, a variety of hypoxia-inducing physiologic mechanisms have been investigated. These models have largely been designed to investigate acute events and have included: partial and complete occlusion of the umbilical cord, placental embolization, and decreased maternal oxygen levels (7,14). These studies have yielded variable results. First, hypoxia alone, with or without hypotension, can lead to permanent brain injury (4). Hypotension appears to worsen the fetal outcome. Second, the hypoxia must be severe (14). Investigators have shown that oxygen volume must drop to approximately 10% of normal before hypoxic brain injury will occur. FHR monitoring abnormalities, such as late decelerations, may be noted at oxygen drops to 40% of normal (14). This level is well above the critical oxygen level. Animal data do not support the concept of "chronic asphyxia" leading to permanent fetal brain injury. Third, the duration of the hypoxic episode affects the fetal outcome: Oxygen volumes at 10% of normal may be endured for more than 30 min with no permanent injury; oxygen volumes at 5% of normal may only be endured 15–20 min (14). Fourth, "fetal reserves" do impact on the degree of insult tolerated by the fetus. For example, growth-restricted fetuses tolerate the same degree of oxygen deprivation for less time than do normal fetuses before they are permanently injured (7,14). Fifth, multiple metabolic factors, such as the presence of free radicals, acid–base status, and the degree of oxygen tension, can affect the degree of neuronal injury. Consequently, postnatal treatment may also affect final neurologic outcome (15).

The fetal physiologic response to hypoxia, as demonstrated by these models, has been well-documented. At higher oxygen volumes (e.g., 10%), a centralization (or shunting) of the fetal circulation occurs, thereby increasing flow to the brain, heart, and adrenals and decreasing flow to less vital organs such as the lungs, kidneys, liver, and gut (7). Such centralization can be maintained for some time without the occurrence of permanent brain injury. Obviously, this will depend on the duration of the insult, the occurrence of hypotension, and the amount of fetal reserve. However, in the face of an even more severe oxygen drop or hypotension, it appears that portions of the brain are uniquely vulnerable to hypoxia-ischemia, and that they may become permanently damaged before other organs show clinical signs of injury. This may occur in the absence of shunting of the fetal circulation. When Myers first looked at animal models in the 1960s, he found that cases of the most severe hypoxia (total occlusion of the umbilical cord) led routinely to mid-brain and brainstem lesions and that partial occlusion led to the more commonly seen cortical injuries with sparing of the central structures (14).

Studying asphyxia in the laboratory differs from studying asphyxial events during human gestation. For example, there are currently no animal models that simulate an antepartum asphyxial episode that produces central nervous system (CNS) injury and then resolves, allowing the gestation to go to term. Furthermore, there is little evidence to determine which of the proposed mechanisms leading to asphyxia are most realistic. Myers' work helped substantiate that complete umbilical cord occlusion does not produce the most common pattern of brain injury, that of diffuse cortical hypoxia-ischemia. Rather, it is likely that other mechanisms are more common because they allow for higher circulating oxygen levels, which are indeed associated with cortical injury patterns. Such observations underscore the probability that the circumstances under which antepartum asphyxial events occur differ from those under which intrapartum asphyxial events occur. A fetus that was injured antepartum and survived to present in labor at term must have undergone an event that resolved itself. Most fetuses who suffer an asphyxial event during labor are monitored and the event recognized, and many of the events causing asphyxia at this time are so catastrophic (e.g., uterine rupture, cord prolapse) that if an immediate cesarean were not performed, the fetus would die.

When we study asphyxiated neonates, some of whom are injured in the past and who yet survived, and some who were injured acutely and likely would have died without intervention, we are likely to be studying neonates who were injured under differing circumstances. This complicates the study situation not only because differences in the presentation of injured neonates may reflect differences in the time of occurrence of the asphyxial episode (i.e., clinical parameters may result from viewing the acute versus resolution phase of injury), but also because differences in neonatal presentation may reflect differences in the severity of the episode; that is, neonates with older lesions may uniformly have less severe asphyxial episodes than those with new, acute lesions who are delivered under catastrophic circumstances. Fetuses who undergo a catastrophic event (such as placental abruption) remote from term would most likely present as a stillborn, and not be included in any study of liveborn children with brain injury. Thus, from an observational point of view, the timing of fetal asphyxial events may be inextricably linked with the physiologic mechanism of the event.

The study of fetal asphyxial brain injury has thus been hampered by not only our lack of knowledge regarding the causes of the hypoxic episode, but also by a lack of ability to classify patients accurately regarding the timing of the insult. Thus, when investigators undertake to study risk factors for fetal asphyxial brain injury, few correlations are identified because neonates injured early in gestation are lumped with neonates injured during the intrapartum period. It is understandable that Apgar scores or cord pH values may differ in these circumstances because in one the asphyxial event has long resolved whereas in the other it is still ongoing. Furthermore, collaboration among the three disciplines of obstetrics, neonatology, and neurology must occur to bring about a better understanding of fetal asphyxial brain injury.

Phelan and Ahn (16) have recently proposed a classification system that separates term neonates with permanent brain injury due to fetal asphyxial events by the timing of the injury. Obviously, this classification system cannot determine the exact moment when injury occurred, but it uses FHR patterns to identify three groups of neonates (16–18): those that were injured prior to presenting in labor, those that were injured during labor acutely, and those that were injured during labor over some period of time. These FHR patterns have been well documented in the obstetrical literature. The first pattern, a nonreactive FHR pattern, is indicative of a prior cerebral insult and is associated with high morbidity and mortality. Early references regarding this type of heart rate pattern date back to 1963, in a paper by Hon and Lee (19). The second pattern, a tachycardic pattern, was also described earlier by Hon (19) and later reconfirmed by Phelan and Ahn (16). Fetuses in this group are admitted in labor with a reactive FHR, indicative of normal neurologic status on admission to the hospital, which subsequently becomes nonreactive and tachycardic and is accompanied by repetitive FHR decelerations and, in most instances, a loss of variability. Such a pattern is indicative of an evolving hypoxic event arising during labor. The third group, the acute group, also presented to the hospital with a normal FHR pattern and underwent a catastrophic event, such as uterine rupture or cord prolapse. These cases were associated with a prolonged FHR deceleration that lasted until delivery and resuscitation of the infant. Using a registry for brain-injured neonates, Phelan and Ahn have described cases with these three FHR patterns, yielding neonatal characteristics for each group that are remarkably consistent with the proposed timing of the injury (16–18). Here we will describe the clinical characteristics of such neonates as classified, if possible, by their FHR groups and focus on hematologic markers and organ status.

NEONATAL pH

A profound metabolic or mixed acidemia at birth, as reflected by an umbilical cord artery pH <7.00, although often a direct result of an hypoxic episode, reflects only the immediate circumstances surrounding birth. Neonates who suffered a hypoxic event prior to labor may show a normal pH, or one that is indeed low because of additional hypoxia experienced after neurologic injury. Furthermore, neonatal outcomes have not been shown to be well predicted by umbilical artery pH (20). This is substantiated by physiologic evidence that oxygen levels must remain severely low for some duration prior to the occurrence of brain injury (4). In terms of pH values, Myers' work demonstrated that animals maintained at a pH of 7.1 showed no hypoxic brain injury, and it also showed that at a pH of <7.0 they could last as long as several hours before they died of cardiac failure (14). Thus, the initial pH that occurs with obstetrical events and FHR patterns is not in and of itself indicative of intrapartum fetal brain injury.

NUCLEATED RED BLOOD CELLS

The presence of nucleated red blood cells (NRBCs), also known as normoblasts, in the cord blood and the neonatal circulation appears to be one of the most valid indicators of previous hypoxemia. Thirty years ago Fox proposed that the number of

NRBCs provided "a rough guide to the degree of oxygen deprivation" a patient has suffered (21). In fact, he was only one of several investigators who suggested that asphyxia induced an increase in the number of NRBC in the circulating blood of newborns. Some of the most intriguing data in support of this proposition came from Soothill et al. (22), who to some degree established a correlation between the number of NRBCs per 100 leukocytes and the severity of fetal hypoxemia experienced by growth-impaired fetuses. Although a few NRBCs may be found in the circulating blood of newborns, it is very unusual to see more than 10 such cells per 100 white blood cells (17,18). When that ratio is exceeded, the most frequent explanations are illustrated in Table 1.

The underlying theory is that the fetus responds to oxygen deprivation not only by diverting blood from less vital organs to the brain, heart, and adrenal glands, but also by stimulating production and release of erythropoietin. The erythropoietin, in turn, speeds up erythropoiesis as a means of improving oxygenation. This stepped-up process results in an increased proportion of immature—and thus nucleated—red blood cells. Indeed, the higher-than-average representation of NRBCs in the blood of asphyxiated newborns may reflect not only hurried erythropoiesis but also asphyxia-induced splenic injury (7) that impairs the ability of that organ to "clear" immature and otherwise suboptimal red blood cells.

Using 46 cases from a national registry of brain-injured neonates, but excluding cases with conditions known to be associated with an elevated NRBC count, Phelan et al. (17) demonstrated that neurologically impaired neonates had significantly higher NRBC than did normal nonasphyxiated newborns (Figure 1). In addition, these investigators were able to show that there were distinct patterns involving maximal NRBC values (Figure 2) and that clearance times (Figure 3) appeared to be associated with the FHR pattern and the timing of fetal hypoxic-ischemic injury. The length of time from identification of normoblasts to their disappearance from the peripheral circulation was determined in 29 of the injured neonates. The mean "clearance time" (18) for these three groups is updated and illustrated in Table 2. Children in the nonreactive group were far more likely than those in the other two groups to maintain NRBCs in their circulation for more than 80 hours after birth.

As the registry data expanded, Korst et al. (18) and later Phelan et al. (23) published a follow-up study on the NRBC values of 153 singleton, term neurologically impaired neonates and were able to correlate the earlier observations (14). First, some

Table 1. The most frequent reasons for elevated nucleated red blood cells

Prematurity: <32 weeks' gestation
Rh sensitization
Uncontrolled maternal diabetes mellitus
Twin–twin transfusion syndrome
Fetal anemia
ABO incompatibility
Intrauterine growth restriction

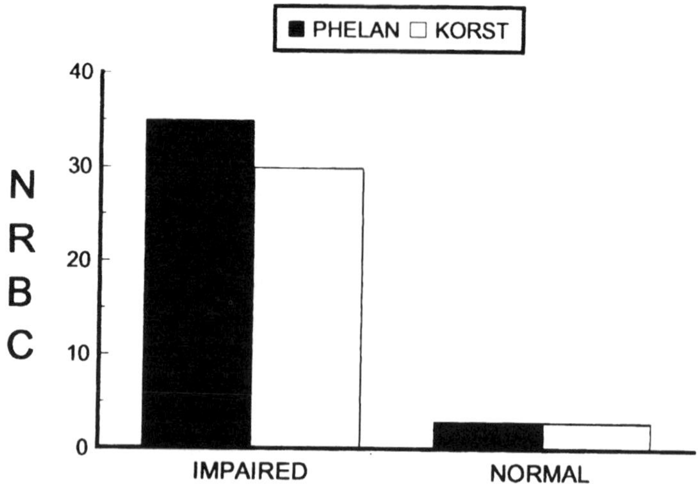

Figure 1. The mean nucleated red blood cell counts (NRBC) of neurologically impaired and normal infants (14).

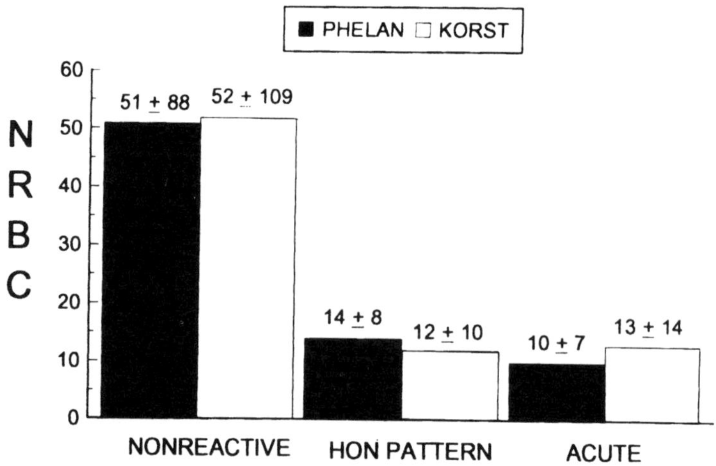

Figure 2. The mean nucleated red blood cell counts of neurologically impaired neonates separated by the intrapartum fetal heart rate (FHR) pattern (14).

infants who have a nonreactive FHR pattern from admission to delivery will have few or no NRBCs in their cord blood or peripheral circulation. This suggests that some CNS insults have occurred so long before delivery that the fetus has had sufficient time before delivery to clear the normoblasts. Second, the initial NRBC count usually is the peak NRBC value, or is very close to that maximum value. When subsequent blood draws show a significant rise in NRBCs, neonatal causes of injury, such as im-

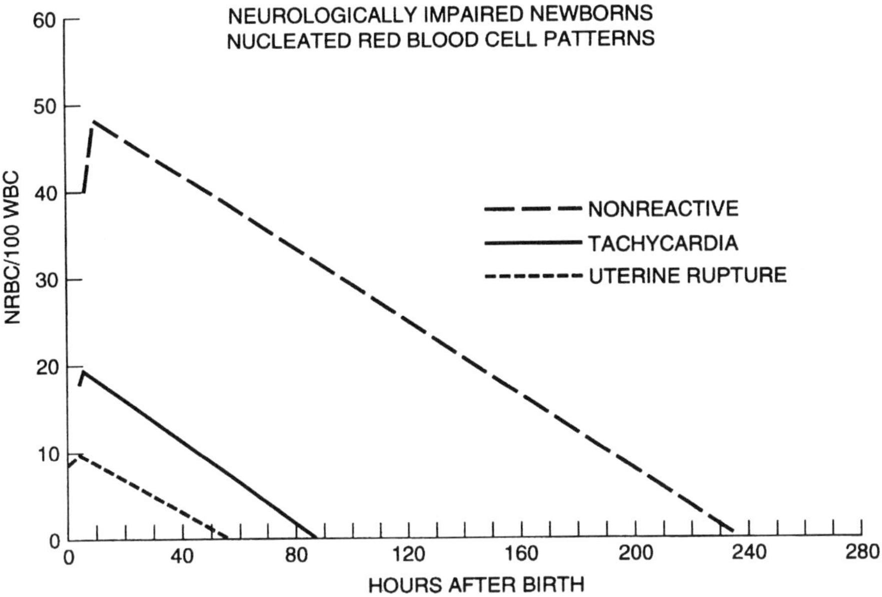

Figure 3. The mean "clearance times" of nucleated red blood cells from the neonatal circulation separated by the fetal heart pattern/timing of the fetal brain injury are presented. (Reproduced with permission from reference 17.)

Table 2. The mean clearance times for the three FHR patterns associated with fetal brain injury (18)

Group	Number	Clearance Time (hours)
Preadmission	39	122 ± 123
Hon pattern	28	52 ± 63
Acute	28	66 ± 66

proper ventilation technique in the neonatal intensive care unit (NICU), may be responsible for the rise.

LYMPHOCYTES

Naeye and Localio (24) first suggested that neonatal lymphocyte counts may be elevated during the first 24 hours following a hypoxic-ischemic injury. Postulating the timing of the injury by maternal history of decreased fetal movement or by catastrophic obstetrical events in 16 patients, they charted lymphocyte counts by the hours post injury and determined for these few patients that lymphocyte counts were elevated above normal values (8000 lymphocytes per mm^3) in the first 24 hours and that all resolved to normal 24 hours after the "injury."

Phelan et al. (23) used cases from their national registry to examine this same question. Eighty-seven neonates were studied: 56 in the nonreactive group and 31 in the acute group. Using linear regression analysis, the authors determined that lymphocyte values declined rapidly within 6, not 24, hours of life and that only data taken in the first few hours of life should be used. In the first 6 hours of life, brain-injured neonates were 25 times more likely to have a lymphocyte count >8000 per mm^3 compared with normal infants: The nonreactive group had a mean ± standard deviation of 11,047 ± 4794 compared with the acute group, which had a mean of 8677 ± 5563. These levels were statistically different from Naeye's normal group (24) as well as statistically different from each other. With one exception, all elevated values dropped to <8000 within 24 hours.

PLATELETS

Hematologic dysfunction can occur as a result of sustained acidosis, hypoxia, and hypotension and may be a manifestation of overt disseminated intravascular coagulation. Decreased platelet values appear to be more evident in cases of pre-admission injury. In the Korst et al. study (25) of 129 term brain-injured infants classified in the three FHR groups, the nonreactive group were eight times more likely than neonates in the Hon and acute groups to have an initial platelet count <150 (1000 per mm^3). Moreover, the mean platelet values for these three groups (Figure 4) illustrate that low platelets are more common in the nonreactive group. Further investigation of patterns of fetal brain injury, the extent of intracerebral bleeding, and the extent of systemic

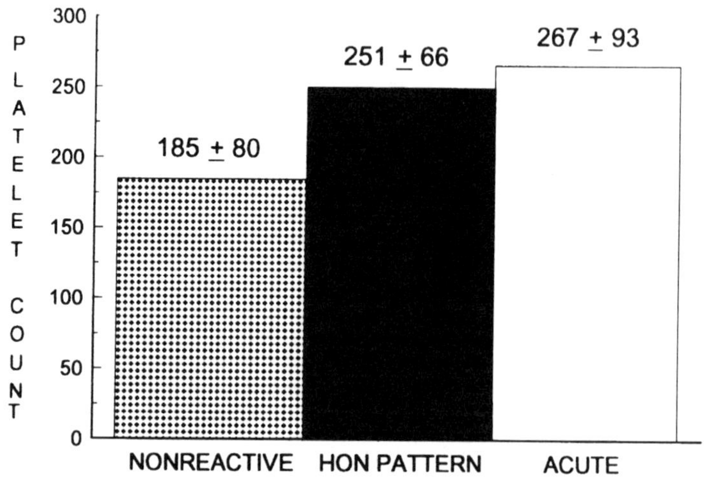

Figure 4. Neonatal platelet counts (number × 1000/mm^3) in neurologically impaired neonates separated by the intrapartum FHR pattern. FHR, fetal heart rate.

vascular endothelial damage are necessary to clarify the physiologic processes leading to the altered platelet counts.

LIVER FUNCTION TESTS

One of the fetal responses to hypoxia is increased shunting of blood through the ductus venosus; subsequent hepatic hypoxia can occur with elevations of liver transaminases. Levels of serum glutamic-oxaloacetic transaminase (SGOT) and glutamic-pyruvic transaminase (SGPT) are considered some of the more specific parameters of liver cell injury and have been suggested as a routine and rapid laboratory test for establishing the presence of hepatic cellular damage following an asphyxial event if centralization of the fetal circulation has occurred (26). Because this injury is highly reversible once the hypoxia has resolved, one would expect that fetuses with preadmission injury may have normal liver transaminases. Fetuses undergoing acute injury may not proceed with the physiologic process of centralizing their circulation, and thus they may also exhibit normal SGOT and SGPT levels (27). Here the circumstances surrounding the timing of the injury must put the liver function tests in the proper context.

CREATININE PHOSPHOKINASE

Hypoxia of cardiac muscle may lead to reduction of cardiac glycogen reserves, resulting in a deficient heart action with decreased stroke volume and cardiac dilatation, leading to systemic hypotension and possibly heart failure or infarction. In animal studies, the degree of myocardial injury has been shown to be directly related to the degree of the asphyxial insult and the survival rates of asphyxiated fetuses (14). Creatinine phosphokinase (CPK) levels should be monitored in neonates suspected of having undergone asphyxial injury during gestation.

RENAL FUNCTION

The combination of ischemia and hypoxemia can cause renal damage. This is manifested in decreased renal function and by the presence of oliguria, hematuria, and proteinuria (28,29). Related hematologic markers that may be useful in determining the physiologic impact of asphyxia on the kidneys are serum creatinine and sodium. Because there is a wide variation in renal composition and output in the immediate neonatal period and because some neonates may show initially high concentrations of serum creatinine due to events and treatment immediately surrounding the birth and immediate neonatal care, a persistently elevated serum creatinine concentration of ≥1.2 mg/dl for 4 or more days after birth appears consistent with severe hypoxic renal damage (30). Earlier resolution of creatinine levels to normal may occur and are likely to reflect less severe injury and less profound centralization of the fetal circulation.

Decreased sodium levels may be noted as a likely result of the syndrome of inappropriate antidiuretic hormone (SIADH) or renal dysfunction (31), and in cases of severe asphyxia these decreased levels may be manifest for several days.

METABOLIC DYSFUNCTION

Although potassium, calcium, and glucose levels are known to be affected by asphyxia (31), they are often documented and/or clinically treated in an inconsistent manner and thus may not be reliable indicators of the occurrence of an asphyxial event.

SUMMARY

In conclusion, for the neonate suspected of having undergone a severe asphyxial episode at some time during gestation, several blood tests may assist in the determination of when and how that episode occurred. The cord blood provides valuable data with the arterial pH, NRBC, lymphocyte, and platelet levels. The NRBC count, SGOT, SGPT, serum creatinine, and serum sodium levels should be monitored for several days if abnormal. CPK levels may indicate the presence of cardiac injury. In the context of the prenatal and intrapartum history and the clinical condition of the neonate, these hematologic markers may provide physicians with information regarding the timing and severity of the fetal asphyxial insult.

ACKNOWLEDGMENT

This project was sponsored in part by the Childbirth Injury Prevention Foundation.

REFERENCES

1. Freeman JM, Nelson KB. Intrapartum asphyxia and cerebral palsy. *Pediatrics* 1988; 82(2):240–249.
2. Naeye RL, Peters EC, Bartholomew M, Landis JR. Origins of cerebral palsy. *Am J Dis Child* 1989;143:1154–1161.
3. Blair E, Stanley FJ. Intrapartum asphyxia: a rare cause of cerebral palsy. *J Pediatr* 1988; 112:515–519.
4. Myers RE. Experimental models of perinatal brain damage: relevance to human pathology. In Gluck L (ed). *Intrauterine asphyxia and the developing fetal brain.* Chicago: Year Book Medical Publishers, 1977;37–97.
5. Myers RE, Valerio MG, Martin DP, Nelson KB. Perinatal brain damage: porencephaly in a cynomolgous monkey. *Biol Neonate* 1973;22:253–273.
6. Brann AW, Myers RE. Central nervous system findings in the newborn monkey following severe in utero partial asphyxia. *Neurology* 1975;25:327–338.

7. Jensen A, Berger R. Fetal circulatory responses to oxygen lack. *J Dev Physiol* 1991;16:181–207.
8. Low JA, Robertson DM, Simpson LL. Temporal relationship of neuropathologic conditions caused by perinatal asphyxia. *Am J Obstet Gynecol* 1989;160:608–614.
9. Morrison I, Olsen J. Weight-specific stillbirths and associated causes of death: an analysis of 765 stillbirths. *Am J Obstet Gynecol* 1985;152:975–980.
10. Kim MS, Elyaderani MK. Sonographic diagnosis of cerebrovascular hemorrhage in utero. *Radiology* 1982;1442:479–480.
11. Chinn DH, Filly RA. Extensive intracranial hemorrhage in utero. *J Ultrasound Med* 1983;2:285–287.
12. Via WF, Churchill JA. Relationships of cerebral disorder to faults in dental enamel. *AMA J Dis Child* 1957;94:137–142.
13. Cohen HJ, Diner H. The significance of developmental dental enamel defects in neurological diagnosis. *Pediatrics* 1970;46:737–747.
14. Myers RE. Two patterns of perinatal brain damage and their conditions of occurrence. *Am J Obstet Gynecol* 1972;112(2):246–276.
15. Vannucci RC. Experimental biology of cerebral hypoxia-ischemia: relation to perinatal brain damage. *Pediatric Res* 1990;27(4):317–326.
16. Phelan JP, Ahn MO. Perinatal observations in 48 neurologically impaired term infants. *Am J Obstet Gynecol* 1994;171:424–431.
17. Phelan JP, Ahn MO, Korst LM, Martin GI. Nucleated red blood cells: a marker for fetal asphyxia? *Am J Obstet Gynecol* 1995;173:1380–1384.
18. Korst LM, Phelan JP, Ahn MO, Martin GI. Nucleated red blood cells: an update on the marker for fetal asphyxia. *Am J Obstet Gynecol* 1996;175:843–846.
19. Hon EH, Lee ST. Electronic evaluation of the fetal heart rate. VIII. Patterns preceding fetal death, further observations. *Am J Obstet Gynecol* 1963;87(6):816–826.
20. Finer NN, Robertson CM, Peters K, Coward JH. Factors affecting outcome in hypoxic-ischemic encephalopathy in term infants. *Am J Dis Child* 1983;137:21–25.
21. Fox H. The incidence and significance of nucleated erythrocytes in the fetal vessels of the mature human placenta. *J Obstet Gynaecol Br Cwlth* 1967;74:40–43.
22. Soothill PW, Nicolaides KH, Campbell S. Prenatal asphyxia, hyperlacticemia, hypoglycemia, and erythroblastosis in growth retarded fetuses. *Br Med J* 1987;294:1051–1053.
23. Phelan JP, Korst LM, Wang YM, Ahn MO. Neonatal nucleated red blood cell and lymphocyte counts in dating fetal neurologic injury [Abstract]. *Am J Obstet Gynecol* 1997; 176(2):S60.
24. Naeye RL, Localio AR. Determining the time before birth when ischemia and hypoxia initiated cerebral palsy. *Obstet Gynecol* 1995;86:713–719.
25. Korst LM, Phelan JP, Wang YM. Neonatal platelet counts and the timing of fetal brain injury [Abstract]. *Am J Obstet Gynecol* 1997;176(2):S61.
26. Zanardo V, Bondio M, Perini G, Temporin GF. Serum glutamic-oxaloacetic transaminase and glutamic pyruvic transaminase activity in premature and full-term asphyxiated newborns. *Biol Neonate* 1985;47:61–69.
27. Phelan JP, Ahn MO, Korst LM, Martin GI, Wang YM. Intrapartum fetal asphyxial brain injury with absent multiorgan system dysfunction. *J Matern Fetal Med* 1998;7(1):19–22.
28. Perlman JM, Tack ED. Renal injury in the asphyxiated newborn infant: relationship to neurologic outcome. *J Pediatr* 1988;113:875–879.

29. Dauber IM, Krauss AN, Symchych PS, Auld PAM. Renal failure following perinatal anoxia. *J Pediatr* 1976;88(5):851–855.

30. Dauber IM, Krauss AN, Symchych MD, Auld PAM. Renal failure following anoxia. *J Pediatr* 1976;88(5):851–855.

31. Fitzhardinge PM. Complications of asphyxia and their therapy. In Gluck L (ed). *Intrauterine asphyxia and the developing fetal brain.* Chicago: Year Book Medical Publishers, 1977;285–292.

11

INTRAVENTRICULAR HEMORRHAGE IN THE PREMATURE INFANT

Jeffrey M. Perlman, M.B.

Department of Pediatrics, University of Texas Southwestern Medical Center, Dallas, Texas

BACKGROUND

Periventricular–intraventricular hemorrhage (PV-IVH) is the most common serious neurologic lesion of the neonatal period occurring predominantly in the premature infant. The routine use of cranial ultrasonography in the early 1980s to visualize the intracranial contents of the premature infant defined the magnitude of the problem. Thus, several large series reported the incidence of PV-IVH to range between 30% and 40% for infants less than 1500 g, with the incidence as high as 50–60% for infants <1000 g and approximately 10–15% for infants between 1001 and 1500 g (1–5). However, recent evidence indicates a declining overall incidence of PV-IVH which appears to be related to both intrapartum and postpartum factors (6,7). In order to understand the complex issues related to PV-IVH, in this chapter the neuropathology, pathogenesis, clinical manifestations, diagnosis, prognosis, and therapies of the lesion will be reviewed.

Asphyxia and Fetal Brain Damage, Edited by Dev Maulik, M.D., Ph.D.
ISBN 0-471-18427-6

Neuropathology

The primary lesion in PV-IVH is bleeding from small vessels in the subependymal germinal matrix. The hemorrhage may be confined to the germinal matrix region, or it may extend and rupture into the adjacent ventricular system or into the periventricular white matter (Figure 1). The germinal matrix, a source of neurons and glia for the developing brain, is a transitional gelatinous region which provides limited support for the vessels that course through it. Over the latter weeks of gestation this matrix becomes less prominent and is essentially absent by term. A luxurious arterial supply to the region is derived from the anterior cerebral artery, via Heubner's artery, and the middle cerebral artery, via the deep lateral striate arteries (8). Further arterial contributions are derived from the penetrating branches of the middle cerebral artery and the internal carotid artery by way of the anterior choroidal artery. The vascular supply to this region is particularly prominent until approximately 32 weeks of gestation (9). This is the period of gestation that the premature infant is most vulnerable to develop a hemorrhage. The rich arterial supply as described above feeds an extensive capillary bed in the matrix. This bed contains irregular vessels that cannot be categorized by light microscopic features as arterioles, capillaries, or vessels (10,11). Thus, these vessels might be expected to be more susceptible to hemorrhage. The rich capillary system is continuous with a well-developed deep venous system. The venous drainage of this region and the cerebral white matter is via the terminal, choroidal, and thalamostriate veins. These vessels course anteriorly to a point of confluence at the level of the head of the caudate nucleus and the foramen of Monroe to form the internal cerebral vein that courses directly posteriorly to join the vein of Galen (10). Therefore, at the usual site of hemorrhage, the blood flow takes a peculiar U-turn,

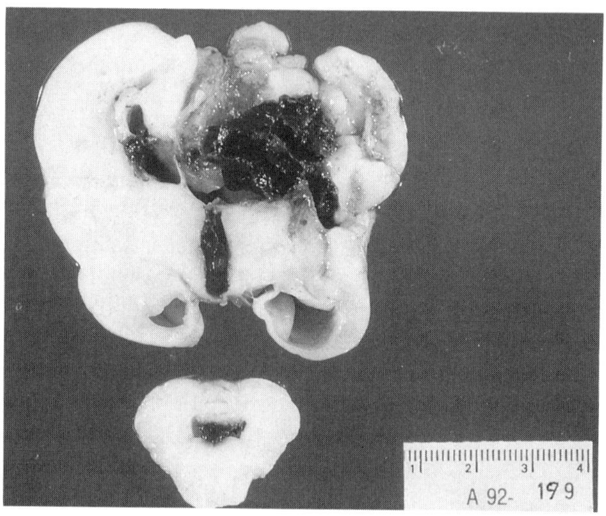

Figure 1. Germinal matrix–intraventricular hemorrhage: coronal section of cerebrum. Note blood in the lateral ventricles, aqueduct of Sylvius, and the fourth ventricle.

suggesting that increases in venous pressure may be equally as important in the pathogenesis of this lesion.

Pathogenesis

When considering the pathogenesis of PV-IVH, the importance of extravascular, vascular, and intravascular factors need to be considered. The genesis of PV-IVH is likely multifactorial; and to varying degrees, different factors may be operative in individual infants. *Intravascular* factors are those that relate primarily to the regulation of cerebral blood flow (CBF) and pressure in the microvascular bed of the germinal matrix. Support for the role of abnormalities of CBF in the genesis of PV-IVH is based in part on experimental studies. Thus, in the beagle puppy, germinal matrix hemorrhage can be produced by systemic hypertension with and without prior hypotension (12,13). This observation has been applied clinically to the premature infant with a germinal matrix where increased cerebral perfusion secondary to elevation in arterial blood pressure is regarded as an important cause of germinal matrix hemorrhage (14). This is more likely to occur in the premature infant, because the cerebral circulation appears to be pressure passive (15,16). Clinically, fluctuations in CBF, particularly in the ventilated preterm infant with respiratory distress syndrome, and increases in CBF as may occur with pneumothorax are considered to be important in the genesis of PV-IVH (17,18). Abrupt elevations in arterial blood pressure may also occur with routine neonatal procedures, such as tracheal suctioning or routine handling, in the infant (14,19–21). Conversely, decreases in CBF occurring either prenatally or postnatally may play an important role in the genesis of PV-IVH in certain infants. A major consequence of the decreased CBF will be injury of germinal matrix vessels that rupture subsequently upon reperfusion (22).

Venous changes such as elevations of venous pressure may also contribute to the occurrence of PV-IVH. Elevations in venous pressure may occur during the labor and delivery process or in association with respiratory distress syndrome and its complications (18, 23). Finally, it is likely that perturbations on both the arterial and venous side of the circulation may act in concert to produce hemorrhage in certain infants (23).

Vascular factors that may predispose to germinal matrix injury include the tenuous capillary integrity and the vulnerability of the matrix capillaries to hypoxic-ischemic injury (9,24).

Extravascular factors that may predispose to injury include the gelatinous supporting matrix (9), an excessive amount of fibrinolytic activity which has been described in the germinal matrix region (25), and a postnatal decrease in tissue pressure commonly observed in the early postnatal period which would lead to an increased pressure gradient across the vessel wall and the potential for capillary rupture (26).

CLINICAL MANIFESTATIONS

Most infants who develop PV-IVH frequently *do not* exhibit overt clinical signs (27). Those infants with more extensive hemorrhage may exhibit a gradual deterioration over several hours characterized by irritability, increasing respiratory distress, occasional pulmonary hemorrhage, increasing respiratory, and/or metabolic acidosis and hyperglycemia. A very small percent of infants exhibit a catastrophic deterioration characterized by acute apnea, hypotonia, and brainstem dysfunction seizures. There is usually an associated bulging fontanel and a fall in hematocrit.

DIAGNOSIS

Real-time cranial ultrasonography is the procedure of choice in the diagnosis of PV-IVH. Ultrasonography is effective in the identification of all degrees of severity of the lesion. The optimal timing of ultrasonography relates to the time of occurrence of PV-IVH. Since approximately 90% of hemorrhage occur by the third day (27,28), the first scan should be performed within this time period in the high-risk infant. Because 20–40% of lesions progress following initial identification, or a small percentage of infants develop IVH beyond the third postnatal day, a second scan should be performed towards the end of the first postnatal week.

Severity of PV-IVH

Cranial ultrasonography has provided a convenient method of defining the severity of PV-IVH. This is of particular relevance since outcome is related to severity of the bleed. The grading sonographic system we use to assess PV-IVH is based on the presence of blood in the germinal matrix and the amount of blood in the lateral ventricles (22,29) (Table 1).

PROGNOSIS

Prognosis can be considered in terms of short-term outcome (i.e., mortality) and the development of posthemorrhagic hydrocephalic (PHH) and long-term outcome (i.e., neurodevelopmental sequelae).

Short-Term Outcome

Mortality. PV-IVH still contributes significantly to the mortality of the very-low-birthweight infant (22,29). However, in recent years, it is the very-low-birthweight infant (i.e., <750 g) that is most vulnerable to large hemorrhage and death.

Table 1. Grading of severity of PV-IVH by cranial ultrasound scan

Grade I:	Germinal matrix blood only
Grade II:	Intraventricular blood (filling <50% of the lateral ventricular area on parasagittal view)
Grade III:	Intraventricular blood (filling >50% of the lateral ventricular area on parasagittal view, the ventricular system is usually dilated)
IPE[a]:	Periventricular echodensity (indicate location and size)

[a]IPE is often referred to as a Grade IV IVH by others.

Hydrocephalus. Posthemorrhagic hydrocephalus complicates approximately 40–50% of cases of severe IVH (30). The evolution of hydrocephalus may be rapid (i.e., days), and in such cases it is usually associated with an elevation in intracranial pressure. Obstruction appears to be secondary to an impairment of cerebrospinal fluid absorption caused by particulate clot usually demonstrated by ultrasound scan. More commonly, a communicating hydrocephalus evolves at 1–4 weeks following the diagnosis of hemorrhage. The hydrocephalus is commonly secondary to an obliterative arachnoiditis in the posterior fossa distal to the outflow of the fourth ventricle. Approximately half the cases of communicating hydrocephalus will resolve spontaneously over the first month. In the remaining infants there is progressive hydrocephalus which may occur in the presence or absence of raised intracranial pressure (31). For those infants who demonstrate progressive increase in ventricular size, therapeutic interventions will depend on the size of the infant, the amount of blood in the ventricles, and the intracranial pressure. Temporizing diversion techniques to control ventricular size include external ventricular drain, serial lumbar punctures, and the use of drugs, namely, acetazolamide and isosorbide (32–35). The prognosis with PHH to a large extent depends on the presence and extent of associated intraparenchymal involvement (33).

Long-Term Outcome

The most critical determinant of long-term neurologic outcome is the degree of parenchymal injury. The size and location of the parenchymal lesion is critical with regard to outcome. Thus, when the IPE is >1cm in diameter and is extensive (i.e., involves frontal–parietal–occipital regions), the mortality is highest (80%) and long-term outcome is universally poor (4,29) (Figure 2). With a smaller lesion (i.e., <1 cm)

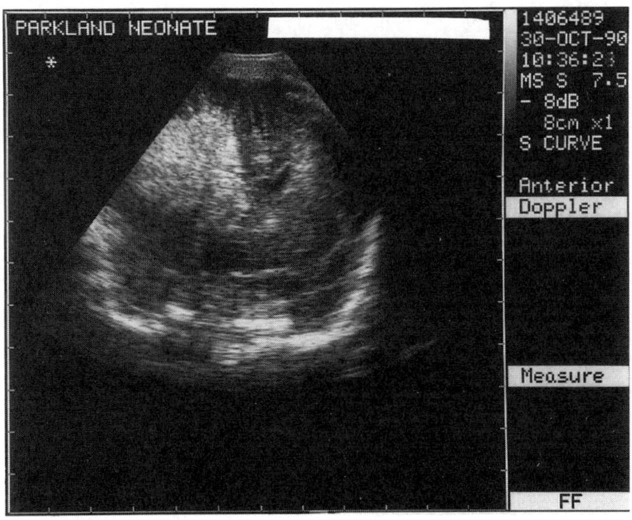

Figure 2. Cranial ultrasound scan: coronal section of brain demonstrating intraventricular blood with dilitation of the lateral ventricle and an associated large right intraparenchymal echodensity.

and localized (i.e., to either frontal, parietal, or occipital regions), the outcome is likely to be more favorable (Figure 3). However, almost two-thirds of such infants will still have an abnormal outcome (4,29).

Prevention. Prevention of PV-IVH is complex and a full discussion is beyond the scope of this presentation. A brief overview is presented below (Table 2).

Prenatal Interventions

GENERAL. Attempts at prevention have focused on (a) identification of women at high risk for premature labor, (b) early detection of premature labor, and (c) early treatment of premature labor with medications (e.g., tocolytic agents). Some of the therapies (i.e., tocolytic agents) have been associated with an increase in PV-IVH (36).

PHARMACOLOGICAL INTERVENTIONS. Several interventions have been evaluated and are briefly reviewed below.

Glucocorticoids. The findings from several studies indicate a significant reduction in the incidence of all PV-IVH as well as the severe form of hemorrhage in preterm infants of mothers administered glucocorticoids (37,40) (Table 3). This is of particular relevance in the smallest of the premature infants (i.e., <750 g). The mechanism(s) of protective action are not clear but may relate to improved respiratory function, more stable blood pressure, and/or a direct effect on germinal matrix maturation (37–39).

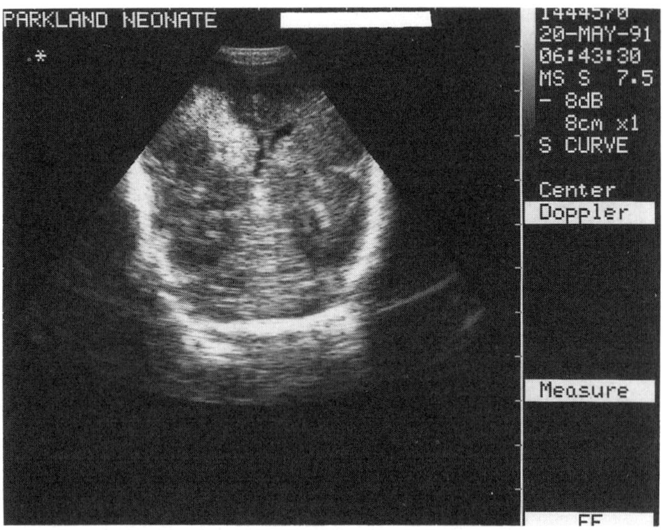

Figure 3. Cranial ultrasound scan: coronal section of brain demonstrating intraventricular hemorrhage and a small right intraparenchymal echodensity.

Table 2. Possible strategies in the prevention of periventricular–intraventricular hemorrhage

Prenatal Interventions	Postnatal Interventions
1. Prevention of premature birth	1. Correction or prevention of major hemodynamic disturbances (e.g., fluctuations in cerebral blood flow)
2. Pharmacologic interventions Glucocorticoids Phenobarbital Vitamin K	2. Pharmacologic interventions Indomethacin Phenobarbital Vitamin E
3. Optimal management of labor and delivery	

Table 3. Antenatal steroid administration and incidence of periventricular–intraventricular hemorrhage (PV-IVH)

Reference	Grade of IVH	Dexamethasone	Placebo
37	1 + 2	9/33 (27%)	10/40 (25%)
	3 + 4	1/33 (3%)	9/40 (22.5%)[a]
38	1 + 2	12/57 (21%)	133/555 (24%)
	3 + 4	1/57 (1.8%)	31/133 (23%)
39	1 + 2	8/77 (10.4%)	18/63 (28.6%)[a]
	3 + 4		

[a]$P < 0.05$ Grade 4 is referred to as an intraparenchymal echodensity in the text.

Phenobarbital. Several randomized controlled studies in which mothers expected to deliver prematurely were administered antenatal phenobarbital suggested a potential benefit—i.e., a reduction in the incidence of PV-IVH as well as the severity of the lesions (41, 42). However, a recent large multicenter randomized study involving approximately 1200 infants failed to demonstrate a protective effect of antenatal phenobarbital therapy on the occurrence of PV-IVH (43).

Vitamin K. The role of vitamin K has also been evaluated in the prevention of PV-IVH. Some of the data suggest a protective role. However, methodological flaws and contradictory effects on the neonatal coagulation profiles hinder interpretation of the data (44,45).

Mode of Delivery. The relationship between PV-IVH and the mode of delivery remains unclear and controversial. Some studies suggest a link between the duration of labor and vaginal delivery and predisposition to hemorrhage, with a protective effect of cesarean section. Others have not found associations between mode of delivery and PV-IVH (46–49).

Postnatal Interventions

CORRECTION OR PREVENTION OF MAJOR HEMODYNAMIC DISTURBANCES. The invariable association between fluctuations in CBFV, subsequent PV-IVH in ventilated premature infants (17), and the demonstration that elimination of these fluctuations reduces the incidence of IVH (50) offers an opportunity to identify and treat a subset of high-risk infants. Since the fluctuations in the systemic and cerebral circulations appear to be related to the mechanics of respiration (51), potential methods of eliminating these fluctuations include optimizing ventilator support or reducing the infant's own respiratory effort with sedatives or paralysis (50). Interestingly, despite the introduction of surfactant replacement therapy to treat preterm infants with respiratory distress syndrome with improvement in respiratory function, the incidence of PV-IVH did not decrease in infants who received the medication compared to control infants (52).

POSTNATAL PHARMACOLOGICAL INTERVENTIONS. A number of interventions have been evaluated in an effort to prevent PV-IVH during the postnatal period. Each is briefly reviewed below.

Phenobarbital. Phenobarbital has been evaluated in several studies as a method of preventing PV-IVH. The proposed *mechanism* of *action* is via dampening of spikes in arterial blood pressure. Initial studies suggested a protective effect (53,54), however, in the largest study, Kuban et al. (55) demonstrated a significantly higher occurrence of all grades of PV-IVH (i.e., 35% versus 19%) as well as of the severe form of the disease (i.e., 13% versus 6%) in phenobarbital versus control infants, respectively ($P < 0.01$) (55).

Indomethacin. Indomethacin has also been evaluated in multiple controlled studies in the treatment of PV-IVH (56–59). The proposed *mechanism* of *action* is via a decrease in baseline CBF as well as attenuation of cerebral hyperemia-induced by asphyxia (60). The cumulative data suggest that the administration of indomethacin therapy on the first day of life reduces the risk of subsequent severe PV-IVH (see Table 4). Current

Table 4. Postnatal indomethacin administration and incidence of periventricular–intraventricular hemorrhage (PV-IVH)[a]

Grade of PV-IVH	Indomethacin ($n = 209$)	Placebo ($n = 220$)
No IVH	184 (88%)	182 (83%)
1	7(3%)	13 (5.9%)
2	15 (7%)	16 (7.3%)
3	2 (1%)	1 (0.5%)
4[b]	1 (0.5%)	10 (4.5%)[c]

[a]Adapted from reference 58.
[b]Grade 4 is referred as an IPE in the text.
[c]$P = 0.03$.

data suggest that the potential neuroprotective role for indomethacin in the prevention of PV-IVH may be greatest in the intubated preterm infant <1000-g birthweight.

Vitamin E. Several studies have evaluated the potential role of vitamin E in the prevention of PV-IVH. One potential mechanism of neuroprotection relates to the antioxidant and free radical scavenger role of vitamin E. No consistent protective effect of vitamin E has been demonstrated. In the largest study to date, a significant reduction in the incidence of PV-IVH was noted (61). However, in a second study, Phelps et al. (62) noted an increased incidence of PV-IVH in infants treated with vitamin E, especially those less than 1000 g, as compared to controls.

SUMMARY

Since the majority of preterm infants (70–75%) do not develop PV-IVH, the risk–benefit ratio of any intervention has to be considered with caution. Currently, there is no specific intervention that appears to consistently prevent PV-IVH. The antenatal use of glucocorticoids (where medically indicated) seems to offer the most promise. In the immediate postnatal period, identifying the infant at greatest risk for subsequently developing PV-IVH (i.e., the intubated infant <1000 g with respiratory distress syndrome requiring surfactant replacement therapy) is important. These infants may benefit from optimal respiratory management and be candidates for possible pharmacologic intervention; for example, as mentioned previously, the use of indomethacin appears to offer the most promise at the current time.

REFERENCES

1. Papillae LA, Burstein J, Burstein R, Koffler H. Incidence and evolution of subependymal and intraventricular hemorrhage: a study of infants with birth weights less than 1,500 gm. *J Pediatr* 1978;92:529–534.
2. Ahmann PA, Lazzara A, Dykes FD, Brann AW, Schwartz JF. Intraventricular hemorrhage in the high-risk preterm infant: incidence and outcome. *Ann Neurol* 1980;7:118–124.
3. Levene MI, Wiggelsworth JS, Dubowitz V. Cerebral structure and intraventricular hemorrhage in the neonate: a real-time ultrasound study. *Arch Dis Child* 1981;56:416.
4. McMenamin JM, Shackelford GD, Volpe JJ. Outcome of neonatal intraventricular hemorrhage periventricular echodense lesions. *Ann Neurol* 1984;15:285.
5. Perlman JM, Volpe JJ. Intraventricular hemorrhage in the extremely small premature infant. *Am J Dis Child* 1986;140:1122.
6. Philips AGS, Allen WC, Tito AM, Wheeler LR. Intraventricular hemorrhage in preterm infants: declining incidence in the 1980's. *Pediatrics* 1989;84:797.
7. Strand C, Laptook AR, Dowling S, et al. Neonatal intracranial hemorrhage. I. Changing pattern in inborn low birthweight infants. *Early Hum Dev* 1990;20:117.
8. DeReuck JL. Cerebral angioarchitecture and perinatal brain lesions in premature and full term infants. *Acta Neurol Scand* 1984;70:391.

9. Hambleton G, Wiggelsworth JS. Origin of intraventricular hemorrhage in the preterm infant. *Arch Dis Child* 1976;51:651.
10. Kuban KC, Gilles FH. Human Diencephalic angiogenesis. *Ann Neurol* 1985;17:539.
11. Larroche KC. *Development pathology of the neonate.* New York: Excerpta Medica, 1977.
12. Goddard-Finegold J, Armstrong D, Zeller RS. Intraventricular hemorrhage following volume expansion after hypovolemic hypotension in the new born beagle. *J Pediatr* 1982;100:796.
13. Kent LR, Stewart WB, Duncan CC, Lambrecht R. Beagle puppy model of interventricular hemorrhage. *J Neurosurg* 1982;57:219.
14. Lou HC, Lassen NA, Friis-Hansen B. Is arterial hypertension crucial for the development of cerebral hemorrhage in premature infants? *Lancet* 1979;1:215.
15. Lou CH, Lassen NA, Friis-Hansen B. Impaired autoregulation of cerebral blood flow in the distressed newborn infant. *J Pediatr* 1979;94:118.
16. Pryds O, Griesen G, Lou H, Friis-Hansen B. Heterogeneity of cerebral vasoreactivity in preterm infants supported by mechanical ventilation. *J Pediatr* 1989;115:638.
17. Perlman JM, McMenamin JB, Volpe JJ. Fluctuating cerebral blood flow velocity in respiratory distress syndrome. Relation to the development of intraventricular hemorrhage. *N Engl J Med* 1983;309:204.
18. Hill A, Perlman JM, Volpe JJ. Relationship of pneumothorax to the occurrence of intraventricular hemorrhage in the premature newborn. *Pediatrics* 1982;69:144.
19. Perlman JM, Volpe JJ. Suctioning in the preterm infant: effects on cerebral blood flow velocity, intracranial pressure and arterial blood pressure. *Pediatrics* 1983;72:329.
20. Goldberg RN, Chung D, Goldman SL, Bancalari E. The associations of rapid volume expansion and intraventricular hemorrhage in the preterm infant. *J Pediatr* 1980;96:1060.
21. Omar SY, Griesen G, lbrahim MM, et al. Blood pressure responses to care procedures in ventilated preterm infants. *Acta Pediatr Scand* 1985;74:920.
22. Perlman JM, Rollins N, Bums D, Risser R. Relationship between periventricular intraparenchymal echodensities and germinal matrix–intraventricular hemorrhage in the very low birth weight infant. *Pediatrics* 1993;91:474.
23. Perlman JM, Volpe JJ. Are venus circulatory changes important in the photogenesis of hemorrhagic and/or ischemic cerebral injury? *Pediatrics* 1987;80:705.
24. Takashima S, Tanaka K. Microangiography and vascular permeability of the subependymal germinal matrix in the premature infant. *Can J Neurol Sci* 1978;5:45.
25. Takashima S, Tanaka K. Microangiography and fibrinolytic activity in subependymal matrix of the premature brain. *Brain Dev* 1972;4:222.
26. Conner ES, Lorenzo AV, Welch K, Dorval B. The role of intracranial hypotension in neonatal intraventricular hemorrhage. *J Neurosurg* 1983;58:204.
27. Perlman JM, Volpe JJ. Cerebral blood flow velocity in relation to intraventricular hemorrhage in the premature infant. *J Pediatr* 1982;100:956.
28. Paneth N, Pinto Martin J, Gardiner J, Wallenstein S, Katsikiosis V, Hegyi T, Hiatt IM, Susser M. Incidence and timing of germinal matrix-intraventricular hemorrhage in low birth weight infants. *Am J Epidemiol* 1993;137:1167.
29. Guzzetta F, Shackelford GD, Volpe S, Perlman JM, Volpe JJ. Periventricular intraparenchymal echodensities in the premature infant: critical determinant of neurologic outcome. *Pediatrics* 1986;78:945.

30. Volpe J. *Neurology of the newborn,* 3rd ed. Philadelphia: WB Saunders, 1995.
31. Hill A, Volpe JJ. Normal pressure hydrocephalus in the newborn. *Pediatrics* 1981;68:623.
32. Dykes FD, Dunbar B, Lazarra A, Ahmann PA. Posthemorrhagic hydrocephalus in high risk preterm infants: Natural history, management and longterm outcome. *J Pediatr* 1989;114:611.
33. Kreusser KL, Tarby TJ, Kovnar E, Taylor DA, Hill A, Volpe JJ. Serial lumbar puncture for at least temporary amelioration of neonatal posthemorrhagic hydrocephalus. *Pediatrics* 1985:75:719.
34. Ventriculomegaly Trial Group. Randomized trial of early tapping in neonatal posthemorrhagic ventricular dilation. *Arch Dis Child* 1990;114:611.
35. Shinnar S, Gammon K, Bergman EW, et al. Management of hydrocephalus in infancy: use of acetazolamide and furosemide to avoid cerebrospinal fluid shunts. *J Pediatr* 1985; 107:31.
36. Groome LJ, Goldenberg RL, Cliver SP, Davis RO, Copper RN. Neonatal periventricular–intraventricular hemorrhage after maternal B-symothamniotic tocolysis. *Am J Obstet Gynecol* 1992;167:837–879.
37. Garite TJ, Rumney PJ, Briggs GC, et al. A randomized placebo controlled trial of betamethasone for the prevention of respiratory distress syndrome at 24–28 weeks gestation. *Am J Obstet Gynecol* 1992;166:646.
38. Jobe AN, Mitchell BR, Gunkel JH. Beneficial effects of combined use of prenatal steroids and postnatal surfactant on preterm infants. *Am J Obstet Gynecol* 1993;168:508–513.
39. Kari MA, Hallman M, Gronen M, Teramo K, Virtanen M, Koivisto M, Ikomen RS. Prenatal Dexamethasone treatment in conjunction with rescue therapy of human surfactant: a randomized placebo-controlled multicenter study. *Pediatrics* 1994;93:730.
40. Crowley P, Chalmers I, Keirse MJNC. The effects of corticosteroid administration before preterm delivery: an overview of the evidence from clinical trials. *Br J Obstet Gynecol* 1990;97:11.
41. Shankaran S, Cepeda EE, Ilagan N, et al. Antenatal phenobarbital for the prevention of neonatal intracerebral hemorrhage. *Am J Obstet Gynecol* 1986;154:53.
42. Morales WJ, Koerton J. Prevention of intraventricular hemorrhage in very low birth weight infants by maternally administered phenobarbital. *Obstet Gynecol* 1986;68:295.
43. Shankaran S, Papile LA, Wright LL, Ehrenkrantz RA, Mele L, et al. The effect of antenatal phenobarbital on neonatal intracranial hemorrhage in preterm infants. *N Engl J Med* 1997;337:466–471.
44. Pomerance JJ, Teal JG, Gogolok JF, et al. Maternally administered antenatal vitamin K: effect on neonatal prothrombin activity, partial prothrombin time and intraventricular hemorrhage. *Obstet Gynecol* 1987;70:235.
45. Kazzi N, Llagan NB, Liang KC, et al. Maternal administration of vitamin K does not improve the coagulation profile of preterm infants. *Pediatrics* 1989;84:1045.
46. Leviton A, Pagano M, Kuban KCK, et al. The epidemiology of germinal matrix hemorrhage during the first half of life. *Dev Med Child Neurol* 1988;33:138.
47. Anderson GD, Bada HS, Shaver BM, et al. The effect of cesarean section on intraventricular hemorrhage in the premature infant. *Am J Obstet Gynecol* 1992;166:1091.
48. Thornburn RJ, Lipscomb AP, Stewart AL, Reynolds EOR, Hope DL. Timing and antecedents of periventricular hemorrhage and of cerebral atrophy in very preterm neonatals. *Early Hum Devel* 1982;151:1022.

49. Strauss A, Kirz D, Mandalou HD, Freeman RK. Perinatal events and intraventricular/ependymal hemorrhage in the very low birth weight infant. *Am J Obstet Gynecol* 1985; 151:1022.

50. Perlman JM, Goodman S, Kreusser KL, Volpe JJ. Reduction of intraventricular hemorrhage by elimination of fluctuating cerebral blood flow velocity in preterm infants with respiratory distress syndrome. *N Engl J Med* 1985;312:1353.

51. Perlman JM, Thack BT. Respiratory origin of fluctuations in arterial blood pressure in premature infants with respiratory distress syndrome. *Pediatrics* 1988;81:399.

52. Jobe AH. Pulmonary surfactant therapy. *N Engl J Med* 1993;328:861–868.

53. Donn S, Roloff DW, Goldstein GW. Prevention of intraventricular hemorrhage in preterm infants by phenobarbitone: a controlled trial. *Lancet* 1981;ii:215.

54. Bedard MP, Shankovan S, Slovis TL, et al. Effect of prophylactic phenobarbital on intraventricular hemorrhage in high risk infants. *Pediatrics* 1984;73:435.

55. Kuban KC, Leviton A, Krishna Moorthy KS, et al. Neonatal intracranial hemorrhage and phenobarbital. *Pediatrics* 1986;77:443.

56. Hanigan WC, Kennedy G, Roemisch F, et al. Administration of indomethacin for prevention of periventricular–intraventricular hemorrhage in high risk infants. *Pediatrics* 1988; 112:931.

57. Bandstra ES, Montalvo BM, Goldberg RN, et al. Prophylactic indomethacin for prevention of intraventricular hemorrhage in premature infants. *Pediatrics* 1988;82:533.

58. Bada HS, Green RS, Pour CY, Rous M, et al. Indomethacin reduces the risk of severe intraventricular hemorrhage. *J Pediatr* 1989;115:631.

59. Ment LR, OH W, Ehrenkranz RA, Philip AGS, et al. Low-dose indomethacin and prevention of intraventricular hemorrhage: a multicenter randomized trial. *Pediatrics* 1994; 94:543.

60. Ment LR, Stewart WB, Duncan CC, et a1. Beagle puppy model of intraventricular hemorrhage; randomized indomethacin trial. *Neurology* 1983;33:179.

61. Sinha S, Davis J, Tonger N, et al. Vitamin E supplementation reduces frequency of periventricular hemorrhage in very preterm infants. *Lancet* 1987;11:466.

62. Phelps DL, Rosenbaum AL, Isenberg J, et al. Tocopherol efficacy and safety for preventing retinopathy of prematurity: a randomized, control double marked masked trial. *Pediatrics* 1987;79:489.

12

FETAL NEUROSONOGRAPHY

Ilan E. Timor-Tritsch, M.D. and Ana Monteagudo, M.D.
Department of Obstetrics and Gynecology, Division of Maternal-Fetal Medicine, New York University Medical Center, New York, New York

INTRODUCTION

Fetal central nervous system malformations are extremely common and rank among the first three in terms of their occurrence considering all fetal anomalies. It is therefore important to scan the CNS extensively, since if such malformations occur, many can be detected as early as 10–11 postmenstrual weeks. To recognize a normal or malformed development of the fetal brain, one has to first be acquainted with the sonographic anatomy as well as with the development of the normal prenatal brain.

Due to the fact that during prenatal life the fetal brain is still in constant development, normal neuroanatomy is different at various gestational ages. The continuous development of certain structures and the time when these achieve the adult appearance should be understood and taken into consideration each time their sonographic examination is undertaken.

Asphyxia and Fetal Brain Damage, Edited by Dev Maulik, M.D., Ph.D.
ISBN 0-471-18427-6

Since the introduction of ultrasound in medicine, it became possible to image the fetal brain using noninvasive technique. With its constant improvement, routine as well as targeted examination of the prenatal brain has become feasible. Soon the more detailed neurosonography may become an integral part of the evaluation of the entire fetal body.

In this chapter, we will not only elaborate on the equipment for the use of fetal neuroscans, but also describe the technique and the concept of how fetal neurosonography should be performed. A special emphasis will be placed upon explaining the importance of emulating the planes used in neonatal neuroscans in order to compare the fetal scans with those performed postnatally and be able to communicate with a pediatric neurologist and neurosurgeon in case of necessity. In the last part of the chapter, the sonographically detectable anomalies of the fetal brain will be discussed.

EQUIPMENT

In spite of the recent and continuous development of ultrasound equipment and more precisely the available transducers, the fetal neuroscan is limited by several physical factors. Among these are the size of the fetal brain (i.e., the gestational age), the available surface or the window through which the transducer can achieve the best image, the fetal presentation and position, and, last but not least, the thickness of the maternal abdominal wall. If all this is understood, it is clear that a variety of transducers with different frequencies and frequency ranges can and should be used and alternated in order to obtain the best images. Since imaging of the fetal brain ultimately depends on the penetration of the sound wave as well as the acoustic impedance of the tissues, it is understood that the gestational age (i.e., the thickening of the fetal skull) with its increasing acoustic impedance will determine in a significant way the types of ultrasound probes employed during the examination. The basic two kinds of ultrasound probes used are the transabdominal and the transvaginal ultrasound probes. In general, the transabdominal probes use lower and the transvaginal probes use higher ultrasound frequencies. During the first half of the pregnancy, high-frequency transvaginal probes can be used. The reasons for this are as follows: At this gestation the fetal skull bones are relatively thin and contain less deposited calcium, and the entire body of the relatively small fetus is closer to the vaginal fornix—that is, the tip of the transvaginal probe. Therefore, it sounds logical that this time is favorable to use higher-frequency probes. This is the reason that almost regardless of fetal position and presentation, the transvaginal probe is the "first line" transducer probe to be employed. If the fetus continues to present with the vertex, there is absolutely no need to relinquish the transvaginal approach. This issue will be discussed later during the chapter. However, if the fetal head cannot be "reached" using the transvaginal route, transabdominal probes will have to be used. The transvaginal ultrasound probes operate typically at frequencies of 5–9 MHz, whereas the transabdominal probes will operate at frequencies of 3.5 to a maximum of 7 MHz. The higher the gestational age, the lower the frequencies to be used in order to penetrate the skull bones, which now have significant amounts of deposited calcium presenting an acoustic impedance seven times that of the water or soft tissues of the fetal body. It should be remembered that even at the very end of the pregnancy, the fetal brain can adequately be imaged through the fontanelle using the transvaginal ultrasound probe, provided that the fetus presents as vertex. At times, we found it valuable to perform external cephalic version in order to better be able to study a suspected anomaly.

CONCEPT AND TECHNIQUE OF FETAL NEUROSONOGRAPHY

The classical planes or coordinates used in imaging of the fetal brain are those used for imaging of other parts of the body, namely, the sagittal, coronal (frontal), and horizontal (axial) planes (Figure 1). The vertical planes are either coronal or sagittal. Only one of the sagittal planes is the median plane. There are, of course, a large number of coronal and sagittal planes, but there is only one median plane. As far as fetal neurosonography is concerned, the coronal and sagittal planes are reached through the anterior fontanelle in the fetus presenting with vertex. Several sections through each plane can be generated. The horizontal (axial) planes are classically achieved by

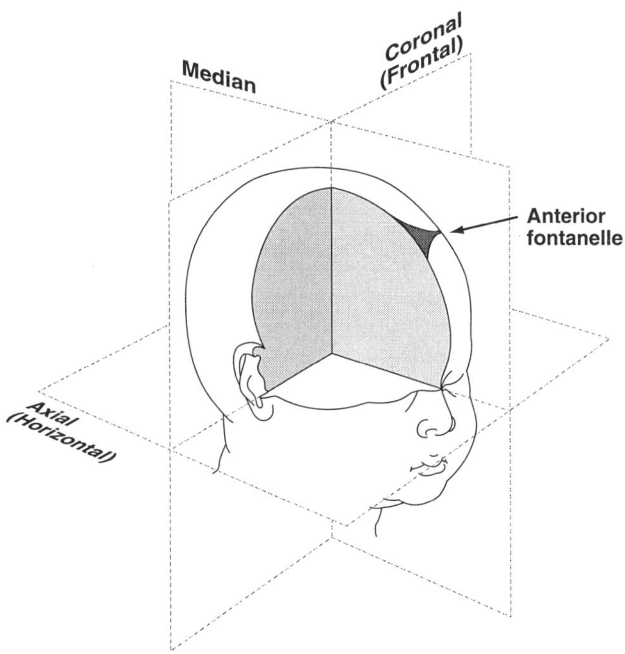

Figure 1. The three classical planes used in imaging the head: axial or horizontal, coronal or frontal, and sagittal. In the sagittal plane, one median and several other paramedian sections are possible.

transabdominal scanning. Transabdominal scanning traditionally uses the thinner temporal bone or temporal fontanelle. However, as pregnancy advances, this becomes less and less favorable. Transvaginal scanning through the anterior fontanelle yields the median and paramedian as well as different coronal and oblique sections, similar to that of the neonatal brain scanning. The tremendous advantage of the transvaginal scanning of the prenatal brain is that the obtained scanning planes are identical, and therefore readily comparable, to those performed in the neonate. The most frequent consultants to the perinatologist in the event of fetal brain malformations are the pediatric neurosurgeons and neurologists. By presenting them with scans that are similar to those used by them, an immediate understanding of the location, extent, and identity of the lesion is obtained.

In addition to the concept of mastering the different anatomical planes used in scanning the fetal brain, a second concept becomes important. This notion is linked to the ability to correctly identify the plane through which the scanning was obtained. This can be facilitated by the knowledge of the orientation, shape, and the anatomy of the ventricular system. As known, the ventricular system is filled with cerebrospinal fluid (CSF), which, of course, on the ultrasound images appears as a sonolucent structure. In the future, three-dimensional ultrasound capabilities may enable us to obtain successive planes or a "sweep" of the sonographic appearance of the brain, stored as a "spacial volume scan." This in turn will enable the user to not only recreate the classical axial, sagittal, and coronal planes, but also obtain other "custom-selected" planes to highlight anatomy and pathology to compare it with any "nonclassical" section of the brain.

At times, when pathology is encountered, it takes some time to recognize its exact nature and location, unless the previously mentioned and compulsively used steps in obtaining the proposed sections are applied. In conclusion, it is important to mentally recreate a three-dimensional picture of the fetal brain. This has to be based upon the planes and the knowledge of the anatomy of normal ventricular system used as points of reference for most of the pictures obtained in different scanning planes.

One can use another, but somewhat more sophisticated, method to identify structures or neuropathology, namely, the study of the arterial and venus network of the fetal brain. These can be studied by the different kinds of color flow studies; however, these in turn require the exact knowledge of the anatomy of these vessels.

As far as the *scanning technique* is concerned, the transabdominal route is well known and employed in all centers and by all the sonographers and sonologists; therefore, we will refrain from describing this technique.

We will, however, place a somewhat larger emphasis on detailing the transvaginal sonographic examination of the brain, which is slowly gaining its deserved place among the scanning options for the fetus. Classically, the transvaginal scan of the fetal brain relies heavily upon the experience gained from the transfontanelle examination of the neonatal brain (1–9). The use of transvaginal sonography in imaging the fetal brain traditionally uses high-frequency ultrasound probes (10–26).

The technique of transvaginal neuroscanning is simple (16,20,22–24). The probe is prepared as usual for transvaginal scanning: Its tip is covered with a clean condom or placed inside a digit of a surgical rubber glove. Recently, specially manufactured pre-gelled vinyl covers have been made available. The patient is then placed in the lithotomy position, and the tip of the probe is slowly advanced to reach the anterior cervical lip. Usually, it is easier to perform fetal neuroscan when the patient's bladder is empty in order to enable the presenting part (i.e., the vertex) to come closer to the tip of the probe. At times, it is necessary to use the abdominal hand to maneuver the head into the most convenient position. The objective is to place the "footprint" of the vaginal probe opposite the anterior fontanelle. By twisting and turning as well as tilting the vaginal probe, the best possible images in each of the coronal and sagittal planes are sought. The abdominally placed second hand of the operator has an important task: stabilizing the fetal head or maneuvering it into the desired position for a clear ultrasound picture.

It is of importance that the machine with which we perform transvaginal fetal brain scanning should have an "end-firing" transducer. This means that there will be a symmetrical picture on both sides of the scanning axis; in other words, the scanning axis and the straight axis of the probe are identical. Use of a non-endfiring out-of-axis vaginal probe makes a perfectly symmetrical imaging of the brain in the coronal planes extremely cumbersome, since the probe itself has to be constantly twisted and tilted into a position to yield the desired symmetrical ultrasound picture.

SCANNING PLANES UNIQUE TO FETAL NEUROSONOGRAPHY

Dependent upon whether transabdominal or transvaginal sonography is used, the sections and the planes will yield different information if fetuses of extremely young ages (i.e., dates to approximately 11 weeks or more mature fetuses) are scanned. The latter is due to the fact that the head follows well-defined and continuing deflection from seven to approximately 11–12 weeks. Scanning the brain before the 12th postmenstrual week is dependent upon the size of the fetus and the resolution of the ultrasound probe. Both of the above determine the "slice thickness" and, hence, the number of sections and the quality of the picture obtained. Scanning at or around 7–8 postmenstrual weeks, one should expect that the only possible "slice thickness" includes almost the entire width of the head, due to the relatively thick imaging slice. At and after the 9th postmenstrual week, due to the somewhat larger headsize, it is possible to obtain several diagnostic quality "slices"—that is, sections. The clear and pretty pictures obtained by Blaas et al. (18,19), who studied the brain structures with extremely high frequency transvaginal probes from 7 to 9 weeks, attest to the feasibility and the importance of fine and resolution-rich "slices." Using such techniques, they were able to show that structures previously described only in embryological studies were readily recognized and imaged. As knowledge as well as the quality of the ultrasound equipment improves in the future, it may be possible to detect deviant development as early as the normal anatomy of the brain is available for sonographic scrutiny.

As pregnancy progresses and reaches 12–13 postmenstrual weeks, the thickening skull bones will progressively attenuate the sound waves, and special approaches as well as lower transducer frequencies are necessary to successfully image the brain. As said before, due to fetal position, the transabdominal sonography is mainly used to achieve the classical axial/horizontal planes. These sections are extremely important since the measurements, which constitute the "gold standard" for determining the size of the lateral ventricles, are performed using these sections. However, if the fetal position enables the transvaginal approach, pictures of extreme resolution and clarity can be obtained. Imaging of the brain structures with high-frequency transvaginal probes is usually done through the anterior fontanelle as an acoustic window. It is very rare to obtain axial or horizontal sections using the transvaginal probe. This may be achieved only if the fetal head is not engaged and is readily movable. Usually and classically, the transvaginal probes will achieve coronal and sagittal planes due to their restricted maneuverability and range of motion determined by the constraints of the introitus and the vagina. It is therefore virtually impossible to obtain *classical* coronal and sagittal sections as used in our anatomic sections by computer tomography or magnetic resonance imaging where the consecutive sections are parallel to each other. Luckily, however, the planes or sections obtained by the transvaginal approach are not only similar but identical to those obtained by the neonatal transfontanelle imaging of the fetal brain (3,4,8,27,28). The similarities between the fetal and the neonatal scanning planes and sections have a practical advantage when prenatal and neonatal brain images have to be compared or a serial follow-up of pathology is compared.

We attempted to standardize the planes and sections obtained by transvaginal fetal neurosonography by anatomic landmarks and by adapting a new nomenclature taking into consideration the fact that the transfontanelle approach is unable to create all the desired classical and parallel to each other anatomic sections. The first premise therefore, using this approach, is the fact that the planes generated are not parallel with each other, and therefore they do not comply with the definitions of the classical planes imaging of the fetal head. In order to be able to realize this, the following paragraph will describe the classical planes with their definitions borrowed from the *Nomina Anatomica* (29).

The *classical planes* consist of two vertical (sagittal and coronal) and one horizontal (axial) planes (Figure 1). In the coronal plane, all sections from the back of the head (occipital) to the anterior pole of the head (frontal) are parallel to each other. The coronal planes can also be called frontal planes. In the sagittal plane, there are differences in the terminology of the specific planes. The "midsagittal" plane is called the median; on each of the two sides of the median, there are right and left paramedian planes. These can be multiple. The term "parasagittal" is incorrect.

The planes described by us using the transvaginal probe diverge in a fan-shaped fashion from a central point which is at the anterior fontanelle. It is therefore incorrect to talk about sagittal planes and coronal planes in the classical sense. Only one section is in the "classical" coronal plane, and only one section is in the "classical" sagittal plane; the rest are really oblique planes. For better understanding and more realistic description, a new nomenclature was therefore proposed (24). To define each of these newly proposed sections, landmark anatomic structures were selected. The combination of the specific landmark structures define every plane.

The landmark structures proposed were: (1) the orbit; (2) the meninges, the falx, and the tentorium cerebelli; (3) ventricles and their connections: the lateral, third, and fourth ventricles, the interhemispheric foramina, the choroid plexus, and the tela choroidea; (4) mid-brain structures such as the corpus callosum, the head of the caudate nucleus, the cavum septi pellucidi and the thalami; (5) infratentorial structures: the cerebellar hemispheres, the vermis, and the cerebellopeduncular cistern (cisterna magna).

The newly proposed planes are the following:

A. *The Coronal Planes* (Figure 2a). These are subdivided into three groups:

1. *The frontal group* consists of two sections: (a) *Frontal-1,* which is also termed "steerhead" configuration, in which the structures seen are the orbits and some facial structures. The homogeneous brain tissue without the tip of the anterior horn of the lateral ventricles is also depicted; however, if the scanning is performed before the sixteenth postmenstrual week, the tips of the anterial horns are still visible using this section. (b) *Frontal-2:* The structures seen are the orbits and the tip of the anterial horns as well as the falx.
2. *The middle group* consists of three sections: (a) *Coronal-1:* The structures seen are the lateral ventricles, the body of the lateral ventricles, the cavum septi pellucidi, corpus callosum, and the head of the caudate nucleus. (b) *Mid-coronal-2:* The structures seen are the lateral ventricles with the choroid plexus entering into the third ventricle through the foramina interventricularis (Monro); the corpus callosum; and the thalamus. (c) *Mid-coronal-3:* The structures seen are the lateral ventricles (atrium) with their choroid plexus; the corpus callosum; and the thalamus.
3. *The occipital group* has two subgroups: (a) *Occipital-1:* The structures seen are the lateral ventricles (posterior horns), cerebellar hemispheres, the vermis, and at times the fourth ventricle. (b) *Occipital-2:* The structures seen are the cerebellar hemispheres, the cerebellar vermis, the tentorium, and the cisterna magna. At times, depending on the angle, the tips of the pointed posterior horns can still be detected.

B. *The Sagittal Planes* (Figure 2b). These are subdivided as follows:

1. *The Median* (previously termed "midsagittal"; as said before, only one median section is possible). The structures are: the entire corpus callosum (before the 18th to the 20th week, only parts of this can be seen); the cavum septi pellucidi; the head of the caudate nucleus; the thalamus; the tela choroidea; midbrain structures such as the corpora quadrigemina, the vermis, the tectum, and the cisterna magna; and the fourth ventricle.
2. *Right and left Oblique-1* (previously called "para-sagittal"). The structures are the anterior horn, atrium, and posterior horn of the lateral ventricles with a choroid plexus "hugging" the thalami. *Note:* The inferior horns should not be visible through these sections since they are lateral to them.
3. *Right and left Oblique-2.* The structures are mostly homogenous texture of the brain tissue with a V-shaped gaping lateral sulcus (the apex of the V-points towards the occiput). The upper arm of the V arises from the temporal lobe and is called parietal operculum. The lower arm of the V is the

temporal operculum. These two structures enclose between them an area called the insula. The insula is "buried" and disappears towards term into the depth through the two closing opercula.

We felt that we made only a very slight deviation from the rigid and classical "anatomic rule" and believe that the clinically applicable gain of this adjustment is well worth the slight bending of the classical rules. Once the meaning of the definitions is known and may be agreed upon, clinical applications may prove useful.

The importance of each of the proposed 10 sections has to be stressed. If the landmarks of each of these sections are known, possible pathology can easily be defined and localized. If, for instance, in the midtrimester, the *Frontal-1* section reveals the anterian horns and the *Occipital-2* shows the dilated posterior horn, one could with good reason suspect a dilatation of the lateral ventricles. In a normal brain none of these sections should contain the anterior and the posterior tips of the lateral ventricles. If, for

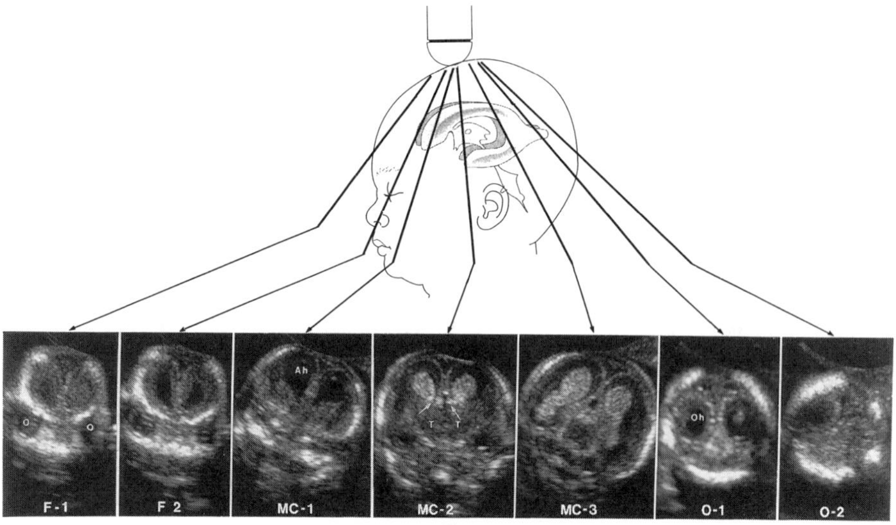

Figure 2. The fetal neuroscan performed with a high-frequency transvaginal probe emulating the neonatal brain scan. This serial scan depicts the brain of a fetus at 16 postmenstrual weeks. **(a)** In the coronal plane, the sections are: the Frontal-1 (F-1) and Frontal-2 (F-2), passing through the white matter and the orbits (O) revealing progressively the anterior horns; MidCoronal-1, -2, and -3 (MC 1–3), revealing the anterior horns (Ah), the antrum with the choroid plexus passing through the interventricular foramina (of Monro) into the third ventricle (*arrows*), the thalami (T), and the midbrain; Occipital-1 and -2 (O-1 and -2) on which the occipital horns (Oh), the tentorium, and the cerebellum with the cisterna magna are seen. **(b)** In the sagittal plane, the sections are as follows: The Median (M) shows that the median surfaces of the hemispheres are still devoid of sulci and gyri. Only the anterior portion (genu) of the corpus callosum is formed (G) with the appropriately small cavum septi pellucidi. Some of the midbrain structures are present. Oblique-1 (Obl-1) depicts the still relatively large anterior horns, the choroid plexus (CP) within the posterior horns, and the thalamus (T). The Oblique-2 (Obl-2) is the most lateral section showing the insular (I) and the closing parietal and temporal opercula (PO and TO).

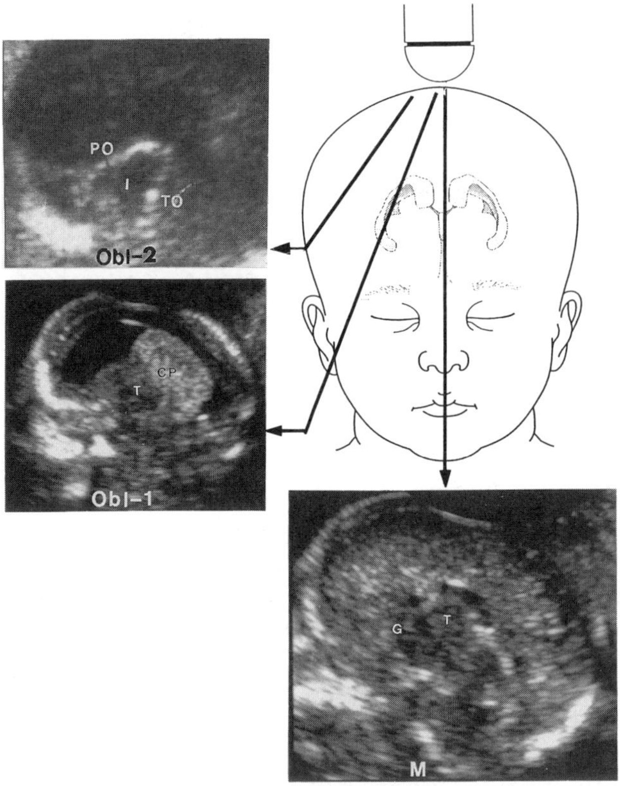

Figure 2. b. *continued*

example, an arachnoid cyst is suspected, this can be precisely localized by the use of all the described sections. If, on the Oblique-1 section, all three horns of the lateral ventricles are seen, dilatation of the lateral ventricles can be diagnosed with great certainty. The different parts of the corpus callosum and their integrity can be followed on the frontal two Midcoronal-1 and -2 as well as -3 sections. One could cite several other examples; however, we are sure that those listed make the necessary point.

We are convinced that because of the systematic way of imaging the fetal brain and because of its simplicity as well as the logic behind it, this method of describing the fetal brain scanned by transvaginal sonography has the potential to become generally accepted as a scanning method. Once again, we have to stress the fact that it emulates the neonatal scanning; therefore the pediatric neurologists and neurosurgeons may be the first to understand its usefulness.

THE DEVELOPING BRAIN AT 6–16 POSTMENSTRUAL WEEKS

Using present ultrasound technology, the first sonolucencies detected within the developing head of the embryo is around the seventh postmenstrual week. At this time, the size of the embryo is about 7–8 mm. The coronal scan of the dorsal aspect of the embryo can yield parallel lines of hyperechoic dots representing the future vertebral column. Blaas et al. (18,19) described in detail the cerebral hemispheres in their development using high-frequency transvaginal ultrasound probes. Starting shortly after the seventh postmenstrual week, the high-frequency transducers can discern between the relatively large rhombencephalon, the diencephalon, and the two tiny cerebral hemispheres. At 8 weeks and several days, the structures such as the cavities and the flexures of the brain appear clearer and better defined. Towards the ninth postmenstrual week and several days past it, several sagittal and coronal sections of the head can be obtained (Figure 3). These reveal the mesencephalon, the rhombencephalon, the budding choroid plexus, the telencephalic vesicles, and the two major flexures: the cephalic and the pontine flexures of the head around which the ventricles are arranged (30–32). Most clinically used ultrasound machines equipped with a transvaginal probe are able to depict these structures and, after 9 weeks, the tortuous string of the sonolucent ventricular system on coronal or axial sections of the fetal head. The falx will become detectable and present throughout the remainder of the pregnancy.

From around 10 postmenstrual weeks, several axial, sagittal, and coronal sections can be obtained; by doing this, we can mentally recreate a three-dimensional picture of the emerging and developing brain structures. At 11–12 postmenstrual weeks, the horizontal section is typical in its appearance since the larger structure (i.e., the symmetrically hyperechoic choroid plexus) is the most prominent structure. "Sand-

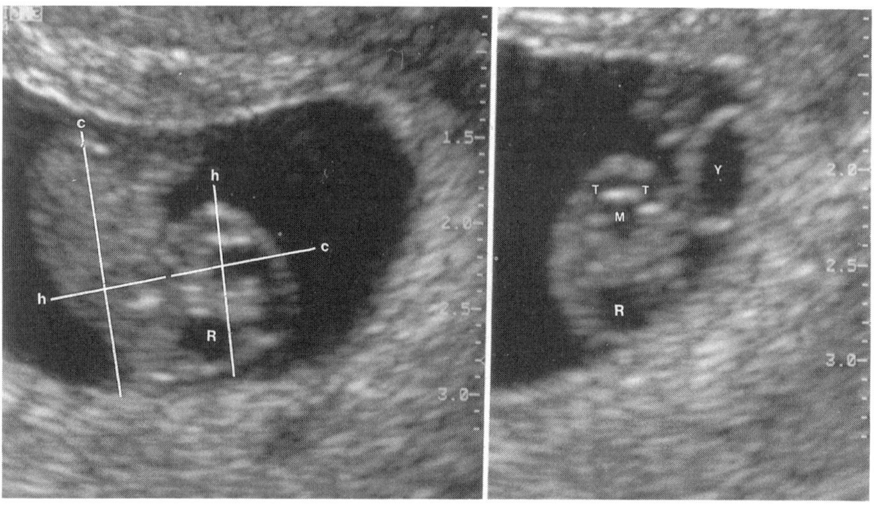

a b

Figure 3. Transvaginal sonogram of a fetus at 9 postmenstrual weeks. **a:** Median (sagittal section) demonstrating the sonolucent "string" of tortuous sonolucent ventricular system of the brain. The most prominent "ventricle" at this time is the rhombencephalon (R). Note that the head is extremely flexed; therefore if shifted towards the fetal body, a horizontal (axial) plane of the head becomes coronal and a coronal plane of the head will intersect the trunk in a horizontal (axial) fashion. **b:** A horizontal section of the fetal head demonstrating the rhombencephalon (R), mesencephalon (M), and telencephalic vesicles (T). Y, yolk sac.

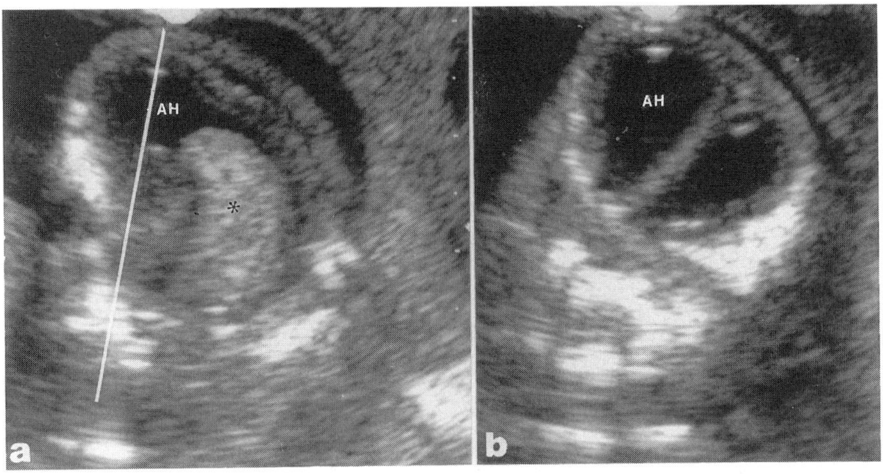

Figure 4. Appearances may be misleading! The relatively large size of the anterior horns of the lateral ventricles are demonstrated at 14 postmenstrual weeks. At this age, this is absolutely normal. **(a)** The paramedian section reveals the anterior horn (AH) and the choroid plexus (*). **(b)** A coronal scan along the white line in part **a** clearly reveals the bilateral and normal anterior horns (AH) at this gestational age. The relative size of the ventricles will decrease at the expense of the progressively thickening cortical mantle and white matter.

wiched" between the two thalami in the midline, the third ventricle appears as a slit-like sonolucent ovoid structure.

It is of practical importance to note that between 11 and 14 to almost 15 postmenstrual weeks, the tip of the anterior horn of the lateral ventricles are extremely prominent and appear as large sonolucent free spaces. This results from the continuous backward "migration" of the choroid plexus into their final position, namely the atria of the lateral ventricles. For a certain time of 2 (maybe 3) weeks, this gradual change leaves the anterior horns relatively large until there is a concomitant gradual increase in the thickness of the white matter and the cortex which slowly reverses the previously high ratio of the ventricle to hemisphere width, resulting in the later almost slit-like size of the anterior horns (Figure 4).

FETAL BRAIN AFTER 15 WEEKS

Around 14–16 postmenstrual weeks, the fetal skull bones grow and become increasingly thick, which in turn prevents the high-frequency sound waves from penetrating and imaging the fetal brain. This is the time to turn to the use of the anterior fontanelle as an acoustic window to be able to scan the fetal CNS. As said before, these sections generated through the anterior fontanelle radiate in a fan-like fashion with their apex originating at the fontanelle. It is possible to generate several sections in the sagittal as well as in the coronal planes.

The scanning planes which are unique to fetal neurosonography were detailed in our prior section. Figure 2A depicts sonographically identifiable anatomic landmarks in the coronal planes, while Figure 2B shows the anatomic landmarks seen by the transvaginal probe through the anterior fontanelle in the sagittal planes.

At times in the early second trimester, we may have the opportunity to scan the fetal head through an axial plane which reveals the classical structures such as the lateral ventricles, the cavum septi pellucidi, and at times the third ventricle. By slightly tilting the scanning plane anteriorly, the anterior horns are visible. The real value of the axial plane is that of interrogating the posterior fossa. This may be done by a slight posterior tilt of the scanning plane (Figure 5). If an "occipital approach" is used, the structures other than those in the posterior fossa may be somewhat blurred. Very important structures in the posterior fossa are: the tentorium, the dumbbell-shaped cerebellum with its hyperechoic cortex, the fourth ventricle, and the vermis, which appears in the midline and is always clearly hyperechoic. The cerebellopeduncular cistern (cisterna magna) is best imaged and measured through an "occipital approach," which also allows the measurement of the bicerebellar distance (Figure 6). The axial picture using the "temporal approach" is also useful for the measurement of the lateral ventricle-to-hemisphere width ratio, which by many is considered to be the gold standard to define ventriculomegaly (33–36).

It is well known that the relative size of the lateral ventricular width decreases from about 70% at 18–20 postmenstrual weeks to about 30% at around 28–29 postmenstrual weeks. Thereafter its size is relatively stable. One of the problems of measuring the ventricular system by TAS is the lack of the measurement standardization as a function of the increasing gestational age. It is also known that the hemisphere close to the transducer is usually "blurred," and therefore the structures are imaged in an ineffective fashion creating clinically undiagnosable inadequate pictures. The graphs and tables as well as nomograms to measure the distance from the medial wall of the lateral ventricle to its lateral wall are of course available (37–40).

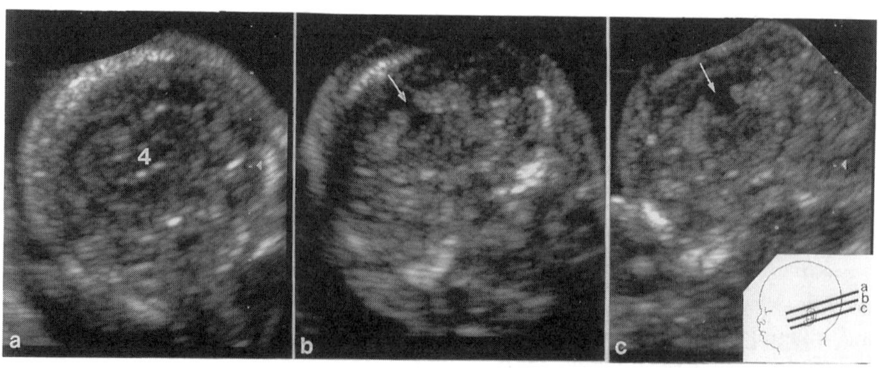

Figure 5. The consecutive axial sections of the posterior fossa at 16 postmenstrual weeks are shown. **(a)** A "high" section passes through the cerebellum with the sonolucent fourth ventricle (4). **(b, c)** These sections reveal the connection between the cisterna magna and the fourth ventricle, called median aperture (of Magendie) (*arrows*).

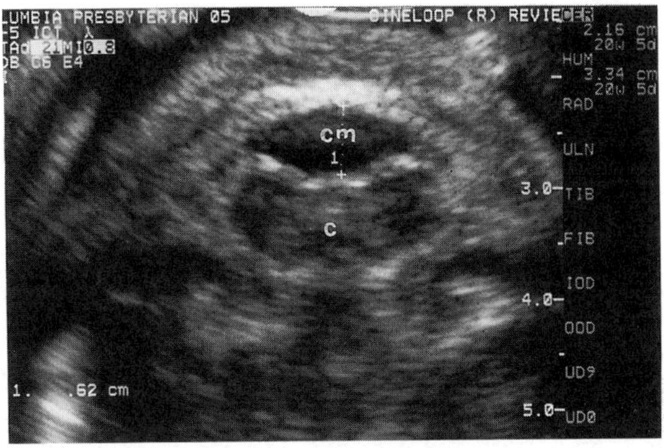

Figure 6. The normal measurement of the cisterna magna (0.62 cm) at 20 postmenstrual weeks is depicted through posterior axial approach. The bicerebellar distance on this picture is 2.1 cm. cm, cisterna magna; c, cerebellum.

Cardoza et al. (41) measured the width of the lateral ventricular atrium as a function of increasing fetal age; however, the value of 7.6 ± 0.6 ml remained relatively constant throughout gestation. This article suggests that the width of the lateral ventricular atrium above 10 ml, which represents four times the standard deviation, should trigger the suspicion of ventriculomegaly.

Campbell (42) suggested measuring the anterior horn–hemispheric widths ratio. This ratio decreases from 60% at 14 postmenstrual weeks to 40% at 21 postmenstrual weeks. The same author proposed that the measurement of the distance between the falx and the lateral wall of the atrium is a sensitive indicator of abnormality. This ratio decreases from 60% to 30% at 15–24 postmenstrual weeks (42). From 27 postmenstrual weeks to term, this same ratio remains constant at 0.56 to 0.51 (43).

Dilatation of the posterior horn (colpocephaly) is probably the most sensitive indicator of ventriculomegaly. If the transvaginal imaging method is used, it is easy to measure the posterior horn (23) using the constructed nomograms (44).

The inferior horn extends from the atrium laterally into the temporal lobe. After 16 weeks, in a normal fetal brain the oblique sections through the anterior and occipital horns do not include the inferior horn, which is found slightly lateral to this plane. Based on our experience, if after 16–18 postmenstrual weeks the anterior, posterior, and inferior horns are imaged on the same Oblique-1 section, ventriculomegaly should seriously be suspected.

The third ventricle is rarely imaged in the late second and third trimester; however, it can readily be depicted in the late first and early second trimesters. It was suggested that the third ventricle may reach transverse diameter of 8.2 mm at term; however, it is unclear whether the choroid plexus is or is not included at the time of the measurement (33).

The fourth ventricle is usually seen on the median plane using the transvaginal probe with a deeper penetrating frequency or on axial sections through an occipital approach (Figure 7). On such a plane, the hyperechoic vermis can also be appreciated.

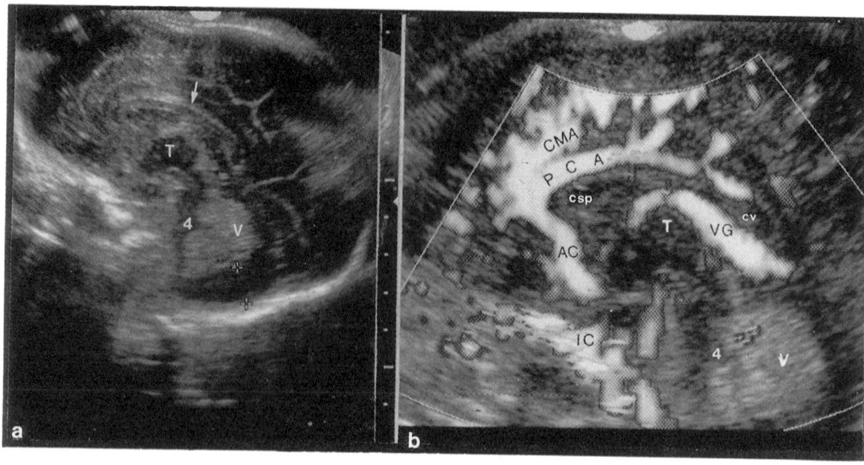

Figure 7. The evaluation of the midline brain structures using the median plane. **(a)** The entire corpus callosum is present (*arrow*). The thalamus (T), the cerebellar vermis (V), the fourth ventricle (4), and the cingulate gyrus and sulcus (CG) following the corpus callosum are the anatomic structures imaged. **(b)** This power color image depicts the following arteries and veins: internal carotid (IC), anterior cerebral artery (AC), pericallosal artery (PCA), calloso-marginal artery (CMA), and vein of galen (VG). The integrity and proper location of these are necessary to complement the gray scale evaluation of a normal midbrain at 20 weeks. csp, cavum septi pellucidi; cv, cavum vergae.

The bilateral and narrow *intraventricular* foramina (of Monro) can be seen thanks to the hyperechoic choroid plexus passing through them from the lateral ventricle into the third ventricle. These paired structures can be detected on the Midcoronal-2 section using the transvaginal scanning approach (Figure 2a, MC 2). Sonographic imaging of the cerebral aqueduct (of Sylvius) which connects between the third and the fourth ventricle were not described using conventional scanning techniques. However, situated in the posterior fossa, the median aperture (of Magendie), a connection between the fourth ventricle and the cisterna magna, can be seen using an axial/occipital approach and is wide open before 16 postmenstrual weeks (Figure 5).

The sonographic evaluation of choroid plexus is attributed increasing importance. It seems that at times this importance is slightly exaggerated. Practically all choroid plexuses present in the brain reside in the lateral ventricles and are the major source of CSF production. Sonographically, the choroid plexes appear as cotton-like structures with irregular borders filling the available space of the lateral ventricles (e.g., the antrum) and are richly supplied by capillaries. The choroid plexes of the lateral ventricles assume their final position at around 18–20 postmenstrual weeks. If they become thin and dangling, they are considered to be sensitive markers of ventriculomegaly. At times, sonography may detect cystic structures within a choroid plexus. These choroid plexus cysts will be discussed in the section on pathology of the brain. The tela choroidea is a thin layer(s) of choroid plexus covering the thalami and can be best imaged on a median section.

The *cavum septi pellucidi* and *cavum vergae* (Figure 7) are not part of the ventricular system, since they do not have connections with the lateral ventricles. However, they are sonographically recognizable fluid-filled midline structures and can be found below the corpus callosum and above the nuclei of the midbrain. The importance of the cava is the fact that they develop parallel with the development of the corpus callosum, and pathology in their development or the lack of their clear imaging is usually associated with extensive developmental pathology of the midbrain.

The corpus callosum (Figure 7) is probably the most important midline structure connecting the right and left hemispheres. It is a relatively late developing structure, starting at around the 12th postmenstrual week and reaching completion at or around the 18th postmenstrual week (45,46).

There are several *subarachnoid spaces and cisterns,* which may be visible using the different approaches and scanning planes. The largest one, the infratentorial cerebellomedullary cistern (cisterna magna), is probably the most important as far as imaging is concerned (Figure 6). At times, the supratentorial quadrigeminal cistern found above the cerebellum and the quadrigeminal plate, has importance, since a large percentage of arachnoid cysts arise from this area.

It is important to know the shape and size of the cisterna magna since its enlargement may lead to detection of pathologies such as the Dandy–Walker malformation or even trisomies. It is considered to be normal when its size is between 3 and 8 mm with a mean value of 4.5 mm (47).

The *posterior fossa* and the upper spinal cord can be the target of transvaginal ultrasound. The most prominent structures of the posterior fossa are the cerebellar hemispheres and their connecting structure, the vermis, and the fluid surrounding the cerebellum. Fine linear echoes of arachnoid are sometimes found in the cisterna magna. The cortex of the cerebellum is hyperechoic due to the fine duplications of the pia mater into the cerebellar gyri, which densely populate the surface of the cerebellum. At times it is necessary to gently manipulate the fetal head into a desirable position through which sound waves can reach the posterior fossa easily. The usual measurements to be taken here are the bicerebellar measurement (48,49) and that of the cisterna magna, measurements which are usually taken on a horizontal section (Figure 6).

The cerebral cortex, where most of the sensory, motor, and intellectual functions are performed, fascinated the imaging specialists, namely the ultrasonographers, for a long time. Neonatal neurosonography, an extremely important imaging field used mainly when the fontanelles are not yet obliterated, contributed valuable information regarding the understanding of the development of the cortex. The present technology (disregarding the advances of the three-dimensional ultrasound for a moment) enable the imaging only of flat surfaces; therefore, the lateral and superior surfaces of the hemispheres can be imaged using tangential planes to image small areas of the cortex. This leaves us with the medial surface of cerebral hemisphere, which usually can be depicted using the median section to image the sulci and gyri and other major structures in this plane. Based on pathological developmental studies, it is clear at 22 postmenstrual weeks that the cerebral hemispheres are still smooth and the lateral sulci on both sides are wide open (Figure 7). By 24 postmenstrual weeks, the lateral sulcus deepens and the cingulate sulcus is also detectable. On the medial surface, the parieto-occipital sulcus and the calcarine fissure (calcar avis) are also present. After 26 postmenstrual weeks, deepening of these fissures and the sulci occur. The biggest increase in the number and the depth of the sulci and gyri take place between 28 and 30 postmenstrual weeks (Figure 8). Slagle et al. (50) describe the developmental steps in the formation of the cingulate gyrus and sulcus in preterm infants and pointed out that this sulcus first becomes continuous and later some of its primary and then secondary branches appear. Finally, during the last weeks of the gestation, other sulci and gyri develop, giving the median surface of the hemisphere a "cobblestone appearance."

Our group studied the development of the cingulate sulcus and gyrus as well as the parieto-occipital and the calcarine fissure in normal fetuses from 14 to 40 postmenstrual weeks and came to the conclusion that the developmental maturation of the normal fetal brain follows a predictable timetable and that this maturation can be fol-

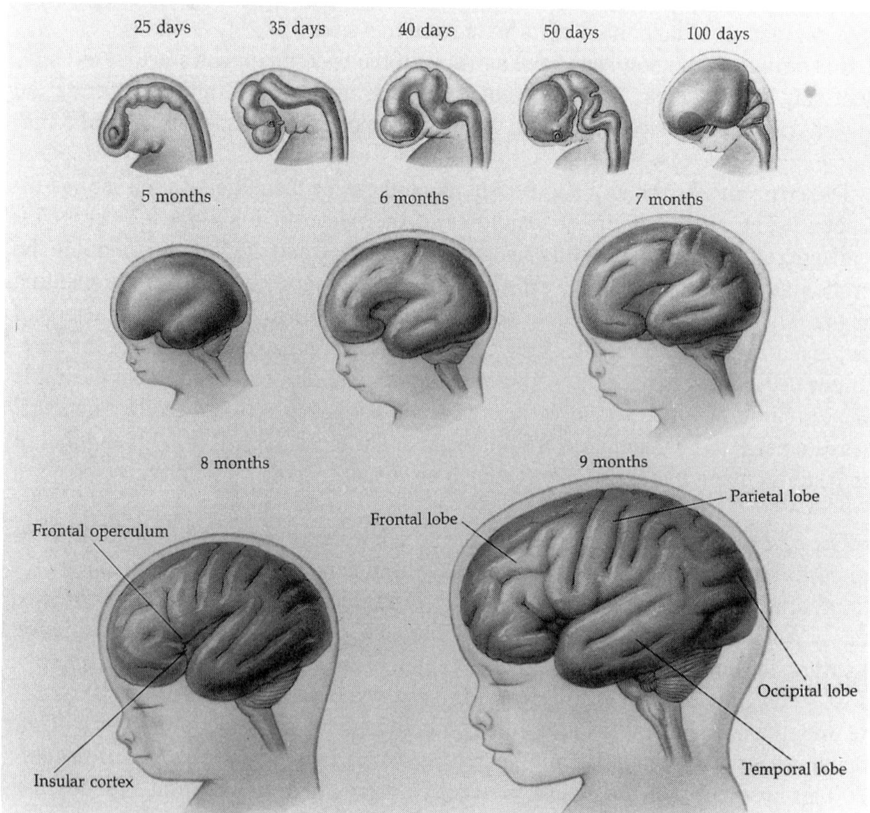

Figure 8. Pictorial representation of the development of the cerebral hemispheres during the embryonic and the fetal period. Note the increase in the sulci and gyri between the ages of 7 months (28 weeks) and 8 months (32 weeks). (Reproduced with permission from Cowan VM. The development of the brain. *Sci Am* 1979;241:112–113.)

lowed by ultrasonography. The sonographic appearance of the fissures, the gyri and sulci, using transvaginal sonographic imaging, lagged behind their anatomic appearance. The greatest discrepancy was regarding the cingulate gyrus, which in the anatomical studies was present by 18 postmenstrual weeks and in our sonographic study was only seen after the 26th postmenstrual week. The callosal sulcus was seen at 14 postmenstrual weeks, both in the sonographic and anatomical studies. We concluded that the recognition of specific structures of the cortical map is possible and that TVS may be used to image some of the developing cortical surfaces. Later on, this can form the basis of clinical application in the diagnosis of certain diseases of the cortical development (26).

Lately it has become evident that it is important to image certain *blood vessels of the fetal brain.* In order to understand the various branches of the supplying arteries and the draining vessels, one should understand the major avenues of the blood supply to the fetal brain.

The brain is supplied mainly by an *anterior* and a *posterior circulation.* The *anterior circulation* originates from the *internal carotid arteries,* while the *posterior* one stems from the vertebral arteries which unite to form a single *basilar artery* in the median plane. Then, they once again give rise to two branches which in turn form the connections with the anterior circulation at the bases of the hemispheres. This hexagonally shaped ring of vessels is known as the circulus arteriosus or hexagon of Willis (Figure 9). It is beyond the scope of this chapter to describe all the arteries and venus drainages of the fetal central nervous system. The interested reader is referred to the

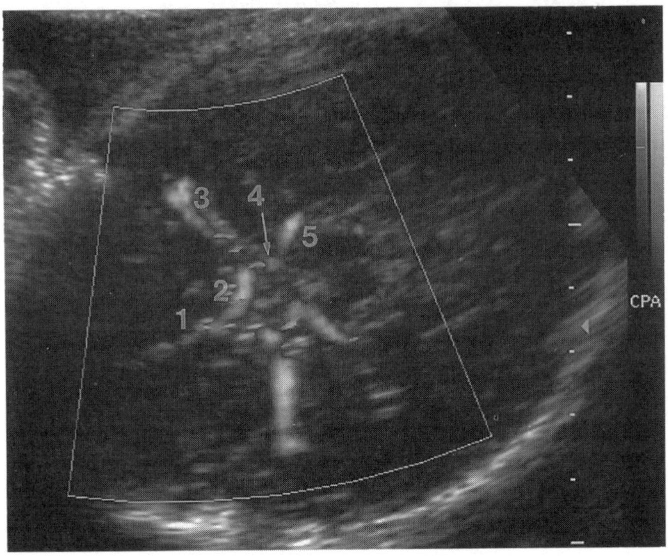

Figure 9. In the axial plane, the arteries forming the hexagon of Willis are imaged using the power color mode at 23 postmenstrual weeks. 1, Anterior communicating artery; 2, anterior cerebral artery; 3, middle cerebral artery; 4, posterior communicating artery; 5, posterior cerebral artery.

classical textbooks or the more targeted anatomic atlases containing details of the circulation of the brain (51).

As far as the sonographic appearance of the cerebral blood vessels are concerned, it should be stated from the outset that the earliest documented discrete pulsations of the brain vessels can be obtained at and immediately after the eighth postmenstrual week (52). These pulsations are visualized with high-frequency transvaginal ultrasound probes. The middle cerebral artery becomes visible in 71% of the cases at 9 postmenstrual weeks; and finally at 11 postmenstrual weeks, in every single case, the cerebral circulation can be depicted (53).

On the horizontal or axial section, the circulus arteriosus of Willis can be sonographically visualized. This hexagonal structure is formed by the posterior cerebral arteries, the posterior communicating arteries, the middle cerebral arteries, the anterior cerebral arteries, and finally the anterior communicating artery, as we proceed from occipital to frontal direction.

The median plane is probably one of the most revealing and clinically important sections to be imaged. On this plane (Figures 7b and 10), we are able to follow the internal carotid artery leading to the anterior cerebral artery. The two main branches of

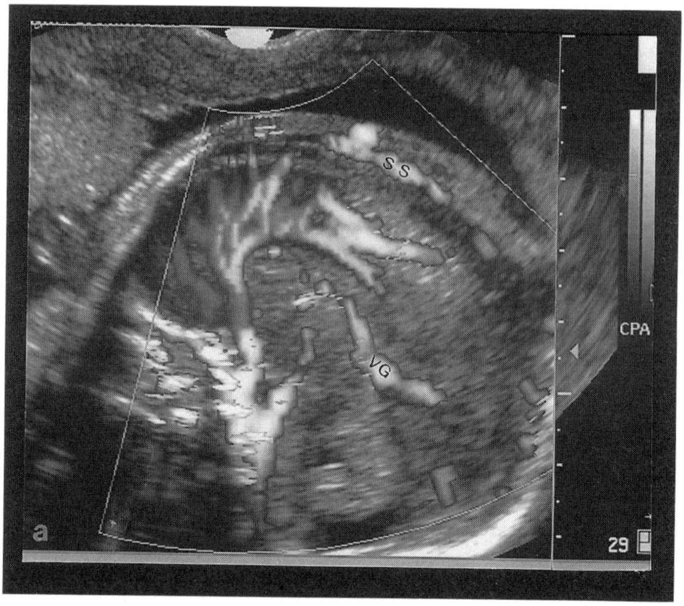

a

Figure 10. Comparison between a normal-appearing and a pathological fetal brain scan in the median plane at 20 weeks is shown. **(a)** Note the anatomic place of the arteries and veins in the normal brain (see legend of Figure 7). SS, superior sagittal sinus; VG, vein of Galen. **(b)** Using a transvaginal probe of a three-dimensional ultrasound system to resolve the size and location of the pericallosal artery, agenesis of the corpus callosum and ventriculomegaly was diagnosed in this fetus. Note the profound differences in the appearance of the arteries imaged in this case. S, sagittal plane; C, coronal plane; H, horizontal plane. The arrow points to the short pericallosal artery.

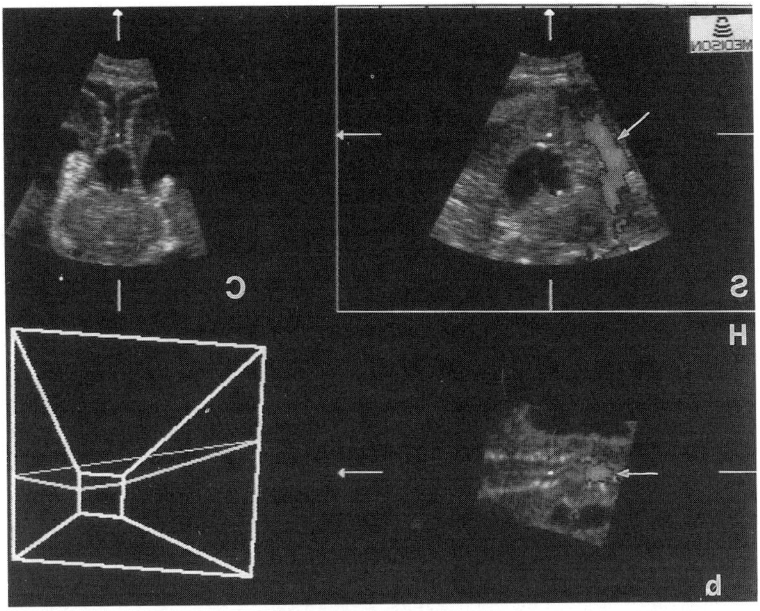

Figure 10. b. *continued*

the latter are the pericallosal artery and the calloso-marginal arteries. These develop together with the corpus callosum, and their presence or absence is a good indicator of the size and the development of the corpus callosum. Other vessels seen on this plane are the superior sagittal and the central draining vein (i.e., the vein of Galen).

If a "coronal plane" is sought, the most revealing may be the Midcoronal-2 section (Figure 11) on which the internal carotid, the midcerebral artery and its small ventriculostriate arteries, the cross section of the pericallosal artery, the arteries of the choroid plexus, and the superior sagittal sinus are evident.

Studies of the middle cerebral arteries with regard to measuring blood flow to the brain of normal as well as grown fetuses can be performed by using transabdominal ultrasound Doppler techniques. During the third trimester, a constant but low-resistance flow in the fetal brain is present. Wladimiroff et al. (54) detected diastolic frequencies in 75% of the fetuses at 18 weeks and in all fetuses after 34 postmenstrual weeks (55). It was found that the PI (pulsatility index) of the middle cerebral artery was higher than that of the internal carotid artery or the anterior cerebral artery (56). Also, the posterior cerebral artery had a lower resistance index than that of the middle and anterior cerebral arteries (57). After 34–36 weeks, there may be a redistribution of fetal circulation with decreased impedance to the flow to the fetal brain, probably to compensate for the progressive decrease in fetal blood pO_2 (58–60). The low cerebral vascular impedance-to-blood-flow at the end of the pregnancy was attributed to the increasing metabolic requirements (61). Meerman et al. (62) published longitudinal studies of fetal and neonatal cerebral blood flow velocities assessed in the middle cerebral artery explaining some of the changes which occur throughout gestation and as transition to the neonatal period.

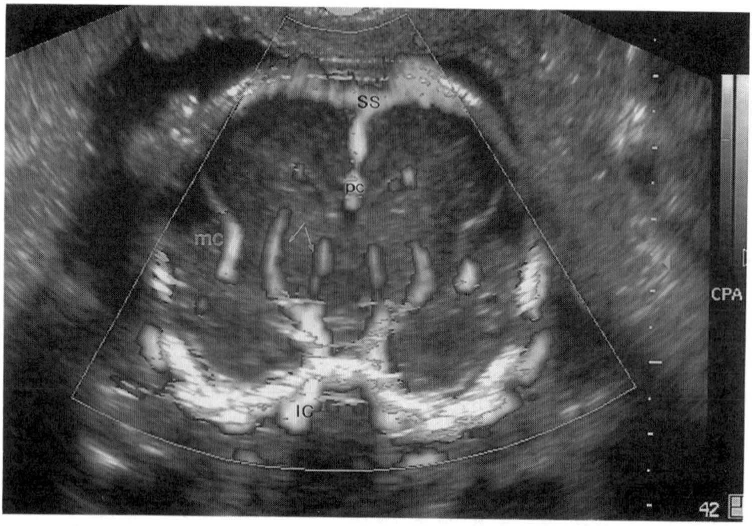

Figure 11. On a Midcoronal-2 section, the arteries highlighted with power color mode are: middle cerebral arteries (mc), internal carotid (IC), pericallosal artery (pc), branches of the arteries supplying the corpus stratum (*arrows*), and the superior sagittal sinus (ss).

It is known that several physiological variables affect the cerebral blood flow in normal pregnancies. These variables, among others, are the fetal heart rate, breathing movements, fetus behavioral states, glucose concentration, head compression, and, last but not least, the labor and delivery. Fetal cerebral blood flow was also studied extensively in pathological states such as fetal anemia, elevated placental restriction in the intrauterine growth restricted fetus, discordant multifetal pregnancies, and increased intracranial pressure.

A detailed discussion of the ultrasonography of the fetal and neonatal cerebral circulation as well as Doppler measurements in various arteries of the fetal brain were eloquently dealt with by Degani et al. (63).

The knowledge of the anatomic location of the major arteries and the venous drainage is important in order to assess normal development of certain structures (i.e., the corpus callosum) or to be able to correctly determine the exact location of the space occupying lesions such as arachnoid cysts. The normal development of the corpus callosum from 12 to 18 weeks can be closely followed by the developing pericallosal artery. If by 18 weeks the entire length of the pericallosal artery (or for that matter, the corpus callosum) is not seen, the diagnosis of partial or total lack of development of the corpus callosum can be made easier.

The clinical importance of sonographic imaging of the venous system is not well-established. Very few anomalies short of that of the vein of Galen were described. Fetal neurosonography is an extremely informative imaging modality which is relatively inexpensive and is definitely noninvasive. Understanding the normal development and the sonoanatomy of the fetal brain, we have an easier task to detect deviant development or pathology and it is easier to localize the lesion using the newly proposed sections of the brain in the sagittal and coronal planes. As said before, the transfer of the information to the pediatrician, neonatal neurologist, and neurosurgeon becomes easier and more fluent, and obviously it is to the advantage of the fetus with brain pathology.

SONOGRAPHICALLY DETECTABLE ANOMALIES OF THE FETAL BRAIN

If any part of the fetal brain deviates from the normal sonographic appearance, we deal with a malformation of the central nervous system (CNS). Since these may (in most of the cases) be present at birth, they are also called congenital brain anomalies. In order to detect and properly diagnose such anomalies, the sonographer/sonologist should be familiar with the development of the fetal brain as described previously. If a CNS anomaly has been found, it is also extremely important to look for other malformations; conversely, if any anomaly is detected in the fetal body, a complete fetal neurosonography should be performed.

Following this, some of the anomalies detectable by ultrasonography during the fetal period will be discussed.

Neural-Tube Defects

A rather short list of neural tube defects will be presented. The normal neural-tube starts to develop at approximately 20 days after ovulation. Fusion of the neural fold or the neural tube starts to occur in the lower regions and proceeds cranially. The completion of this neural-tube formation occurs at or slightly prior to 32 post-ovulatory days. Neural-tube defects (NTDs) result from a failure to close this neural tube. Lesions of the head and the neck area for various severities occur if the anterior neuropore is not closed, and defects that arise from disraphic conditions affecting the lower sacral or coxigeal areas result in various degrees of overt or occult dysraphic defects.

The incidence of NTDs in the United States is about 2 per 1000 births; however, if one parent has an NTD, the risk increases to 5%. If a previous sibling was affected, the recurrent risk is approximately 2%; and if two previous offspring are affected, the risk in the subsequent one becomes 6–10% (64).

The *anencephaly/exencephaly sequence* is a malformation where there is an absence of the fetal cranium. This can be of various degrees. It is a lethal condition, and almost three-fourths of the fetuses are stillborn. Such NTDs are complex developmental malformations affecting the production of the mesenchyme (65,66). There are three phases in the development of anencephaly: The first is dysraphia, which is a failure of closure of the region of the calvarium (67,68). The second is exencephaly, or total exposure of the formed brain, which is found uncovered by the skullbones, even during the embryonic period. The third is the anencephaly, which is a total disintegration of the exposed brain (23–26). Bronshstein and Ornoy (69) reported on the development of anencephaly from exencephaly which they followed looking at several anencephalic fetuses from early gestation. Anencephaly or exencephaly can be detected reliably from about the 10th or 11th postmenstrual week (70).

Our group contributed observations as to the fact that anencephaly results from a progressive "rubbing off" of exposed brain tissue. Amniocentesis was performed in anencephalic fetuses at different and successive gestational ages. Free-floating neuronal cells were detected in the amniotic fluid (71,72).

Exencephaly/anencephaly sequence is relatively easy to detect, and this is the reason that the first fetal malformation detected by transabdominal ultrasound was that of an anencephalic fetus done by transabdominal sonography (73). Usually, if the fetus is scanned at around 11 or 12 postmenstrual weeks, the typical picture of exencephalic/anencephalic fetus is that of a fetal head much wider than usual and the crown rump length lags several millimeters behind the expected measurement at the specific gestational age (Figure 12).

Anencephaly can be of two types: The first type is called *holoacrania,* in which the entire calvarium is missing. This is the easiest to recognize sonographically. Various degrees of spinal rachischisis spanning over several vertebrae may be present (Figure 13). The second type is termed *merocrania,* in which there is partial or incomplete median cranial defect with parts of the brain uncovered by the skull. In most cases, polyhydramnios is also seen.

Iniencephaly

Iniencephaly is a complex and lethal malformation with three distinguishable features: (a) a defect in the formam magnum and the occiput, (b) spinal retroflection, and (c) various degrees of open spinal defects. As in anencephaly, most of the affected fetuses are female. Its reported incidence is 1–6 per 10,000 births. There are

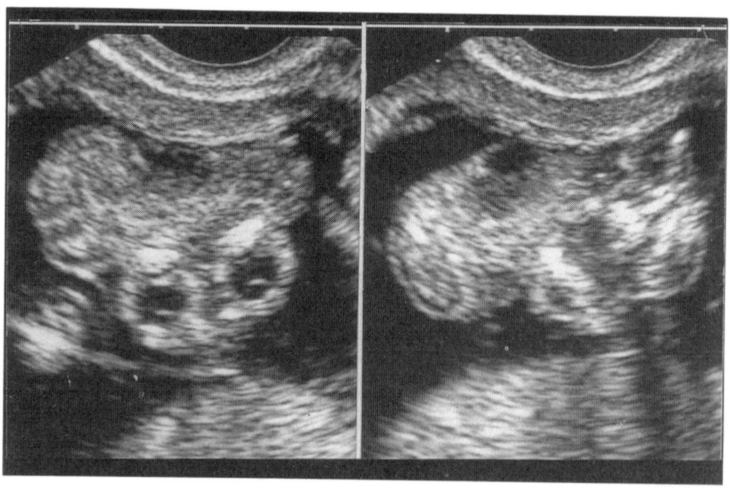

Figure 12. Exencephaly at 12 postmenstrual weeks. Note the lack of the bony skull.

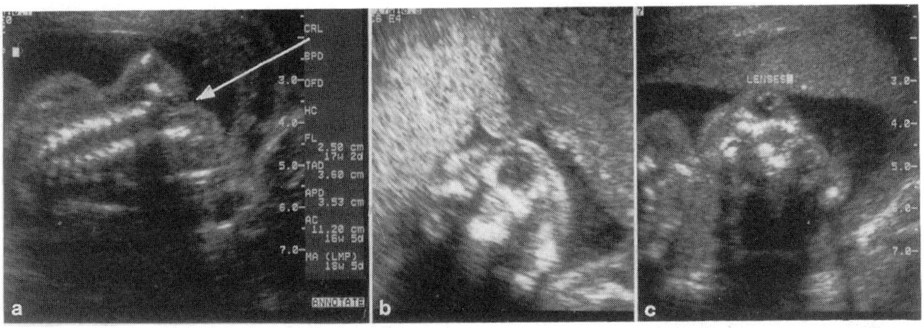

Figure 13. At 18 postmenstrual weeks, anencephaly and rachischisis are imaged. **(a)** The arrow points to the cervical rachischisis. **(b)** The median section clearly shows the lack of the bony skull. **(c)** A coronal section confirms no skull above the orbits.

two subtypes: the closed type and the open type (74,75). Its association with open malformation is as high as 84%.

The sonographic diagnosis is relatively simple, and it is based on imaging the head in fixed retroflection and imaging the spine in a lordotic position. As said, various degrees of posterior cephalocele or protrusion of brain tissue in the occipital area is seen as well as other anomalies such as rachischises and omphalocele (76,77) (Figure 14). Using TVS iniencephaly has been diagnosed as early as the 12th postmenstrual week of gestation (78). Malformations such as hydrocephalus, microcephaly, agenesis of various parts of the brain, and deformities of the thorax, the face, and the abdominal wall are found.

Cephaloceles

Cephaloceles are brain bulges through cranial defects pushing the meninges in front of the brain tissue. At times, only the meninges are bulging, and this is termed *meningocele*. If the defect contains brain tissue, it is called *meningo-encephalocele.* Its incidence ranges from 1 in 3500 to 1 in 5000 live births. The cephalocele may emerge from the occipital, ethmoidal, temporal, and parietal regions of the fetal head. Geographical or regional differences in their incidence were described (79–88). *Occipital cephaloceles* occur more commonly in females than in males. Using TVS, occipital cepholoceles have been diagnosed as early as 12 weeks of gestation (83). Their sizes may range from extremely small to sizes equaling the fetal skull.

Choroid Plexus Cysts

These fluid-filled cysts of the choroid plexus have an approximate incidence of 0.95%. Usually they are benign and asymptomatic and disappear by the 24th postmenstrual week. They may be associated with an abnormal fetal karyotype.

The sonographic approach is simple: These cysts have a sonolucent structure of various sizes, are uni- or bilateral, and have various shapes (Figure 15). Choroid plexus cysts can be detected using TVS as early as the 11th–12th weeks of the gestation.

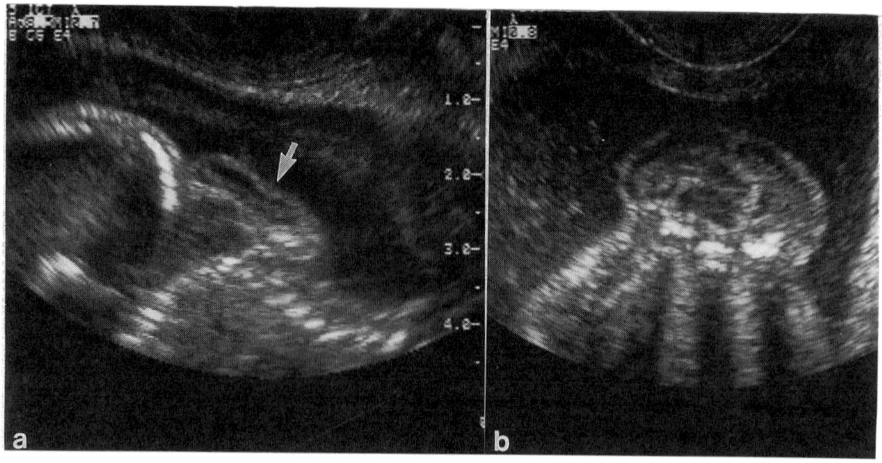

Figure 14. Transvaginal images of a fetus at 20 postmenstrual weeks with iniencephaly. **(a)** The occipital segment of the skull and upper thoracic spine are imaged. Note the virtually nonexistent cervical vertebrae and the upper thoracic spina bifida (*arrow*) and meningocele. **(b)** Cross section at the level of the spinal defect.

Various associations of the choroid plexus cysts were described and published including chromosomal aneuploides (89–98). We defer from discussing these aspects of the choroid plexuses.

Ventriculomegaly and Hydrocephalus

These two terms are at times used interchangeably; however, ventriculomegaly is a dilatation of the lateral ventricles when there is normal intraventricular pressure of the CSF. As opposed to this, hydrocephalus is more than just ventriculomegaly, since there is an increased amount of pressure exerted by the CSF causing increasing fetal head size and thinning of the brain tissue. The incidence of hydrocephalus in live births is 0.5–3 in 1000 (99). Usually, hydrocephalus is divided into noncommunicating and communicating hydrocephalus. The noncommunicating hydrocephalus is caused by aqueductal stenosis, Dandy–Walker malformation or various space-occupying masses exerting pressure upon the aqueduct. The second kind of hydrocephalus is the communicating hydrocephalus, which can occur as a result of or in association with Arnold–Chiari malformation, encephalocele, congenital absence of arachnoid granulations, inflammatory processes, lissencephaly, and so on (100,101).

Aqueductal stenosis may develop at around 15–18 postmenstrual weeks of gestation (Figure 16). In almost three-fourths of the cases, the reason for the obstruction of the flow through the aqueduct can be found. In about 2% of all cases, the disease may be inherited—that is, an X-linked disorder affecting males transmitted through female carriers (102,103).

Early diagnosis of ventriculomegaly or hydrocephalus is, and probably will remain, a challenge to the ultrasonographer (20,23,104–106). Very early in the second trimester in a normal fetus the size of the lateral ventricle is relatively large. However,

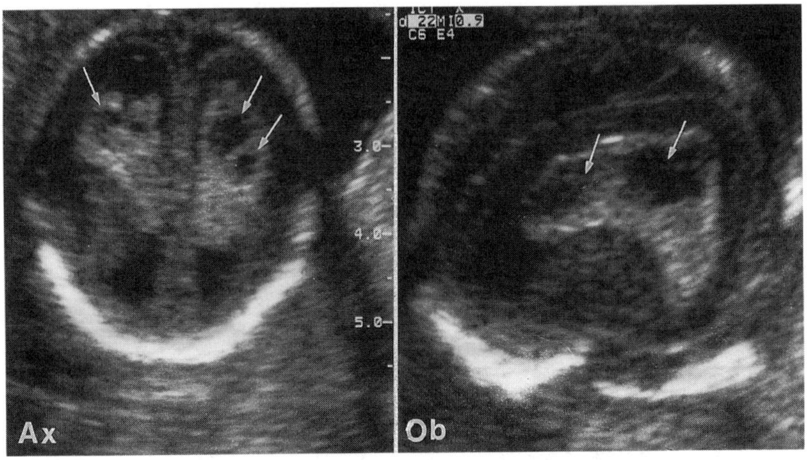

Figure 15. At 16 postmenstrual weeks, an axial and an oblique plane show bilateral choroid plexus cysts (*arrows*) on the axial (Ax) and the Oblique-1 planes (Ob).

during the gestation, the ratio of the hemispheric width to the ventricular width progressively diminishes, and at around 28 weeks it stabilizes and occupies about one-third of this distance. Employing ultrasonography, the lateral ventricles within the fetal brain can be assessed qualitatively and quantitatively (104–110).

Qualitative ways to assess the size of the ventricular dilatation are as follows:

1. *The gestalt approach,* where the sonographer and the sonologist appraise the degree of dilatation by relying on their experience and the appearance of the anomaly.
2. Relying on indirect signs of looking at the results of the dilatation of the ventricles. Some of these indirect signs are the shape of the lateral ventricles, the thickness of the surrounding brain parenchema (Figure 16 b–d), and the mobility of structures or parts of the lateral ventricle on sections that should not normally be present—that is, detection of the temporal horn on an oblique scan, which usually has to contain only the anterior and the posterial horns.
3. *Looking at shape and the mobility of the choroid plexus* (Figure 16d). If the choroid plexus is extremely thin and if it is seen "dangling" or "floating" freely within the dilated ventricle, this signifies a significant dilatation (105,109).
4. *Examining the third ventricle.* Any time this structure is seen on an axial or a Midcoronal section, the suspicion of its dilated nature should be raised.
5. *Looking at the shape of the skull.* If the diagnosis is Arnold–Chiari Type II malformation, developing at a time when the skull is still malleable, the bitemporal depression will create the "lemon-shaped" skull. The impaction of the cerebellum in the posterior fossa will result in its "banana-shaped deformity" (Figure 17).

Quantitative methods to assess the size of the lateral ventricles obviously depend upon their direct measurements (107,108,110).

The "gold standard" of measuring the size of the lateral ventricles is that performed on the axial section. Here, the distance between the midline and the inner

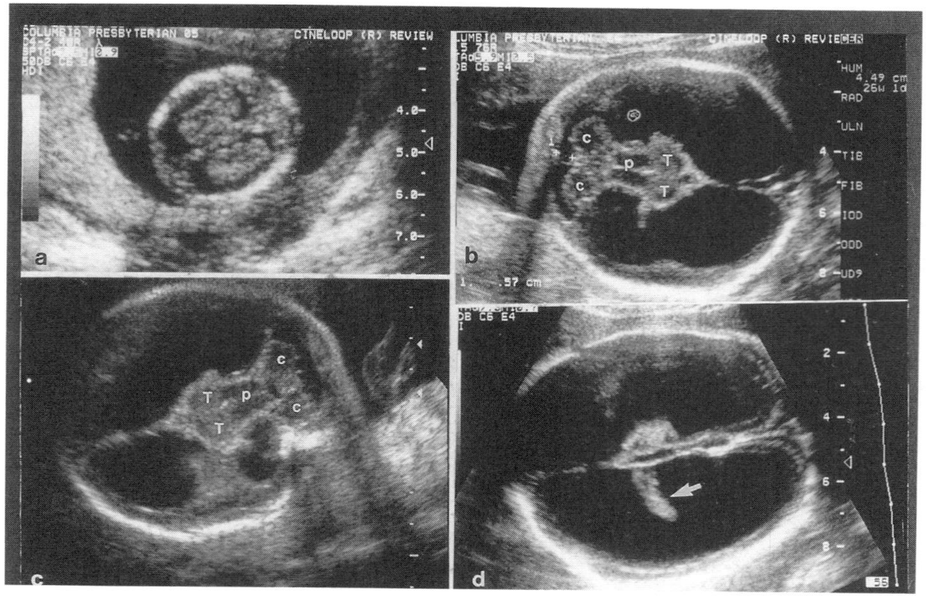

Figure 16. Several scans of a fetus with ventriculomegaly which developed during the late second trimester. **(a)** At 14 postmenstrual weeks, no sonographic signs of ventricular dilatation are present. **(b, c)** High axial sections show normal appearing brain stem and posterior fossa. However, the brain parenchyma is thin. c, cerebellum; p, pedunculi; T, thalamus. **(d)** High axial section demonstrating extreme loss of cortical mantle and dangling choroid plexus (*arrow*).

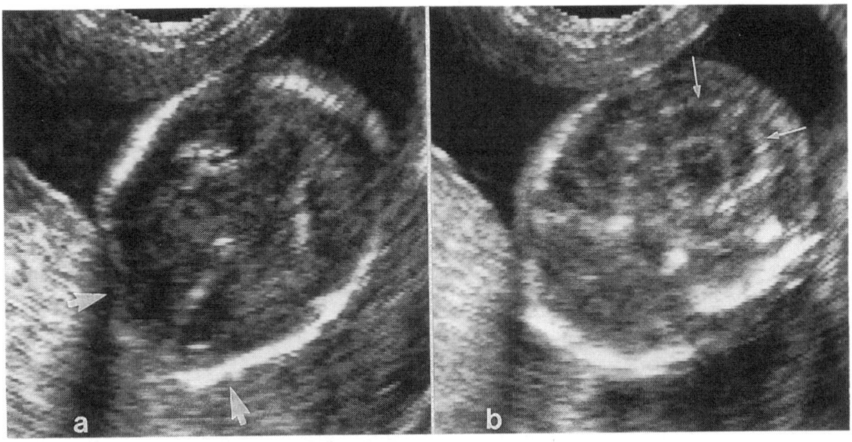

Figure 17. Arnold–Chiari type II malformation in a fetus at 17 postmenstrual weeks. **(a)** This high axial section demonstrates the depression of the frontal bones creating the "lemon sign" of the skull (*arrows*). **(b)** A lower axial section demonstrates the disappearance of the cisterna magna as a result of the impacted and "banana-shaped" cerebellum (*arrows*). This fetus had a lumbar spina bifida and meningocele.

bony skull representing the hemispheric widths is compared to the measurement from the midline to the lateral wall of the lateral ventricles. As said before, this ratio decreases from about 70% at 20 weeks to about 28–30% at around 30 weeks' gestational age. Thereafter it is extremely stable to term.

The normal LVW/HW ratio at 15 weeks is about 71%, and by 37 weeks it is 29%; this reflects the rapid growth of the cerebral hemispheres as pregnancy progresses. The diagnosis of intrauterine hydrocephalus is relying upon a BPP greater than 11 cm or a head-to-abdomen ratio greater than 2.0. Nomograms for evaluation of the lateral ventricular width to the hemispheric widths ratio are available.

In addition to the ventricle-to-hemisphere ratio, the anterior horn of the lateral ventricles can also be measured. The portion of the anterior horn found anterior to the interventricular foramen can also be measured. Its relative size is decreasing with advanced gestational age. Nomograms of the cerebral frontal horn distance throughout the pregnancy are also available and may indicate a ventriculomegaly.

The atrium of the lateral ventricles can also be measured on the axial plane used for the measurement of the BPD. This can be recognized by the echogenic choroid plexus within it. Measurements such as the cerebral atrial distance, the atrial width/hemispheric width ratio, and the atrial width/cerebral atrial distance ratio throughout pregnancy were determined and are available. These measurements can be considered an indication of the dilatation of the lateral ventricles in the fetus.

The increase in the size of the posterior occipital horn of the lateral ventricles may be the most indicative of ventriculomegaly. These can be imaged on a horizontal plane that is normally used for the measurement of the BPD.

Our group developed nine nomograms to define the lateral ventricles between 14 and 40 weeks' gestation using transvaginal sonography. A total of seven measurements of the fetal lateral ventricles were used to generate these nomograms (106,110).

The earliest changes in the size of the lateral ventricle during the formation of the ventriculomegaly or hydrocephalus are the dilatation of the posterior horns and the compression or the thinning of the choroid plexus. The change in size or the increase in the posterior horn can be detected on the longitudinal and coronal sections of the ultrasound picture. When a fetus suspected of having ventriculomegaly is scanned using TVS, the most useful and efficient section to obtain is the right or the left Oblique-1 section. On this picture, the thickness of the choroid plexus as well as the size of the posterior horn can be easily measured. The ratio of the choroid plexus to the height of the posterior horn is the most sensitive measure of the coloprocephaly or dilatation of the posterior horns.

If prenatal diagnosis of ventriculomegaly and hydrocephalus are made, this should prompt a careful sonographic evaluation of the fetus as well as chromosomal studies to rule out or to make a diagnosis of diseases associated with chromosomal anomalies. About 70–80% of fetuses with hydrocephalus will have associated anomalies. About 60% of these are extracranial, cardiac, or renal anomalies. The mortality rate of fetuses with a detectable hydrocephalus ranges from 60% to 74%, with an approximate survival rate of 30% (111–113). The association of hydrocephalus with chromosomal abnormalities has been reported to range between 4% and 28%. Recently an increasing concern over the significance of mild or borderline cases of fetal ventriculomegaly has emerged. The most important issue considering the mild dilatation of the lateral ventricles in the fetus is that of the agreement of how it is measured and what the cut of measurement is. It is now considered that an 11 to 13-mm size of the lateral ventricle measured on an axial picture is considered a small dilatation of the ventricles.

If only a mild dilatation of the lateral ventricles is observed in an isolated fashion (i.e., no other malformations of chromosomal aneuploides are detected), this enables the counselors to quote a normal 70% survival rate (114–116).

It seems that the most important prognostic factors in the outcome of in utero-detected hydrocephalus are (a) the presence or absence of associative anomalies, (b) associated chromosomal anomalies, and (c) the amount of residual brain tissue around the lateral ventricles.

Holoprosencephaly

Holoprosencephaly has an approximate incidence of 1 in 1600 births; however, it is presumed that this anomaly is associated with high percentage of earlier midtrimester pregnancy loss, and therefore ultrasound scans performed at these early gestational ages may encounter this anomaly more frequently (117). Holoprosencephaly may occur as an isolated anomaly; however, at times, chromosomal abnormalities are associated with it. Autosomal dominant transmission and its association with syndromes were also described. Holoprosencephaly is often associated with facial anomalies. By their appearance and anatomic presentation, holoprosencephaly may be classified as *alobar, semilobar,* and *lobar holoprosencephaly* (118–120).

Alobar holoprosencephaly demonstrates a totally absent interhemispheric fissure and corpus callosum, the thalami are fused in the midline, and there is an absence of the third ventricle. In the *semilobar type,* the two cerebral hemispheres are partially split or separated, above which there is a singular ventricular cavity. In addition, a separation of the hemispheres in the occipital area and a partial development of the posterior and the inferior horns is also seen. This configuration renders the ventricles a teardrop shape on the axial section.

The sonographic features of a lobar holoprosencephaly are important and they usually show a complete division of the two hemispheres. The cavum septi pellucidi is absent. The corpus callosum is usually absent (121). It may be accompanied by the presence of a single eye or a single orbit and a prominent proboscis found above the eye socket. The face may contain a midline cleft lip and palate (122). It is often associated with trisomy 13. Over 60% of the infants with trisomy 13 also have holoprosencephaly. Conversely, 20% of the cases of holoprosencephaly are associated with trisomy 13. Almost all types of holoprosencephaly are associated with microcephaly. However, at times, if hydrocephalus is also present, there may be head enlargement present. The sonographic diagnosis of holoprosencephaly was reported as early as 12 weeks and was based upon the lack of development of the falx and the fusion of the thalami (123). At times, lipomas of the corpus callosum can be detected (124).

The sonographic prenatal diagnosis of lobar holoprosencephaly is quite difficult and it is usually based upon the absence of a septum pellucidum and the communication between the frontal horns and the third ventricle as well as the wedge-shaped separation of the thalami.

Since the pericallosal artery is also missing, this can be used as a reliable sign of the disease (125,126).

The differential diagnosis of lobar holoprosencephaly is *septo-optic displasia,* which is quite a rare anomaly characterized by the absence of the septum pellucidum and the hypoplasia of the optic disks. The antenatal picture of septo-optic displasia is almost identical to that of lobar holoprosencephaly. The definitive diagnosis is usually made after birth when the vision of the newborn can be tested. If blindness is observed, the diagnosis is septo-optic displasia (123).

Agenesis of the Corpus Callosum

Situated in the midline, the corpus callosum with its four segments (genu, rostrum, truncus, and splenium) constitute the largest collection of fibers connecting the different areas of the cerebral cortex situated in the opposite hemispheres. Total or partial lack in the development of this midline structure is termed agenesis of the corpus callosum (ACC) or partial agenesis of the corpus callosum (PACC) depending upon the extent of the missing part. If PACC is the case, usually the splenium and part of the truncus is missing. The incidence in the general population is thought to be 0.3–0.7% (119,120); however, there is a higher incidence in the neurologically impaired patient population (121).

A variety of etiological factors in its development are sought, the most important factor being the genetic factor. Syndromes with Mendelian and/or X-linked dominant inheritance were also described as well as sporadic occurrence (123).

The sonographic diagnosis in the fetus is based upon the total or partial (usually posterior) lack of the sonolucent structure connecting the hemispheres in the midline. On coronal sections, the lateral ventricles appear separated and displaced upwards because the horizontally situated fibers of the corpus callosum are missing. It appears that the third ventricle is directly communicating with the unusually wide interhemispheric fissures. On an axial section, due to the more prominent dilatation of the occipital horns (colpocephaly) compared to those of the anterior horns, a teardrop configuration of the lateral ventricles results. The walls of the frontal horns may be so close to each other that a peculiar parallel double line appears which is termed "railroad tracks." On the median section, the normal appearance of the cavum septi pellucidi flanked from above by the "C"-shaped corpus callosum and cingulate sulcus, cingulate gyrus, and the pericallosal artery (on color coded flow studies) is absent. Instead, the high position of the third ventricle and the radial (sunburst) appearance of the gyri and sulci become relatively easily diagnosed. At times, lipomas were observed to appear at the location of the corpus callosum (124). They appear as echogenic structures; however, it is rare to see them in the second trimester.

The diagnosis of total or partial agenesis of the corpus callosum is not hard if a targeted fetal neuroscan is performed. It should, however, be noted that on axial scans the diagnosis is significantly harder to make than on coronal or median scanning planes. It is therefore stressed here that if any suspicion of this developmental disorder arises, TVS should be performed. We found it worthwhile to vert fetuses from breech to vertex presentation to be able to apply the coronal and the sagittal planes to rule out or to establish the diagnosis.

Another useful way to make the diagnosis is to follow the semicircular course of the pericallosal artery (Figures 7B and 10). Normally this artery follows the superior surface of the corpus callosum. If the entire corpus callosum or parts of it are missing, the artery will also be shorter, indicating the extent of the anomaly (125).

Chromosomal anomalies are often (about 20%) present in cases of ACC (126). The most encountered chromosomal aneuploidies are trisomy 18, 13, and 8.

Dandy–Walker Malformation

This complex spans over a number of varieties from mild to severe. The diagnosis of the more severe malformation—that is, the Dandy–Walker malformation (D-WM)—is made based upon an enlarged cisterna magna, a significant hypoplasia of the cerebellum, absence of the cerebellar vermis, and enlarged fourth ventricle; and, at times, it is associated with various degrees of ventriculomegaly of the lateral ventricles and/or agenesis of the corpus callosum and even haloprosencephaly. The diagnosis of the less severe form—that is, the Dandy–Walker variant (D-WV)—demonstrates mild dilatation of the cisterna magna and a small defect in the cerebellar vermis without dysplastic cerebellar hemispheres. It is customary to make the diagnosis of D-WV if the posterior fossa, the fourth ventricle, and the cerebellar hemispheres are normal, but the fourth ventricle visibly communicates with the cerebellopeduncular cistern.

The diagnosis can be reliably made starting the 14th week; however, it was detected even earlier using TVS. A cisterna magna of 10 mm or more should trigger serious investigation.

The incidence of D-WM at birth is about 1 in 38,000 live births; however, it may be present in as many as 12% of all cases of infants with hydrocephalus (127). The pathogenesis of D-WM is not yet fully elucidated. One of the theories is that of an imbalance in the production of the CSF between structures below and above the aqueduct (of Sylvius) (128).

The numbers of abnormalities associated with D-WM are vast: autosomal recessive diseases such as Walker–Warburg syndrome, Ellis–van Creveld syndrome, and Meckel–Gruber syndrome; X-linked dominant syndromes such as Aicardi's syndrome; a long list of chromosomal abnormalities; environmental factors such as infections, alcohol, and diabetes; and multifactorial diseases such as neural-tube defects and congenital heart disease. It may occur sporadically as in holoprosencephaly, deLange's syndrome, kidney, facial, and digital abnormalities, and Goldenhar syndrome, among others (129).

Mortality rates are reported to be high in infants; however, due to the low incidence of this anomaly, only limited series were published. The mental capacity of survivors is low in the majority of the cases (127,129–131).

Arachnoid Cysts

Most subarachnoid cysts are located above the tentorium; however, they may also occur below the tentorium. They consist of CSF-filled spaces, which do not connect with the cerebral ventricles. Arachnoid cysts are space-occupying lesions of various sizes and are benign in nature (Figure 18). Sonographically, their borders are smooth and the content is sonolucent. The left side of the brain is more commonly affected. More than half are located in the middle cranial fossa; about 10% are in a potentially dangerous area, namely the suprasellar cistern; about 10% grow in the quadrigeminal cistern; only about 5–10% are seen in the posterior fossa (132). The ones in the posterior fossa have to be differentiated from the D-WM. At times, the differential

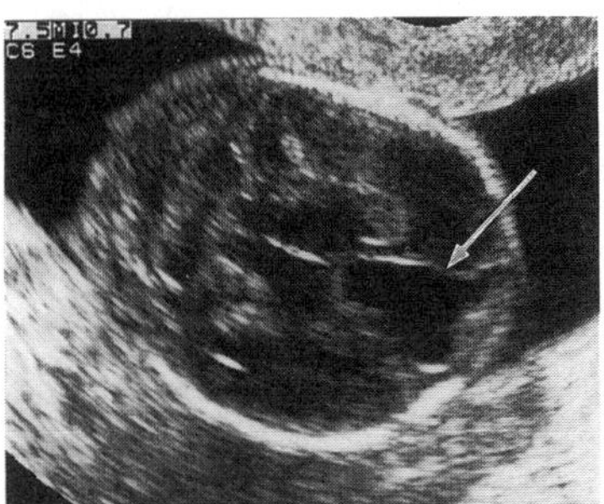

Figure 18. Arachnoid cyst (*arrow*) situated in the interhemispheric fissure.

diagnosis of arachnoid cysts presents problems: Large choroid plexus cysts, porencephalic cysts, and vein of Galen malformations have to be considered. Its association with chromosomal syndromes is rare; however, arachnoid cysts may occur with other CNS or non CNS anomalies. If the cyst is "strategically" located to block CSF circulation, it may cause hydrocephalus.

The long-term prognosis is dependent upon its location; however, it is generally considered to be good. If they are located on the convexity of the brain (e.g., temporal lobe) the outcome is considered good (133). The treatment is surgical: excision, shunting, or creating an escape for the fluid in the cyst into the arachnoid space (134).

As in any other CNS anomaly, genetic counseling and testing should be offered to the patient.

Porencephaly

This term refers to a sonolucent cystic structure amidst the substance of the fetal brain resulting, most probably, from an extensive destruction of the brain, communicating with the ventricles. Porencephalic cysts may be solitary or multiple and usually have irregularly shaped walls as well as some "debris" within the cavity (Figure 19). Neurological deficit in the newborn or infant is usually the rule.

Schizencephaly

As opposed to the arachnoid cyst, with no connection to other structures and the porencephaly with connection only to the ventricles, schizencephaly is a CNS malformation in which the lateral brain ventricles communicate with the subarachnoid space and are lined with gray matter covered with pia-ependymal layer. Sonographically, they appear wedge-shaped with their apex pointing towards the periphery. They

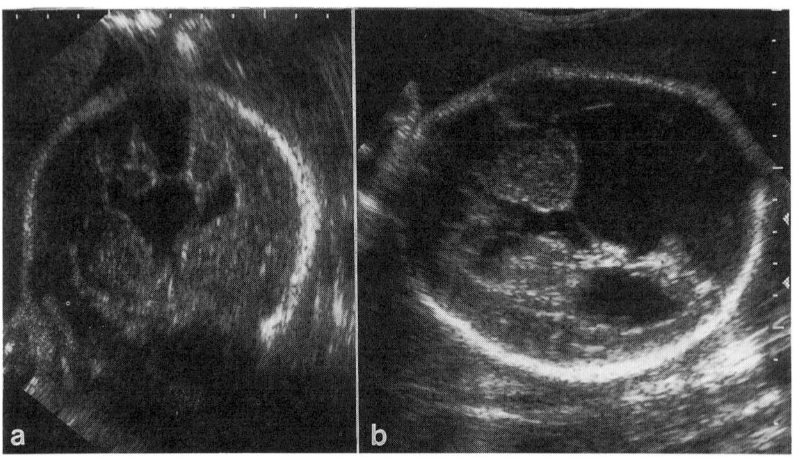

Figure 19. Porencephalic cyst at 34 postmenstrual weeks. **(a)** Midcoronal-1 section. **(b)** Horizontal section.

may be unilateral or bilateral and appear along the course of the middle cerebral artery—that is, the lateral sulcus. The occlusion of this artery may play a role in the generation of this cleft (135).

The differential diagnosis includes holoprosencephaly arachnoid cysts (bilateral) and hydranencephaly. It can be associated with ventriculomegaly, AGCC, absent cavum septi pellucidi, and septo-optic dysplasia.

The prognosis is dependent upon the type and the extent of the lesion.

Lissencephaly and Pachygyria

Lissencephaly (agyria) or smooth brain surface is a rare anomaly which is a neuronal migrational disorder occurring together with pachygyria or macrogyria consisting of wide and large, but few, gyri (136–138).

Sonographically, the diagnosis not only is hard to establish, but, if feasible, is accomplished late in gestation (26–28 postmenstrual weeks). This is due to the fact that normal development of the gyration occurs towards the end of the second trimester.

Clinical syndromes associated with these abnormalities of the cortical surface of the brain are Miller–Diecker syndrome, Norman–Roberts syndrome, chromosomal abnormalities, Walker–Warburg syndrome, and Fukuyama congenital muscular dystrophy, among others (139–141).

The outcome in this disease is generally very poor. Depending on the syndrome of which this disorder is part of, the outcome may also be lethal.

Tumors of the Brain

Tumors of the fetal brain are rare. At birth, they represent less than 1% of all tumors. Most of them are teratomas, craniopharyngiomas, and hemangioblastomas (133). The teratomas of the fetal brain usually arise from the pineal gland and distort the third ventricle. Hydrocephalus is the rule, since the space occupying lesion obliterates the flow of the CSF. Sonographically, they may appear as cystic with hyperechoic areas or foci.

Fetal intracranial teratomas have been detected by sonography (142–150). At times, it is hard to identify the structures in general or the midline structures which usually present the point of reference in the localization of pathological structures in the brain. This is due to the distortion created by the tumor. At times, distortion of the skull, the face, and the orbits may also be seen. Fetal hydrops and high-output cardiac failure were also described (149).

The prognosis for the fetus/neonate with teratoma of the brain is hopeless. Some infants survived up to one and a half years of age, but severe neurological impairment and, later, demise was unavoidable. The prognosis for the neonate depends upon the size of the tumor, the extent of brain destruction, the degree of hydrocephalus, and other associated effects of the tumor itself.

Choroid I plexus papillomas are benign tumors of the choroid plexus and fortunately are quite rare (151,152). This tumor may cause hydrocephalus due to its space-occupying nature. However, overproduction of the CSF alone may also lead to dilatation of the ventricles. Sonographic examination is usually able to localize, and therefore determine the nature of, the lesion originating from within the ventricles.

Intracranial Hemorrhage

Intracranial hemorrhage rarely occurs in utero. It may be caused by hypoxemia, congenital vascular defects, blood clotting defects, ingestion of drugs, maternal complications, and thrombosis of the umbilical cord or its entanglement (153–158). At times, trauma may also result in intracranial hemorrhage (159,160).

Periventricular hemorrhage may also occur in utero; however, its incidence is not known.

The end result of intracranial hemorrhage may be porencephaly. Grant (161) published the transformation of hemorrhage in the intrapareuchimal brain tissue into porencephalic cysts.

The neurodevelopmental prognosis of fetuses with intracranial hemorrhages is grossly unknown, and it is related to the severity and the location of the hemorrhage.

Intracerebellar hemorrhage was also reported (162,163). These appear as echogenic masses in the posterior fossa, namely the area of the cerebellum. Their differential diagnosis is a tumor in the posterial fossa. Unfavorable outcome of all the cases published in the literature is evident.

Subdural hemorrhages have been reported and connected to trauma sustained during the prenatal period (164,165).

Infections of the Fetal Brain

Infection reaches the fetal CNS usually through a transplacental passage. Toxoplasmosis, rubella, cytomegalovirus, and herpes are the most prominent and documented infections. The intracranial sonographic findings of infections are microcephaly, hydrocephalus, intracranial hyperechogenicities (calcifications?), cerebellar hypoplasia, an enlarged cerebellopeduncular cistern, periventricular cysts, and ischemic destructive sequelae, such as porencephaly, hydroanencephaly, and polymicrogyria (166–172). It is interesting to state that these intracranial, hyperechoic foci, or calcifications do not cast an acoustic shadow (173).

Prenatal diagnosis of fetal CMV infection should rely on a combination of diagnostic tests such as serology, amniotic fluid, cultures, and ultrasonography. Although sonographic diagnosis is feasible, this may not be obvious before the second trimester, at which time the lesions within the liver should also be looked for.

The intracranial sonographic findings of fetal *toxoplasmosis* include the intracranial calcifications, hydrocephalus, microcephaly, brain atrophy, and hydranencephaly (174). It should be noted that hydrocephaly is present in almost 75% of the cases; however, intracranial calcifications are present in a minority of the cases (less than 20%). If they are present, the intracranial calcifications are multifocal and located in the periventricular area, the white matter, the cortex, and the basal ganglia. One may consider other extracranial sonographic findings such as a thick placenta, liver echogenicities, hepatomegaly, ascites, and pericardial or pleural effusion (172,175).

Congenital *rubella* may also cause sonographically detectable pathology in the fetal brain. These are subependymal dependable cysts in the caudate nucleus, echogenic foci in the basal ganglia, and microcephaly (176,177).

It should be noted that the infections create subtle changes in the fetal brain tissue, in which case high-frequency transducers (i.e., TVS) may be of real value. Other indirect signs such as dilatation of the ventricles or microcephaly can be detected using high TAS.

SUMMARY AND CONCLUSIONS

Fetal neuroscan in general and using TVS in particular can detect the overwhelming majority of early developing structural anomalies of the CNS. As structures develop, this imaging modality can also diagnose those pathologies which occur later in gestation.

To achieve a high-level diagnostic performance, one must renew the basic knowledge in anatomy and development of the fetal brain and employ high-resolution ultrasound machines operated by skillfully trained sonographers and sonologists.

The time of the "one shot" axial plane by TAS as the "gold standard" of "evaluating the fetal brain" is long over!

REFERENCES

1. Babcock DS, Han BK, LeQuesne GW. B-mode gray scale ultrasound of the head in the newborn and young infant. *AJR* 1980;134:457–468.
2. Johnson ML, Rumack CM. Ultrasonic evaluation of the neonatal brain. *Radiol Clin North Am* 1980;18:117–131.
3. Ben-Ora A, Eddy L, Hatch G, et al. The anterior fontanelle as an acoustic window to the neonatal ventricular system. *J Clin Ultrasound* 1980;8:65–67.
4. Dewbury KC, Aluwihare APR. The anterior fontanelle as an ultrasound window for study of the brain: a preliminary report. *Br J Radiol* 1980;53:81–84.
5. Grant EG, Schelligner D, Borts FT, et al. Real-time sonography of the neonatal and infant head. *AJR* 1981;136:265–270.
6. Slovis TL, Kuhns LR. Real-time sonography of the brain through the anterior fontanelle. *AJR* 1981;136:277–286.
7. Edwards MK, Brown DL, Muller J, et al. Cribside neurosonography: real-time sonography for intracranial investigation of the neonate. *AJR* 1981;136:271–276.
8. Richardson DJ, Grant EG. Scanning techniques and normal anatomy. In Grant GE (ed). *Neurosonography of the preterm neonate.* New York: Springer-Verlag, 1986:1–24.
9. Naidich TP, Yousefzadeh DK, Gusnard DA. Sonography of the normal neonatal head. Supratentorial structures: state of the art imaging. *Neuroradiology* 1986;28:408–427.
10. Timor-Tritsch IE, Farine D, Rosen MG. A close look at early embryonic development with the high-frequency transvaginal transducer. *Am J Obstet Gynecol* 1988;159:676–681.
11. Kushnir U, Shalev J, Bronshtein M, et al. Fetal intracranial anatomy in the first trimester of pregnancy: transvaginal ultrasonographic evaluation. *Neuroradiology* 1989;31: 222–225.

12. Timor-Tritsch IE, Monteagudo A, Warren WB. Transvaginal ultrasonographic definition of the central nervous system in the first and early second trimesters. *Am J Obstet Gynecol* 1991;164:747–753.
13. Warren WB, Timor-Tritsch IE, Peisner DB, et al. Dating the early pregnancy by sequential appearance of embryonic structures. *Am J Obstet Gynecol* 1989;161:747–753.
14. Timor-Tritsch IE, Peisner DB, Raju S. Sonoembryology: an organ-oriented approach using a high-frequency vaginal probe. *J Clin Ultrasound* 1990;18:286–298.
15. Timor-Tritsch IE, Blumenfeld Z, Rottem S. Sonoembryology. In Timor-Tritsch IE, Rottem S (eds). *Transvaginal sonography,* 2nd ed. New York: Chapman & Hall, 1991:241.
16. Timor-Tritsch IE, Monteagudo A. Transvaginal sonographic evaluation of the fetal central nervous system. *Obstet Gynecol Clin North Am* 1991;18:713–748.
17. Achiron R, Achiron A. Transvaginal ultrasonic assessment of the early fetal brain. *Ultrasound Obstet Gynecol* 1991;1:336–344.
18. Blaas HG, Eik-Nes SH, Kiserud T, et al. Early development of the forebrain and midbrain: a longitudinal ultrasound study from 7 to 12 postmenstrual weeks of gestation. *Ultrasound Obstet Gynecol* 1994;4:183–192.
19. Blaas HG, Eik-Nes SH, Kiserud T, et al. Early development of the hindbrain: a longitudinal ultrasound study from 7 to 12 weeks of gestation. *Ultrasound Obstet Gynecol* 1995;5:151–160.
20. Monteagudo A, Reuss ML, Timor-Tritsch IE. Imaging the fetal brain in the second and third trimesters using transvaginal sonography. *Obstet Gynecol* 1991;77:27–32.
21. Blaas HG, Eik-Nes SH, Kiserud T, et al. Three-dimensional imaging of the brain cavities in human embryos. *Ultrasound Obstet Gynecol* 1995;5:228–232.
22. Monteagudo A, Timor-Tritsch IE, Reuss ML, et al. Transvaginal sonography of the second and third trimester fetal brain. In Timor-Tritsch IE, Rottem S (eds). *Transvaginal sonography,* 2nd ed. New York: Chapman & Hall, 1991:393–425.
23. Monteagudo A, Timor-Tritsch IE, Moomjy M. Nomograms of the fetal lateral ventricles using transvaginal sonography. *J Ultrasound Med* 1993;5:265–269.
24. Timor-Tritsch IE, Monteagudo A. Transvaginal fetal neurosonography: standardization of the planes and sections by anatomic landmarks. *Ultrasound Obstet Gynecol.* 1996; 8:42–47.
25. Malinger G, Zakut H. The corpus callosum: normal fetal development as shown by transvaginal sonography. *AJR* 1993;161:1041–1043.
26. Monteagudo A, Timor-Tritsch IE. Development of fetal gyri, sulci and fissures: a transvaginal sonographic study. *Ultrasound Obstet Gynecol* 1997;9:222–228.
27. Cohen HL, Ziprkowski M. New diagnostic insight in pediatric neurosonography. *Diagn Imag* 1991;13:142–146.
28. Grant E, Richardson J. Infant and neonatal neurosonography technique and normal anatomy. In Taveras J (ed). *Radiology diagnosis–imaging–intervention,* vol 3. Philadelphia: Lippincott, 1994:1–7.
29. *Nomina anatomica,* 6th ed. Authorized by the 12th International Congress of Anatomists, London, 1985. Edinburgh: Churchill Livingstone, 1989.
30. O'Rahilly R, Müller F. Ventricular system and choroid plexuses of the human brain during the embryonic period proper. *Am J Anat* 1990;189:285–302.
31. O'Rahilly R, Müller F. Embryonic length and cerebral landmarks in stages human embryos. *Anat Rec* 1984;209:265–271.

32. Westergard E. The lateral cerebral ventricles of human fetuses with a crown rump length of 26–178 mm. *Acta Anat* 1971;409–421.
33. Denkhaus H, Winsberg F. Ultrasonic measurement of the fetal ventricular system. *Radiology* 1979;131:781–787.
34. Jeanty P, Dramaix-Wilmet M, Delbeke D, et al. Ultrasonic evaluation of fetal ventricular growth. *Neuroradiology* 1981;21:127–133.
35. Pretorious DH, Rose JA, Manco-Johnson ML. Exclusion of fetal ventriculomegaly with a single measurement of the width of the lateral ventricular atrium. *Radiology* 1988; 169:711.
36. Lustig-Gillman I, Snyder JR, Silverman F, et al. Sonographic anatomy of the fetal cerebral ventricles, with reference to the early diagnosis of hydrocephaly. *J Pernat Med* 1984;12:185–191.
37. Goldstein I, Reece EA, Pilu G, et al. Sonographic evaluation of the normal developmental anatomy of fetal cerebral ventricles. I. The frontal horn. *Obstet Gynecol* 1988;72:588–592.
38. Pilu G, Reece EA, Goldstein I, et al. Sonographic evaluation of normal developmental anatomy of the fetal cerebral ventricles. II. The atria. *Obstet Gynecol* 1989;73:250–256.
39. Goldstein I, Reece EA, Pilu G, et al. Sonographic evaluation of the normal developmental anatomy of the fetal cerebral ventricles. IV. The posterior horn. *Am J Perinatol* 1990;7:79–83.
40. Goldstein I, Reece EA, Pilu G, et al. Sonographic assessment of the fetal frontal lobe: a potential tool for the prenatal diagnosis of microcephaly. *Am J Obstet Gynecol* 1988; 158:1057–1062.
41. Cardoza JD, Goldstein RB, Filly RA. Exclusion of fetal ventriculomegaly with a single measurement of the width of the lateral ventricular atrium. *Radiology* 1988;169:711.
42. Campbell S. Diagnosis of fetal abnormalities by ultrasound. In Milunsky A (ed). *Genetic disorders and the fetus*. New York: Plenum, 1979:431–467.
43. Hadlock FP, Deter RL, Park SK. Real-time sonography: ventricular and vascular anatomy of the fetal brain in utero. *AJR* 1981;136:133–137.
44. Monteagudo A, Timor-Tritsch IE, Moomjy M. In utero detection of ventriculomegaly during the second and third trimesters by transvaginal sonography. *Ultrasound Obstet Gynecol* 1994;4:193–198.
45. Lemire RJ, Loeser JD, Leech RW, et al. *Normal and abnormal development of the human nervous system*. New York: Harper & Row, 1975:260–277.
46. Pilu G, Sandri R, Perolo A, et al. Sonography of fetal agenesis of the corpus callosum: a survey of 35 cases. *Ultrasound Obstet Gynecol* 1993;3:318–329.
47. Laing FC, Stamler CE, Jeffrey BR. Ultrasonography of the fetal subarachnoid space. *J Ultrasound Med* 1983;2:29–32.
48. Goldstein I, Reece EA, Pilu G, et al. Cerebellar measurements with ultrasonography in the evaluation of fetal growth and development. *Am J Obstet Gynecol* 1987;156:1065–1069.
49. Hill LM, Guzick D, Fried J, et al. The transverse cerebellar diameter in estimating gestational age in the large-for-gestational-age fetus. *Obstet Gynecol* 1990;75:983–992.
50. Slagle TA, Oliphant M, Gross SJ. Cingulate sulcus development in preterm infants. *Pediatr Res* 1989;26:598–602.
51. Martin JH (ed). *Neuroanatomy: text and atlas*. New York: Elsevier, 1989.

52. Predanic M, Zudenigo D, Funduk-Kurjak B, et al. Assessment of early normal pregnancy. In Kuriak A (ed). *An atlas of transvaginal color doppler: the current state of the art.* London: Parthenon Publishing, 1994:51–69.
53. Van den Wijngard JAG, Groanengerg IAL, Wladimiroff JW, et al. Cerebral Doppler ultrasound of the human fetus. *Br J Obstet Gynaecol* 1989;96:845–849.
54. Wladimiroff JW, van den Wijngaard JAGW, Degani S, et al. Cerebral and umbilical arterial blood flow velocity waveforrns in normal and growth-retarded pregnancies. *Obstet Gynecol* 1987;69:705–709.
55. Vyas S, Nicolaides KH, Bower S, et al. Middle cerebral artery flow velocity waveforms in fetal hypoxemia. *Br J Obstet Gynaecol* 1990;97:797–803.
56. Mari G, Moise KJ, Deter RL, et al. Doppler assessment of the pulsatility index in cerebral circulation of the human fetus. *Am J Obstet Gynecol* 1989;160:698–703.
57. Hata K, Hata T, Makihara K, et al. Fetal intracranial arterial hemodynamics assessed by color and pulsed Doppler ultrasound. *Int J Gynecol Obstet* 1991;35:139–145.
58. Ferrazi E, Gementi P, Bellotti M, et al. Doppler velocimetry: critical analysis of umbilical cerebral and aortic reference values. *Eur J Obstet Gynecol Reprod Biol* 1991;38:189–196.
59. Satoh S, Kojanagi T, Hara K, et al. Developmental characteristics of blood flow in the middle cerebral artery in the human fetus in utero, assessed using the linear assay-pulsed Doppler method. *Early Hum Dev* 1988;17:195–203.
60. Veille JC, Hanson R, Tatum K. Longitudinal quantitation of middle cerebral artery blood flow in normal human fetuses. *Am J Obstet Gynecol* 1994;169:1393–1398.
61. Mari G, Deter RL. Middle cerebral artery flow velocity waveforms in normal and small-for-gestational-age fetuses. *Am J Obstet Gynecol* 1992;166:1262–1270.
62. Meerman RJ, Van Bel F, Van Zuiten PH, et al. Fetal and neonatal cerebral blood velocity in the normal fetus and neonate. *Early Hum Dev* 1990;24:209–217.
63. Degani S, Lewinsky R. Fetal and neonatal circulation in ultrasonography of the prenatal and neonatal brain. In Timor-Tritsch IE, Monteagudo A, Cohen H (eds). *Ultrasonography of the prenatal and nenonatal brain.* Stamford, CT: Appleton & Lange, 1996: 347–402.
64. American College of Obstetricians and Gynecologists (ACOG). Alpha-fetoprotein. Washington, DC: ACOG, 1991. ACOG technical bulletin 154.
65. O'Rahilly R, Müller F. The nervous system. In *Human embryology & teratology.* New York: Wiley-Liss, 1992.
66. Marin-Padilla M. Cephalic axial skeletal–neural dysraphia disorders: embryology and pathology. *Can J Neural Sci* 1991;18:153–169.
67. Müller F, O'Rahilly R. Cerebral dysraphia (future anencephaly) in a human twin embryo at stage 13. *Teratology* 1984;30:167–177.
68. Müller F, O'Rahilly R. Development of anencephaly and its variants. *Am J Anat* 1991;190:193–218.
69. Bronshtein M, Ornoy A. Acrania: anencephaly resulting from secondary degeneration of a closed neural tube: two cases in the same family. *J Clin Ultrasound* 1991;19:230–234.
70. Rottem S, Bronshtein M, Thaler I, et al. First trimester transvaginal sonographic diagnosis of fetal anomalies. *Lancet* 1989;1:444–445.
71. Greenebaum E, Mansakhani MM, Heller DS, Timor-Tritsch IE. Open neural tube defects: immunocytochemical demonstration of neuroepithelial cells in amniotic fluid. *Diagn Cytopathol* 1997;16(2):143–144.

72. Timor-Tritsch IE, Greenebaum E, Monteagudo A, Baxi L. The exencephaly–anencephaly sequence: proof by ultrasound imaging and amniotic fluid cytology. *Matern Fet Med* 1996;5:182–185.

73. Campbell S, Johnstone FD, Holt EM, et al. Anencephalus: early ultrasonic diagnosis and active management. *Lancet* 1972;2:1226.

74. Rodriguez MM, Reik RA, Carreno TD, et al. Cluster of iniencephaly in Miami. *Pediatr Pathol* 1991;11:211–221.

75. Aleksic SN, Budzilovich GN. Iniencephaly. In Myrianthopoulos NC (ed). *Handbook of clinical neurology,* vol 6. Amsterdam: Elsevier, 1987:129–136.

76. Foderaro AE, Abu-Yousef MM, Benda JA, et al. Antenatal ultrasound diagnosis of iniencephaly. *J Clin Ultrasound* 1987;15:550–554.

77. Shoham (Schwatz) Z, Caspi B, Chemke J, et al. Iniencephaly: prenatal ultrasonographic diagnosis—a case report. *J Perinat Med* 1988;16:139–143.

78. Bronshtein M, Timor-Tritsch IE, Rottem S. Early detection of fetal anomalies. In Timor-Tritsch IE, Rottem S (eds). *Transvaginal sonography.* New York: Chapman & Hall, 1991: 327–371.

79. Icenogle DA, Kaplan AM. A review of congenital neurologic malformations. *Clin Pediatr* 1981;9:565–576.

80. Hidalgo H, Bowie J, Rosenberg ER, et al. In utero sonographic diagnosis of fetal cerebral anomalies. *AJR* 1982;139:143–148.

81. Chervenak FA, Isaacson G, Mahoney MF, et al. Diagnosis and management of fetal cephalocele. *Obstet Gynecol* 1984;64:86–90.

82. Naidich TP, Altman NR, Braffman BH, et al. Cephaloceles and related malformations. *Am J Neuroradiol* 1992;13:655–690.

83. Fleming AD, Vintzileos AM, Scorza WE. Prenatal diagnosis of occipital encephalocele with transvaginal sonography. *J Ultrasound Med* 1991;10:285–286.

84. Goldstein I, Reece EA, Pilu G, et al. Sonographic evaluation of the normal developmental anatomy of the fetal cerebral ventricles. IV. The posterior horn. *Perinatology* 1990; 7:79–83.

85. Monteagudo A, Timor-Tritsch IE. Cephalocele, anterior. *Fetus* 1992;2:(4):1–4.

86. Brown MS, Sheridan-Pereira M. Outlook for the child with a cephalocele. *Pediatrics* 1992;90:914–919.

87. Cullen MT, Athanassiadis AP, Romero R. Prenatal diagnosis of anterior parietal encephalocele with transvaginal sonography. *Obstet Gynecol* 1990;75:489–491.

88. Yokota A, Kajiwara H, Kohchi M, et al. Parietal cephalocele: clinical importance of its atretetic form and associated malformations. *J Neurosurg* 1988;69:545–551.

89. Nadel AS, Bromley BS, Frigoletto FD, et al. Isolated choroid plexus cysts in the second trimester fetus: Is amniocentesis really indicated? *Radiology* 1992;185:545–548.

90. Gabrielli S, Reece EA, Pilu G, et al. The clinical significance of prenatally diagnosed choroid plexus cysts. *Am J Obstet Gynecol* 1989;160:1207–1210.

91. Achiron R, Barkai G, Katzenelson B, et al. Fetal lateral ventricle choroid plexus cysts: the dilemma of amniocentesis. *Obstet Gynecol* 1991;78:815–818.

92. Chinn DH, Miller EI, Worthy LM, et al. Sonographically detected fetal choroid plexus cysts: frequency and association with aneuploidy. *J Ultrasound Med* 1991;10:255–258.

93. Gross ST, Shulman LP, Tolley EA, et al. Isolated fetal choroid plexus cysts and trisomy 18: a review and meta-analysis. *Am J Obstet Gynecol* 1995;172:83–87.

94. Hertzberg BS, Kay HH, Bowie JD. Fetal choroid plexus lesions. Relationship of antenatal sonographic appearance to clinical outcome. *J Ultrasound Med* 1989;8:77–82.

95. Kupferminc MJ, Tamure RK, Sabbagha RE, et al. Isolated choroid plexus cyst(s): an indication for amniocentesis. *Am J Obstet Gynecol* 1994;171:1068–1071.

96. Porto M, Murata Y, Warneke LA, et al. Fetal choroid plexus cysts: an independent risk factor for chromosomal anomalies. *J Clin Ultrasound* 1993;21:103–108.

97. Platt LD, Carlson DE, Medearis AL, et al. Fetal choroid plexus in the second trimester of pregnancy: a cause for concern. *Am J Obstet Gynecol* 1991;164:1652–1656.

98. Sarno AP, Polzin WJ, Kalish VB. Fetal choroid plexus cyst in association with cri du chat (5p-) syndrome. *Am J Obstet Gynecol* 1993;169:1614–1615.

99. Habib Z. Genetics and genetic counselling in neonatal hydrocephalus. *Obstet Gynecol Surv* 1981;36:529.

100. Mealy J Jr, Gilmor RL, Bubb MP. The prognosis of hydrocephalus overt at birth. *J Neurosurg* 1973;39:348–355.

101. Burton BK. Recurrence risks for congenital hydrocephalus. *Clin Genet* 1979;16:47.

102. Friedman JM, Santos-Ramos R. Natural history of X-linked aqueductal stenosis in the second and third trimesters of pregnancy. *Am J Obstet Gynecol* 1984;150:104–106.

103. Brocard O, Raggage C, Vilbert M, et al. Prenatal diagnosis of X-linked hydrocephalus. *J Clin Ultrasound* 1993;21:211–214.

104. Benacerraf BR, Birnholz JC. The diagnosis of fetal hydrocephalus prior to 22 weeks. *J Clin Ultrasound* 1987;15:531–536.

105. Bronshtein M, Ben-Schlomo I. Choroid plexus dysmorphism: a sonographic sign of fetal hydrocephalus. *J Clin Ultrasound* 1991;19:547–553.

106. Monteagudo A, Timor-Tritsch IE, Moomjy M. In utero detection of ventriculomegaly during the second and third trimesters by transvaginal sonography. *Ultrasound Obstet Gynecol* 1994;4:193–198.

107. Pretorius DH, Drose JA, Manco-Johnson ML. Fetal lateral ventricular ratio determination during the second-trimester. *J Ultrasound Med* 1986;5:121–124.

108. Cardoza ID, Goldstein RB, Filly RA. Exclusion of fetal ventriculomegaly with a single measurement of the width of the lateral ventricular atrium. *Radiology* 1988;169:711–714.

109. Cardoza JD, Filly RA, Podrasky AE. The dangling choroid plexus: a sonographic observation of value in excluding ventriculomegaly. *AJR* 1988;151:767–770.

110. Monteagudo A, Timor-Tritsch IE, Moomjy M. Nomograms of the fetal lateral ventricles using transvaginal sonography. *J Ultrasound Med* 1993;5:265–269.

111. Pretorius DH, Davis K, Manco-Johnson ML, et al. Clinical course of fetal hydrocephalus: 40 cases. *AJR* 1985;144:827–831.

112. Nyberg AD, Mack LA, Hirsch J, et al. Fetal hydrocephalus: sonographic detection and clinical significance of associated anomalies. *Radiology* 1987;163:187–191.

113. Hudgins RJ, Edwards MSB, Goldstein R, et al. Natural history of fetal ventriculomeagaly. *Pediatrics* 1988;82:692–697.

114. Mahony BS, Nyberg DA, Hirsch JH, et al. Mild idiopathic lateral cerebral ventricular dilatation in utero: sonographic evaluation. *Radiology* 1988;169:715–721.

115. Bromley B, Frigoletto FD, Benacerraf BR. Mild fetal lateral cerebral ventriculomegaly: clinical course and outcome. *Am J Obstet Gynecol* 1991;164:863–867.

116. Achiron R, Schimmel M, Achiron A, et al. Fetal mild idiopathic lateral ventriculomegaly: Is there a correlation with fetal trisomy? *Ultrasound Obstet Gynecol* 1993;3:89–92.

117. Matsunaga E, Shiota Y. Holoprosencephaly in human embryos: epidemiological studies of 150 cases. *Teratology* 1977;16:261.

118. Pilu G, Sandri F, Perolo A, et al. Prenatal diagnosis of lobar holoprosencephaly. *Ultrasound Obstet Gynecol* 1992;2:88.

119. Grogono JL. Children with agenesis of the corpus callosum. *Dev Med Child Neurol* 1968;10:613.

120. Jellinger F, Gross H, Kaltenback E. Holoprosencephaly and agenesis of the corpus callosum frequency of associated malformations. *Acta Neurol Pathol* 1981;55:1–10.

121. Jeret JS, Serur D, Wisniewiski K, et al. Frequency of agenesis of the corpus callosum in the developmentally disabled population as determined by computerized tomography. *Pediatr Neurosci* 1986;12:101.

122. DeMyer W, Zeman W. Alobar holoprosencephaly (arhinencephaly) with median cleft lip and palate: clinical electroencephalographic and nosologic considerations. *Confin Neurol* 1963;23:1.

123. Pilu G, Perolo A, David C. Midline anomalies of the brain. In Timor-Tritsch IE, Monteagudo A, Cohen HL (eds). *Ultrasonography of the prenatal and neonatal brain.* Stamford, CT: Appleton & Lange, 1996:241–258.

124. Mulligan G, Meier P. Lipoma and agenesis of the corpus callosum with associated choroid plexus lipomas. In utero diagnosis. *J Ultrasound Med* 1989;8:583.

125. Baarsma R, Martijn A, Okken A. The missing pericallosal artery on sonography. A sign of agenesis of the corpus callosum in the neonatal brain? *Neuroradiology* 1987;29:47.

126. Pilu G, Sandri F, Perolo A, et al. Sonography of fetal agenesis of the corpus callosum: a survey of 35 cases. *Ultrasound Obstet Gynecol* 1993;3:318–329.

127. Osenback RK, Menezes AH. Diagnosis and management of the Dandy–Walker malformation: 30 years of experience. *Pediatr Neurosurg* 1991;18:179.

128. Gardner E, O'Rahilly R, Prolo D. Dandy–Walker and Arnold–Chiari malformations: clinical, developmental and teratological considerations. *Arch Neurol* 1975;32:393–407.

129. Murray JC, Johnson JA, Bird RD. Dandy–Walker malformation: etiologic heterogeneity and empiric recurrence risk. *Clin Genet* 1985;28:272.

130. Sawaya R, McLaurin RL. Dandy–Walker syndrome: clinical analysis of 23 cases. *J Neurosurg* 1981;55:89.

131. Hirsch JF, Pierre Kahn A, Reiner D, et al. The Dandy–Walker malformation. A review of 40 cases. *J Neurosurg* 1984;61:515.

132. Osborn AG. Miscellaneous tumors, cysts and metastases. In *Diagnostic neuroradiology.* St. Louis: Mosby-Year Book, 1994:639–642.

133. Richard KE, Dahl K, Sanker P. Long-term followup of children and juveniles with arachnoid cysts. *Childs Nerv Syst* 1989;5:184–187.

134. Marinov M, Undjian S, Wezka P. An evaluation of the surgical treatment of intracranial cysts in children. *Childs Nerv Syst* 1989;5:177–1893.

135. Messer J, Haddad J, Casanova R. Transcranial Doppler evaluation of cerebral infarction in the neonate. *Neuropediatrics* 1990;22:147–151.

136. Dobyns WB, Kirkpatrick JB, Hittner HM, et al. Syndromes with Lissencephaly. II. Walker–Warburg and cerebro-oculo-muscular syndrome and a new syndrome with type II lissencephaly. *Am J Med Genet* 1985;22:157–195.

137. Banna M, Malabarey T. Lissencephaly and pachygyria. *Can J Assoc Radiol* 1989;40: 156–158.

138. Dobyns WB, Greenberg F. Syndromes with lissencephaly type I: Miller–Dierker and Norman–Roberts syndromes and isolated lissencephaly. *Am J Med Genet* 1984;18: 509–526.

139. Volpe JJ. Neuronal proliferation, migration, organization and myelination. In Volpe JJ (ed). *Neurology of the Newborn,* 3rd ed. Philadelphia: WB Saunders, 1995:97–98.

140. Byrd SE, Osborn RE, Bohan TP, et al. The CT and MR evaluation of migrational disorders of the brain. *Pediatr Radiol* 1989;19:151–156.

141. Dobyns WB. Developmental aspects of lissencephaly and the lissencephaly syndromes. *Birth Defects* 1987;23(1):225–241.

142. Wakai S, Arai T, Nagai M. Congenital brain tumors. *Surg Neurol* 1984;21:597–609.

143. Hoff NR, Mackay IM. Prenatal ultrasound diagnosis of intracranial teratoma. *Clin Perinatol* 1979;6:293–319.

144. Kirkinen P, Suramo I, Jouppila P, et al. Combined use of ultrasound and computed tomography in the evaluation of fetal intracranial abnormality. *J Perinat Med* 1982;10: 257–265.

145. Paes BA, DeSa DJ, Hunter DJ, et al. Benign intracranial teratoma—prenatal diagnosis influencing early delivery. *Am J Obstet Gynecol* 1982;143:600–601.

146. Smith WL, Menezes A, Franken EA. Cranial ultrasound in the diagnosis of malignant brain tumors. *J Clin Ultrasound* 1983;11:97–100.

147. Cappe IP, Lam AH. Ultrasound diagnosis of chorioid plexus papilloma. *J Clin Ultrasound* 1985;13:121–123.

148. Ferreira J, Eviatar L, Schneider S, et al. Prenatal diagnosis of intracranial teratoma. Prolonged survival after resection of a malignant teratoma diagnosed prenatally by ultrasound: a case report and literature review. *Pediatr Neurosurg* 1993;19:84–88.

149. Sherer DM, Abramowicz JS, Eggeres PC, et al. Prenatal ultrasonographic diagnosis of intracranial teratoma and massive craniomegaly with associated high-output cardiac failure. *Am J Obstet Gynecol* 1993;168:97–99.

150. Ulreich S, Hanieh A, Furness ME. Positive outcome of fetal intracranial teratoma. *J Ultrasound Med* 1993;3:163–165.

151. Gradin WC, Taylon C, Fruin AH. Choroid plexus papilloma of the third ventricle: case report and review of the literature. *Neurosurgery* 1983;12:217–220.

152. Hawkins JC. Treatment of choroid plexus papilloma in children: a brief analysis of twenty years' experience. *Neurosurgery* 1980;6:380.

153. Martin R, Roessman U, Fanaroff A. Massive intracerebellar hemorrhage in low birth weight infants. *J Pediatr* 1976;89:290–293.

154. Zalneraitis EL, Young RSK, Krishnamoorthy KS. Intracranial hemorrhage in utero as a complication of isoimmune thrombocytopenia. *J Pediatr* 1979;95:611–614.

155. Jackson JC, Blumhagen JD. Congenital hydrocephalus due to prenatal intracranial hemorrhage. *Pediatrics* 1983;72:344–346.

156. Lustig-Gillman I, Young BK, Silverman F, et al. Fetal intraventricular hemorrhage: sonographic diagnosis and clinical implications. *J Clin Ultrasound* 1983;11:277–280.

157. Achiron R, Pinchas OH, Reichman B, et al. Fetal intracranial hemorrhage: clinical significance of in utero ultrasonographic diagnosis. *Br J Obstet Gynaecol* 1993;100:995–999.

158. Haidi HA, Finley J, Mallette JQ, et al. Prenatal diagnosis of cerebellar hemorrhage: medicolegal implications. *Am J Obstet Gynecol* 1994;170:1392–1395.

159. Portman M, Brouillette RT. Fetal intracranial hemorrhage complicating amniocentesis. *Am J Obstet Gynecol* 1982;144:731–735.

160. Knuppel RA, Salvatore DLD, Agarwal R, et al. Documented fetal brain damage resulting from a motor vehicle accident. *J Ultrasound Med* 1994;13:402–404.

161. Grant EG. Neurosonography: germinal matrix-related hemorrhage. In Grant EG (ed). *Neurosonography of the pre-term neonate.* New York: Springer-Verlag, 1986:31–68.

162. Fogarty K, Cohen HL, Haller JO. Sonography of fetal intracranial hemorrhage: unusual causes and a review of the literature. *J Clin Ultrasound* 1989;17:366–370.

163. Portman M, Brouillette RT. Fetal intracranial haemorrhage complicating amniocentesis. *Am J Obstet Gynecol* 1982;144:731–735.

164. Rotmensch S., Grannum PA, Nores JA, Hall C, Keller MS, McCarthy S, Hobbins AJC. In utero diagnosis and management of fetal subdural hematoma. *Am J Obstet Gynecol* 1991;164:1246–1248.

165. Kawabata I, Imai A, Tamaya T. Antenatal subdural hemorrhage causing fetal death before labor. *Int J Gynecol Obstet* 1993;43:57–60.

166. Shackelford GD, Fulling KH, Glasies CM. Cysts of the subependedymal germinal matrix: sonographic demonstration with pathologic correlation. *Radiology* 1983;149: 117–121.

167. Mittlemann-Handwerker S, Pardes JG, Post RC, et al. Fetal ventriculomegaly and brain atrophy in a woman with intrauterine cytomegalovirus infection. A case report. *J Reprod Med* 1986;11:1061–1064.

168. Butt W, Machkay RD, de Crespingy LC, et al. Intracranial lesions of congenital cytomegalovirus infection detected by ultrasound scanning. *Pediatrics* 1984;73:611–614.

169. Twickler DM, Perlman J, Maberry MC. Congenital cytomegalovirus infection presenting as cerebral ventriculomegaly on antenatal sonography. *Am J Perinatol* 1993;10:404–406.

170. Tassin GB, Maklad NF, Stewart RR, et al. Cytomegalic inclusion disease: intrauterine sonographic diagnosis using findings involving the brain. *Am J Neuroradiol* 1991;12: 117–122.

171. Achiron R, Pinchas-Hamiel O, Lipitz S, et al. Prenatal Ultrasonographic diagnosis of fetal cerebral ventriculitis associated with asymptomatic maternal cytomegalovirus infection. *Prenat Diagn* 1994;14:523–526.

172. Hohlfeld P, Mac Aleese J, Capella-Pavlovski M, et al. Fetal toxoplasmosis: ultrasonographic signs. *Ultrasound Obstet Gynecol* 1991;1:241–244.

173. Fakhry J, Khoury A. Fetal intracranial calcifications. The importance of periventricular hyperechoic foci without shadowing. *J Ultrasound Med* 1991;10:51–54.

174. Becker LE. Infections of the developing brain. *Am J Neuroradiol* 1992;13:537–549.

175. Blaakaer J. Ultrasonic diagnosis of fetal ascites and toxoplasmosis. *Acta Obstet Gynecol Scand* 1986;65:653–654.

176. Osborn AG. Infections of the brain and its linings. In *Diagnostic neuroradiology*. St. Louis: Mosby-Year Book, 1994.

177. Ayamashita Y, Matsuishi T, Murkmi Y, et al. Neuroimaging findings (ultrasonography, CT, MRI) in 3 infants with congenital rubella syndrome. *Pediatr Radiol* 1991;21: 547–549.

13

THE BRAIN-DAMAGED BABY: FETAL HEART RATE LESSONS FROM THE DATA BANK

Jeffrey P. Phelan, M.D. and Myoung Ock Ahn, M.D., Ph.D., M.P.H.

Department of Obstetrics and Gynecology, Pomona Valley Hospital Medical Center, Pasadena, California (JPP); and Department of Obstetrics and Gynecology, Cha Women's Hospital, Seoul, Korea (MOA)

INTRODUCTION

Since the introduction of electronic fetal heart rate monitoring (EFM), EFM has become an invaluable adjunct in the assessment of antepartum and intrapartum fetal well-being (1–5). The goal of EFM is to continuously assess fetal health during labor and to permit the early detection of intrapartum fetal distress. In the past, the presence of contraction-mediated fetal heart rate (FHR) decelerations such as repetitive late decelerations has served as the basis for intervention. If traditional maneuvers failed to relieve the "fetal distress" such as maternal position change, oxygen administration, intravenous fluid administration, and/or discontinuation of oxytocin after a reasonable period of time, expedited delivery would be indicated. With the increasing use of continuous EFM, intrapartum fetal death rates declined throughout the United States (6).

Asphyxia and Fetal Brain Damage, Edited by Dev Maulik, M.D., Ph.D.
ISBN 0-471-18427-6

But the question remains, Does early identification of "intrapartum fetal distress" prevent fetal neurologic injury, or is the FHR pattern merely a manifestation of underlying fetal neurologic injury? For example, as pointed out by Perkins (7), "the number of infants injured during labor is highly overestimated and the number injured prior to labor is highly underestimated."

Though Perkins' view is probably accurate, the prevailing medical and societal view is that fetal neurologic impairment occurs as a consequence of labor or events surrounding birth. This popular misconception has resulted in tremendous amounts of litigation and the belief that the obstetrician not only was responsible for a child's cerebral palsy but also could have prevented it. However, a large percentage of fetal central nervous system (CNS) injuries are unrelated to intrapartum care (8–10). Nevertheless, the intrapartum FHR tracings have been used as evidence to establish noncompliance with accepted standards of obstetrical care. The primary basis for this perception has been that changes in the FHR preceded neurologic impairment of the fetus. But, do fetuses undergo brain injury in such a manner? As suggested by several investigators (8,10–12), the FHR pattern may demonstrate underlying fetal neurologic impairment and may be more useful in identifying those fetuses who have already sustained CNS injury prior to labor.

Therefore, the purpose of this chapter is fourfold. First, we will attempt to update the literature on electronic fetal monitoring and the role of the fetal admission test to guide patient care and time fetal neurologic injury. Second, we will review the FHR patterns associated with CNS injury in the term fetus. Third, these FHR patterns will help to serve as a basis for providing intrapartum management recommendations. Fourth, we must emphasize that these FHR patterns apply to term and postdate pregnancies and may not necessarily apply to preterm or twin pregnancies. Finally, the recommendations, contained herein, do not imply or infer a standard of care for the management of intrapartum obstetrical patients. Rather, this chapter represents only a single piece of the cerebral palsy puzzle.

BACKGROUND

The assessment of fetal status with electronic EFM on admission to the hospital has been referred to as the fetal or labor admission test (13). With the use of the fetal admission test, outpatient and inpatient fetal monitoring principles are applied to the laboring patient. Here, the principal goals of the labor admission test are to identify those fetuses at high risk for intrapartum fetal distress and to reassign risk of those patients alleged to be at either a high or low risk before labor to a different risk category soon after admission to labor and delivery.

The fetal admission test in early labor using either an initial fetal monitoring period (14–16) or the fetal response to acoustic or scalp stimulation (17,18) is a more active management approach to labor than the one that waits for the fetus to dictate intervention. With this approach, the fetal admission test serves as a form of intrapartum risk assessment and provides an immediate evaluation of current fetal condition. This permits reallocation of the patient's risk status to high or low risk depending on the fetal admission test result (13). Thus, patients deemed to be at high risk upon admission to the hospital could be reassigned to low risk in the face of a normal or reactive fetal admission test. Conversely, those fetuses considered low risk on admission to the hospital could be reallocated to a high-risk category based on a suspicious or nonreactive fetal admission test result. Regardless of the patient's prior risk status, the initial admission test period redefines that risk status and can also be used to estimate when or how a fetus might be injured during a given labor.

THE REACTIVE FETAL ADMISSION TEST

A reactive admission test is associated with a low probability of an adverse fetal outcome during labor (13–18). For example, Krebs et al. (14) were able to show an inverse relationship between the number of FHR accelerations and fetal outcome (Figure 1). In that study, the presence of three or more FHR accelerations in a 30-minute window was associated with a less than 3% risk of an adverse event arising during that labor. An adverse event included, but was not limited to, umbilical cord prolapse, placental abruption, delivery-related events such as shoulder dystocia or forcep injury, or the development of an abnormal FHR pattern during labor. The likelihood of an abnormal intrapartum FHR pattern developing in labor after a reactive admission test was only 1.4% (Figure 2). Moreover, the type of fetal distress that developed in this group was characteristically acute.

A reactive FHR pattern obtained on admission to the hospital or anytime during labor is not only a sign of fetal well-being but also a sign of normal fetal acid–base status and the absence of fetal asphyxia (19–21). As demonstrated in Figure 3, fetuses

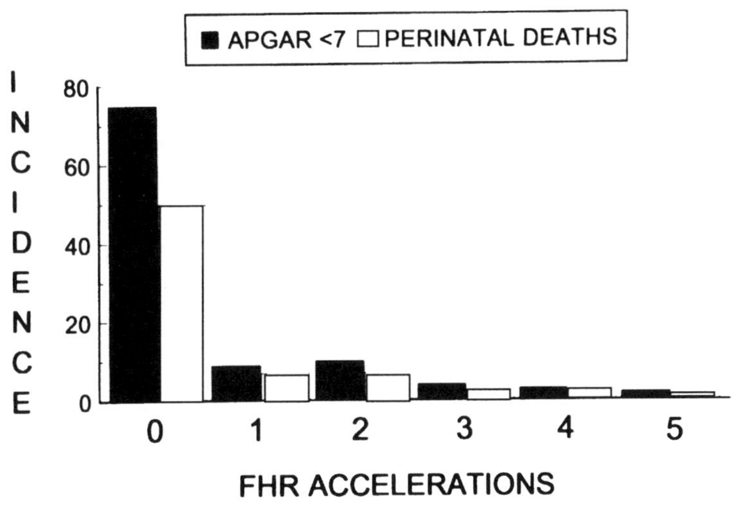

Figure 1. Perinatal outcome based on the number of fetal heart rate accelerations on admission to the hospital. (Reproduced with permission from reference 13.)

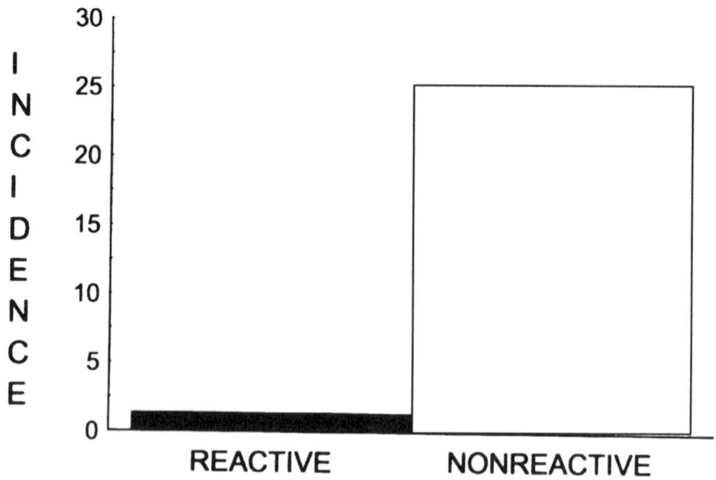

Figure 2. The incidence of intrapartum fetal distress based on the admission fetal heart rate pattern (14–16).

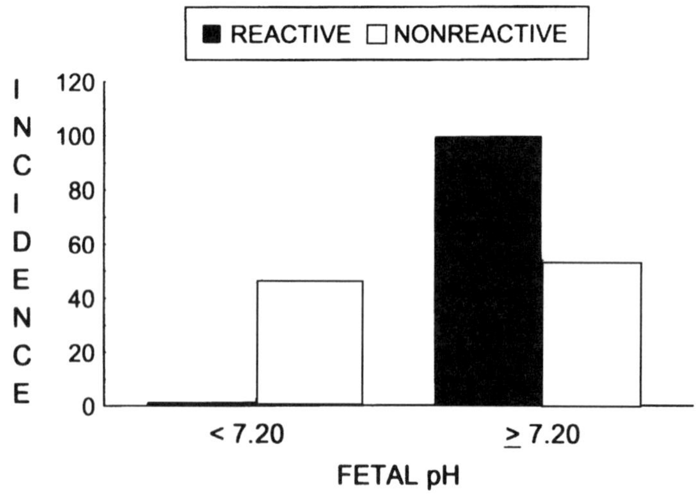

Figure 3. The relationship between intrapartum fetal acid–base status and the reactivity of the fetal heart rate (19–21).

with the ability to accelerate their heart rate were significantly more likely to have a pH of 7.20 or higher. Moreover, normal fetal acid–base status was observed regardless of whether the acceleration was spontaneous (22) or induced (19–21). Thus, a reactive FHR pattern found on admission to the labor and delivery unit signifies a lower probability of fetal distress developing during labor.

THE NONREACTIVE FETAL ADMISSION TEST

The absence of FHR accelerations (Figure 1) or fetal nonreactivity on admission to the hospital is associated with a greater probability of an adverse fetal outcome (14). In addition, there is an inverse relationship between the number of FHR accelerations, oligohydramnios (23,24), FHR decelerations (23), meconium-stained amniotic fluid (23), intrapartum fetal distress (13–16,24–26) (Figure 2), and long-term neurologic impairment (8,12,27,28). For example, if fetal nonreactivity is present for more than 120 minutes, higher rates of operative intervention, perinatal mortality, and long-term neurologic impairment are observed (13,24–26).

FHR OBSERVATIONS IN THE NEUROLOGICALLY IMPAIRED INFANT

The fetal admission test permits the clinician to assess fetal status on admission to the hospital and to place patients into groups based on their risk status that will facilitate patient management during labor. This categorization based on the fetal admission test also enables the clinician to better understand the pathogenesis of fetal neurologic injury. For example, the admission and final FHR patterns of 300 brain-damaged infants in our national registry of brain-damaged babies established in 1991 are illustrated in Figure 4 (8,27). Of these, 135 (45%) and 152 (51%) fetuses exhibited a nonreactive or reactive fetal admission test, respectively. In the remaining 13 (4%) patients, a persistent prolonged FHR deceleration or "bradycardia" from admission to

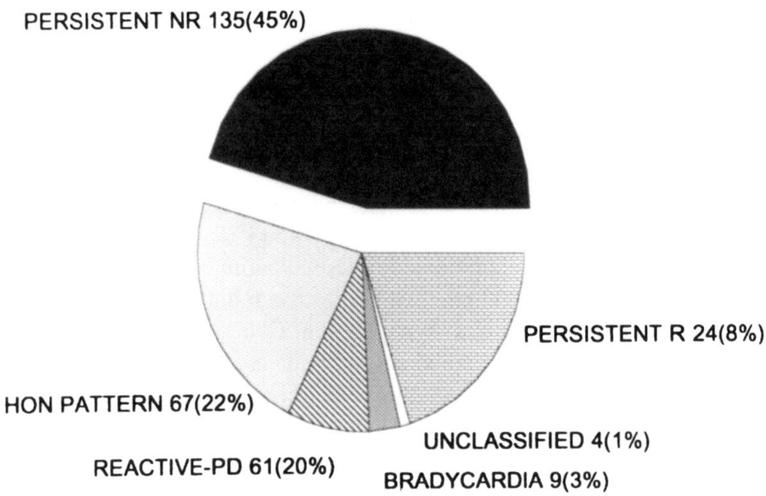

Figure 4. The admission and subsequent FHR patterns of 300 neurologically impaired neonates (FHR, fetal heart rate; PD, prolonged FHR deceleration; R, reactive; NR, nonreactive). [(Reproduced with permission from reference 27.)

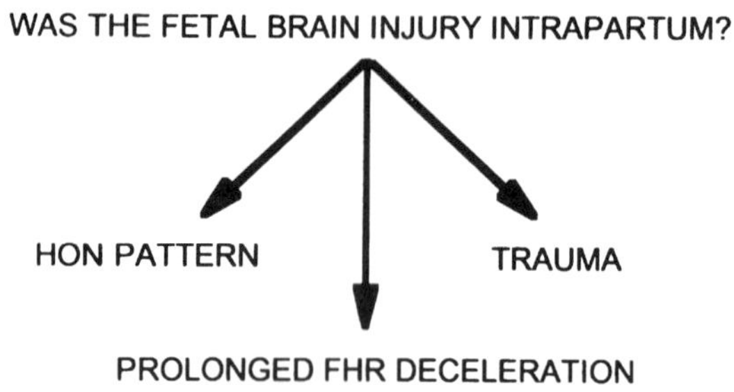

Figure 5. When a fetus has a reactive fetal admission test, fetal brain injury during labor appears to occur in one of three ways (FHR, fetal heart rate).

delivery was observed [9 (30%)] or the FHR pattern could not be classified [4 (1%)]. After admission, those patients with a reactive admission test exhibited one of the following FHR patterns giving rise to their neurologic injury: (1) a Hon FHR pattern of intrapartum asphyxia or (2) a prolonged FHR deceleration. In addition, 24 (8%) patients remained reactive throughout the course of labor and were not asphyxiated during labor (28). In contrast, the fetus with a nonreactive admission test remained nonreactive with or without FHR decelerations until delivery. Thus, a clinician with a patient who has a reactive admission test is in a better position clinically to anticipate how a fetus might be injured during a given labor (Figure 5). To better understand these principles, we will address each group individually.

THE BRAIN-DAMAGED INFANT AND THE REACTIVE FETAL ADMISSION TEST

On admission to the hospital, the overwhelming number of obstetrical patients will have a reactive FHR pattern (Figure 6). Of these, more than 98% will go through labor uneventfully and most will deliver vaginally. In the few patients (typically 1–2%) that develop intrapartum fetal distress, the type of fetal distress is characteristically, but not always, acute and manifested by a sudden prolonged FHR deceleration. Of these, an even smaller number of fetuses will ultimately manifest CNS injury.

Patients who had a persistent reactive FHR pattern during labor (Figure 4) and who are later found to have an underlying form of CNS injury represent 8% of the term brain-damaged infants we have studied (28). These fetuses were found to have sustained an early pregnancy (usually <24 weeks' gestation) insult such as lissencephaly or a postnatal insult (such as Group B streptococcal infection). In the absence of a postnatal insult, the neonatal course of those infants with an early pregnancy brain insult is usually uncomplicated and the baby and mother typically go home from the hospital at the normal time.

In contrast with the persistent reactive FHR group, fetal CNS injury in the fetus with a reactive fetal admission test may arise, in the absence of trauma, as a result of

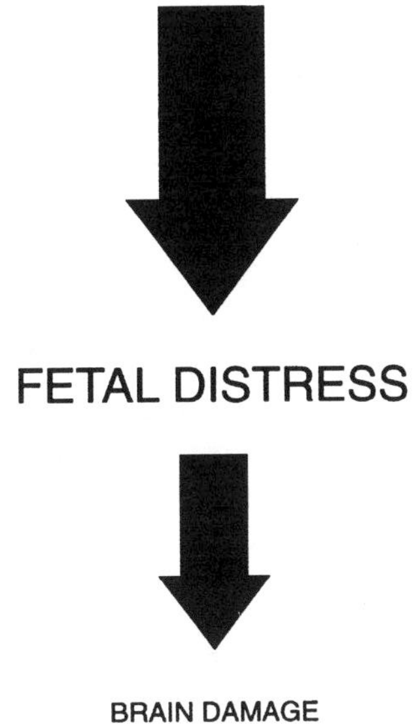

Figure 6. With a reactive fetal admission test, the likelihood of intrapartum fetal distress is less than 2% and the likelihood of fetal brain damage is even smaller (14).

a prolonged FHR deceleration or a Hon pattern of intrapartum asphyxia (Figure 5). In the former group, the FHR pattern is reactive; and, as a result of a sudden catastrophic event (Table 1), a sudden prolonged FHR deceleration to approximately 60 beats per minute (bpm) occurs and lasts until the time of delivery. As illustrated in Table 1, the prolonged FHR deceleration is associated with a wide array of patient groups such as uterine rupture, placental abruption, and cord prolapse. Given the acute nature of this FHR pattern, limited time is available to preserve normal CNS function.

Based on our experience, the timing of neurologic injury in this group depends on four factors (Table 2). First, the admission FHR pattern provides an indicator of fetal status prior to the catastrophic event. If, for example, the FHR pattern is reactive on admission and a sudden prolonged FHR deceleration occurs, the neurologic insult is most likely acute. In contrast, a prolonged FHR deceleration that follows a persistent nonreactive FHR pattern is most likely consistent with a post-asphyxial insult and represents a preterminal pattern (12).

Second, the fetal growth pattern at the time of presentation to the hospital also plays a role in the timing of fetal neurologic injury. Fetal growth, to a large extent, is dependent on the functional placental surface area (29). As such, infants who are small-, appropriate-, or large-for-gestational-age will have different functional placental surface areas available to them. As a consequence, the time interval to injury in an acute asphyxial event will depend to a large extent on the ability of the maternal–fetal unit to maintain placental exchange. For example, in infants with intrauterine growth retardation or who are small-for-gestational-age, the time to CNS injury

Table 1. Some of the catastrophic events that give rise to a sudden prolonged fetal heart rate deceleration

Uterine rupture
Cord prolapse
Fetal exsanguination
Maternal arrest

Table 2. The clinical factors to consider when determining the timing of fetal neurologic injury in situations of a sudden catastrophic event resulting in a sudden prolonged FHR deceleration[a]

Prior FHR pattern
Fetal growth pattern
Duration of the FHR deceleration
Intactness of the placenta

[a]FHR, fetal heart rate.

will be less than that for an appropriate- or a large-for-gestational-age infant. In essence, fetal growth is a reflection of either (a) the functional placental surface area available to each fetus or (b) the ability to withstand a catastrophic event for a longer period of time.

The remaining two factors in Table 2, namely, the duration of the prolonged FHR deceleration and the intactness of the placenta, are intertwined. Thus, in cases of a complete placental separation, the onset of the prolonged FHR deceleration to fetal injury interval will be shorter than if the placenta were intact. Based on the Leung study (30) in cases of uterine rupture, the interval to CNS injury was less than 18 min. Our experience (27) would suggest an even shorter time to neurologic injury of 16 minutes whenever the placenta has completely separated. If the placenta remains intact, a longer period of time appears to be available before the onset of CNS injury.

In contrast to the acute asphyxial group, the Hon pattern of intrapartum asphyxia is uniquely different and evolves over a period of time (8,27). Similar to the acute group, the Hon pattern begins with a reactive fetal admission test. Subsequently during labor, the fetus develops a nonreactive FHR pattern or a loss of reactivity (8). As the labor continues, a substantial rise in baseline heart rate from admission (135 ± 9.7 bpm) to a mean maximum (186 ± 14.5 bpm) baseline heart rate is observed (8,27). The range is 155 bpm to 220 bpm. This constitutes a 38.5 ± 13.4% mean percent rise in baseline heart rate from admission. This percent rise in baseline FHR ranges from 17% to 82%. This rise in baseline FHR is usually not accompanied by maternal pyrexia. When a substantial rise in baseline fetal heart rate is encountered, the FHR pattern is also associated with repetitive FHR decelerations and ultimately a loss of FHR variability (Figure 7) (8,27). "As labor progresses and the fetus nears death, the slope becomes progressively less steep until the FHR does not return to its baseline rate and ultimately terminates in a profound bradycardia" (12) or stairsteps-to-death

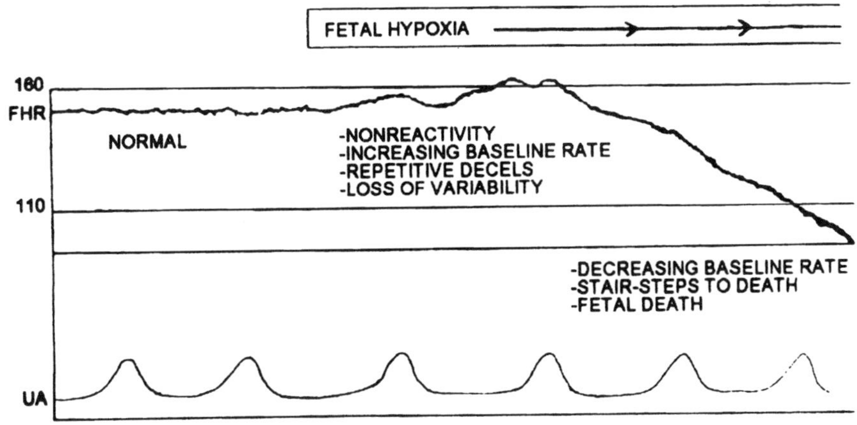

Figure 7. The characteristics of Hon's intrapartum FHR pattern are presented.

pattern (8,27). Of note, while not all fetuses will manifest an FHR tachycardia (>160 bpm), all fetuses will manifest the other changes of repetitive FHR decelerations and loss of variability (8,27).

Thus, the development of a persistent, nonreactive FHR pattern in a patient with previously reactive FHR pattern and no fever in conjunction with a substantial rise in baseline FHR, an FHR tachycardia, and repetitive FHR decelerations would appear to be consistent with Hon's theory of intrapartum asphyxia.

In summary, the patient who presents with a reactive fetal admission test is at low risk for intrapartum fetal distress during labor. The likelihood of intrapartum fetal distress in that patient is less than 2%. The probability of fetal brain damage arising out of that labor is even smaller (Figure 6). But, should intrapartum fetal distress occur, the fetus will fall into the catastrophic event category (Figure 5) manifested by a sudden prolonged FHR deceleration or the Hon group.

Thus, the intrapartum management of patients with a reactive fetal admission test is to focus on the changes in the baseline fetal heart rate. Does the FHR rise in keeping with Hon's pattern of intrapartum asphyxia or does it drop as we see in a sudden, catastrophic event. If the patient develops a loss of reactivity and a substantial rise in baseline fetal heart rate in association with repetitive FHR decelerations in the absence of maternal pyrexia (8,27), assessment of fetal acid–base status and/or consideration for delivery depending on the circumstances would appear to be reasonable. While the Hon pattern takes time to evolve, the sudden prolonged FHR deceleration group has a shorter time to CNS injury. Given the likelihood of neurologic injury arising at some time after the onset of the prolonged FHR deceleration, limited time is available to attempt remedial measures and/or intrauterine fetal resuscitation (31,32) before resorting to operative intervention. Since this CNS injury is quite rapid and most, if not all, hospitals in the United States are not technically capable of responding fast enough to deliver the fetus in this circumstance, this form of fetal CNS injury is probably not preventable.

THE PERSISTENT NONREACTIVE FHR PATTERN

The persistent nonreactive FHR pattern group accounts for 45% of the FHR patterns observed in the brain-damaged baby population (Figure 4) (27). This population is characterized by the presence of reduced fetal activity prior to admission to the hospital, male fetuses, old meconium, meconium sequelae such as meconium aspiration syndrome and persistent pulmonary hypertension, and oligohydramnios (8). The typical FHR pattern is nonreactive with a fixed baseline that normally does not change from admission until delivery (8,27).

When looking at the admission FHR pattern, the persistent nonreactive FHR pattern group can be divided into three phases (Table 3). These three phases, in our opinion, represent a post-CNS insult compensatory response in the fetus. Moreover, this FHR pattern, in our opinion, does not represent ongoing asphyxia or worsening of the CNS injury (8). For a fetus to have ongoing fetal asphyxia, an FHR pattern similar to that of Hon would have to be seen. There, a progressive and substantial rise in baseline heart rate is observed in response to ongoing fetal asphyxia. In contrast, the FHR baseline in the nonreactive group remains fixed and an FHR tachycardia is usually not seen. Thus, the fetal FHR phase, I, II or III, on admission to the hospital appears to equate with the length of time from the fetal CNS insult. Thus, Phase I would appear to be closer to the time of the insult, and Phase III would appear to be more distant in time from the injury-producing event.

As previously noted, these pregnant women typically complain of reduced or absent fetal activity prior to arrival to the hospital or describe fetal movement that is different or has changed (8). In contrast with the reactive fetal admission group where the fetal activity is characterized as normal, the typical maternal history, herein, is one of a sudden burst of fetal activity followed by quiescence. When the burst of fetal activity occurs, the mothers have described the fetal movement as if the fetus is going to jump out of her abdomen. Upon arrival to the hospital, the fetus is usually in one of the recovery phases, I, II, or III. Neurologic injury in this circumstance typically occurs at or around the time of the burst in fetal activity or soon thereafter (33).

In our opinion, the persistent nonreactive FHR pattern represents a group of fetuses with a static encephalopathy and is not a sign of ongoing fetal asphyxia (8,12,27). Thus, earlier intervention in the form of a cesarean on admission to the hospital would not, in our opinion, substantially alter neonatal outcome.

Table 3. Fetuses with preadmission central nervous system injury exhibit a persistent nonreactive FHR pattern intrapartum (8) and can be divided into three phases based on the baseline FHR and the FHR variability[a,b]

Phase	Baseline Rate (bpm)	Variability	Incidence (%)
I	>160	Diminished	19
II	110–160	Diminished	39
III	110–160	Average	43

[a]Data from reference 27.
[b]FHR, fetal heart rate.

When a persistent nonreactive FHR pattern is encountered in a term or postdate pregnancy, we believe the pregnant woman should not be sent home, but should be kept on continuous EFM until the fetal status has been clarified. The duration of nonreactivity before fetal assessment with scalp or acoustic stimulation, a biophysical profile, a contraction stress test, or fetal pulse oximetry will depend on the circumstances, and will be influenced by a number of factors beyond the scope of this chapter. However, as previously noted, persistent nonreactivity lasting in excess of 90–120 minutes in a term fetus should prompt other tests to establish fetal status. To remove any ambiguity, practitioners should consider the establishment of a protocol to address the nonreactive FHR admission test result in their hospitals.

In addition, the pregnant woman should be advised of the FHR pattern and its potential clinical significance. The subsequent management with respect to the route of delivery will depend on the discussion with the patient and the clinical findings.

SUMMARY

Neurologically impaired infants can present with either a reactive or nonreactive fetal admission test. Those infants who arrive with a reactive fetal admission test appear to be normal neurologically at the time of admission and later sustain neurologic injury during the course of labor through the development of a Hon FHR pattern or a catastrophic event such as a uterine rupture. In contrast, the persistent nonreactive group probably represents a preadmission neurologic insult that antedates arrival to the hospital. Whether antepartum fetal surveillance in this population can alter the outcome is less certain. But clearly, this is an area of future investigation.

In those patients with a reactive fetal admission test, the primary focus during labor is on the changes in the baseline fetal heart rate. In contrast, the nonreactive patient poses a medical, legal, and ethical dilemma. This is because the finding of a persistent nonreactive FHR pattern and an unchanging fixed baseline fetal heart rate from admission until delivery suggests a static encephalopathy that antedated the patient's arrival to the hospital (8,10–12,27). In this population, earlier intervention in the form of a cesarean would not, in our opinion, substantially alter neonatal outcome. Thus, open discussion with the family prior to delivery would appear to be beneficial.

ACKNOWLEDGMENT

This project was sponsored in part by the Childbirth Injury Prevention Foundation.

REFERENCES

1. Hon EH (ed). *An atlas of fetal heart rate patterns.* New Haven, CT: Hardy Press, 1968.
2. Hon EH, Quilligan EJ. Electronic evaluation of the fetal heart rate. *Clin Obstet Gynecol* 1968;11:145–167.

3. Albers LL, Krulewitch DJ. Electronic fetal monitoring in the United States in the 1980s. *Obstet Gynecol* 1992;82:1:8–10.
4. Freeman RK. Contraction stress testing for primary fetal surveillance in patients at risk for utero-placental insufficiency. *Clin Perinatol* 1982;9:265–270.
5. Phelan JP. The nonstress test: a review of 3000 tests. *Am J Obstet Gynecol* 1981;139:7–10.
6. Yeh SY, Diaz F, Paul RH. Ten year experience intrapartum fetal monitoring in Los Angeles County/University of Southern California Medical Center. *Am J Obstet Gynecol* 1982;143:496–500.
7. Perkins RP. Perspectives on perinatal brain damage. *Obstet Gynecol* 1987;69:807–819.
8. Phelan JP, Ahn MO. Perinatal observations in forty-eight neurologically impaired term infants. *Am J Obstet Gynecol* 1994;171:424–431.
9. Menticoglou SM, Manning FA, Harman CR, Morrison I. Severe fetal brain injury without evident intrapartum trauma. *Obstet Gynecol* 1989;74:457–461.
10. Shields JR, Schifrin BS. Perinatal antecedents of cerebral palsy. *Obstet Gynecol* 1988;71:899–905.
11. Van der Moer P, Gerretsen G, Visser G. Fixed heart rate pattern after intrauterine accidental decerebration. *Obstet Gynecol* 1985;65:125–127.
12. Hon EH, Lee ST. Electronic evaluation of the fetal heart rate: VIII. Patterns preceding fetal death, further observations. *Am J Obstet Gynecol* 1963;87:814–826.
13. Phelan JP. Labor admission test. *Clin Perinatol* 1994;21:879–885.
14. Krebs HB, Petres RE, Dunn LJ, et al. Intrapartum fetal heart rate monitoring. VI. Prognostic significance of accelerations. *Am J Obstet Gynecol* 1982;142:297–305.
15. Sarno AP, Phelan JP, Ahn MO. Relationship of early intrapartum fetal heart rate patterns to subsequent patterns and fetal outcome. *J Reprod Med* 1990;35:239–242.
16. Ingemarsson I, Arulkumaran S, Paul RH, et al. Admission test: a screening test for fetal distress in labor. *Obstet Gynecol* 1986;68:800–806.
17. Ingemarsson I, Arulkumaran S, Paul RH, et al. Fetal acoustic stimulation in early labor in patients screened with the admission test. *Am J Obstet Gynecol* 1988;158:70–74.
18. Sarno AP, Ahn MO, Phelan JP, et al. Fetal acoustic stimulation in early labor in patients screened with the admission test. *Am J Obstet Gynecol* 1990;162:762–767.
19. Clark SL, Gimovsky ML, Miller FC. Fetal heart rate response to scalp blood sampling. *Am J Obstet Gynecol* 1982;144:706–708.
20. Clark SL, Gimovsky ML, Miller FC. The scalp stimulation test: a clinical alternative to fetal scalp blood sampling. *Am J Obstet Gynecol* 1984;148:274–277.
21. Smith CV, Nguygen HN, Phelan JP, Paul RH. Intrapartum assessment of fetal well-being: a comparison of fetal acoustic stimulation with acid–base determinations. *Am J Obstet Gynecol* 1986;155:726–728.
22. Shaw K, Clark SL. Reliability of intrapartum fetal heart rate monitoring in the post term fetus with meconium passage. *Obstet Gynecol* 1988;72:886–889.
23. Rutherford SE, Phelan JP, Smith CV, et al. The four quadrant assessment of amniotic fluid volume: an adjunct to antepartum fetal heart rate testing. *Obstet Gynecol* 1987;70:353–356.
24. Leveno KJ, Williams ML, DePalma RT, Whalley PJ. Perinatal outcome in the absence of antepartum fetal heart rate acceleration. *Obstet Gynecol* 1983;61:347–355.
25. Devoe LD, McKenzie J, Searle NS, Sherline DM. Clinical sequelae of the extended nonstress test. *Am J Obstet Gynecol* 1985;151:1074–1078.

26. Brown R, Patrick J. The nonstress test: How long is long enough? *Am J Obstet Gynecol* 1981;141:646–651.
27. Phelan JP, Ahn MO. Fetal heart rate observations in 300 term brain damaged infants. *J Mat Fetal Invest* 1998;8:1–5.
28. Ahn MO, Phelan JP. Normal fetal heart rate patterns in the term brain damaged infant: a failure of intrapartum fetal monitoring? *J Mat Fetal Invest* 1998;8:58–60.
29. Molteni RA, Stys SJ, Battaglia FC. Relationship of fetal and placental weight in human beings: fetal/placental weight ratios at various gestational ages and birthweight distributions. *J Reprod Med* 1978;21:327–332.
30. Leung A, Leung EK, Paul RH. Uterine rupture after previous cesarean delivery: maternal & fetal consequences. *Am J Obstet Gynecol* 1993;169:945–950.
31. Ingemarsson I, Arulkumaran S, Ratnam SS. Single injection of terbutaline in term labor. II. Effect on uterine activity. *Am J Obstet Gynecol* 1985;153:865–869.
32. Strong TH Jr. Amnioinfusion. *J Reprod Med* 1995;40:108–114.
33. Naeye RL, Localio AR. Determining the time before birth when ischemia and hypoxemia initiated cerebral palsy. *Obstet Gynecol* 1995;86:713–719.

14

COMPUTERIZED APPROACHES TO FETAL SURVEILLANCE

Lawrence D. Devoe, M.D.

Department of Obstetrics and Gynecology, Medical College of Georgia, Augusta, Georgia

INTRODUCTION

Detection of the fetus who is likely to suffer perinatal asphyxia has been a constant goal of antepartum surveillance methods. Pathophysiologic observations, such as abnormal baseline fetal heart rate (FHR), are imprecise markers for asphyxia, even in advanced active labor (1). This is an unfortunate state of affairs since obstetricians are typically held accountable for adverse neurologic outcomes in term infants whose intrapartum monitoring records display *any* abnormality whatsoever (2). Because it is now recognized that conventional antepartum modalities for evaluating fetal condition have limited sensitivity and predictive accuracy for predicting risk of asphyxia, investigators have sought other aids to improve this situation.

Virtually all conventional assessment approaches require the clinician to perform a series of routine tasks to gather data relevant to the immediate and projected fetal status:

1. Assemble a current pregnancy dataset containing historical, physical and laboratory information.

Asphyxia and Fetal Brain Damage, Edited by Dev Maulik, M.D., Ph.D.
ISBN 0-471-18427-6

2. Identify the presence of significant pregnancy risk factors.
3. Stratify the estimated level of risk for perinatal asphyxia/death.
4. Select antepartum evaluation strategy for antenatal evaluation, based on the best testing method(s) for the risks previously identified.
5. Conduct and analyze the test(s), integrate their results into the current clinical context, and refine the presumed level of fetal risk accordingly (post-test likelihood).
6. Devise a clinical strategy least likely to result in premature obstetric intervention or excessive delay of delivery.

In the conventional world, however, real obstacles are placed in front of achieving the best clinical performance. Clinicians are likely to base fetal assessment on their prior experience with specific obstetric problems and their related testing methods. Clinicians' responses are colored by estimates (accurate or otherwise) of the likelihood of asphyxia or death for infants of specific gestational age or birthweight delivered at that precise moment in time. These responses are further limited by the actual amount of clinical data known for a specific patient. Standard antepartum tests are subject to erroneous or factitious outcomes which may stem from observer variation or technical problems. Optimal clinical practice should be steered by the best available data obtained from appropriate clinical trials in a specific domain—for example, evidence-based medicine (3). In the realm of fetal testing, however, few methods have received the sufficiently sized prospective, randomized, controlled trials needed to establish best practice recommendations (4).

What are the ideal characteristics of tests used for antepartum prediction of perinatal asphyxia? In general, they should possess the following properties:

1. Reliable, reproducible, objective measures for predicting presence or absence of risk.
2. Readily accessible schemes which incorporate clinical features to identify fetuses at such high risk for asphyxia that labor should be avoided.
3. Translatability into model systems usable to forecast fetal intrapartum outcomes long before the onset of active labor.

The shortcomings of current antepartum assessment tests for satisfying these goals are evident. Devoe et al. (5) analyzed individually the most common tools for routine fetal surveillance, the nonstress test, amniotic fluid assessment, and umbilical arterial Doppler velocimetry. They concluded that for the conditions most commonly encountered in testing (i.e., maternal hypertension, diabetes mellitus, postdatism, and intrauterine growth restriction), the individual tests provided limited "stand alone" power. Their screening performance was strongly influenced also by specific testing indication which, in turn, was associated with prevalence of perinatal asphyxia. More specifically, Visser et al. (6) showed in a selected population of fetuses with intrauterine growth restriction undergoing cordocentesis that FHR baseline characteristics such as absent accelerations, decreased variation, and apparent decelerations were highly (> 60%) correlated with fetal acidemia.

More sophisticated measures of fetal well-being, as represented by multiple parameter biophysical profile (BPP) testing, have been evaluated against fetal acid-base balance. Vintzileos et al. (7) correlated results of a BPP score of fetuses delivered without labor and their subsequent umbilical arterial pH values. They found a 90% sensitivity for acidemia when the BPP score was below 7. Manning et al. (8) correlated BPP scores with fetal umbilical venous pH obtained through cordocentesis; a stepwise linear relationship was observed between BPP score and umbilical venous pH. Devoe et al. (9) confirmed the implications of both reports showing a linear correlation of computerized BPP and umbilical artery pH at delivery. Fetal umbilical artery Doppler velocimetry showing absent or reversed end-diastolic velocity has been correlated with fetal acid–base balance. Nicolaides et al. (10), among others, have shown a high correlation (80%) of absent end-diastolic velocities with hypoxia but much lower correlation (50%) with fetal acidosis as determined from cordocentesis samples obtained in such pregnancies.

In summary, these background observations suggest that while antepartum fetal markers may exist for perinatal asphyxia, conventional antepartum testing does not predict this condition consistently or sufficiently early to alter outcome. It should be recalled that the populations included in these studies are usually highly selected and overrepresented with profoundly growth-restricted infants, and thus these observations may not be readily generalized to other populations. Systematic studies looking at serial observations in human subjects are quite limited, giving further limitation to the prognostic implications of sequential assessment tests (11). Finally, and more importantly, the events leading to hypoxia and asphyxia in the intrapartum period may stem from intrapartum events which cannot be predicted prior to labor. While the potential benefits from optimal antenatal screening may be limited to a small subset of the population at risk for asphyxia, such benefits could be maximized through the use of improved antenatal analytic systems.

COMPUTERIZATION AND FETAL ASSESSMENT: BACKGROUND

The history of computerization and fetal assessment can be traced to the 1970s when early generation electronic fetal monitors (EFMs) were interfaced with mainframe computers (12). In the following decade, EFMs were linked to desktop personal computers (PCs); and software for archival/retrieval, analysis, and remote transmission were developed (13–15). More recently, clinical trials have been conducted on the various aspects of computerized analysis of the FHR baseline, including comparisons with human observers and application to antepartum testing. These latter reports will provide the focus for a subsequent section. While other aspects of fetal biophysical testing, including the biophysical profile and fetal vascular Doppler velocimetry, have been subjected to computerized analyses, this chapter will deal principally with approaches used to address computer applications to the investigation of the resting FHR as a window into prediction of fetal hypoxia and asphyxia.

The most important issues, which computerized FHR analysis needs to address, stem from the observation that the functionality of EFM has changed little since the appearance of the first analog systems. Visual displays of FHR, fetal activity artifacts, and uterine contractions are neither explained nor analyzed by these systems. Further, the data array presented to observers is vast and changes rapidly. Most users of fetal monitoring systems are not domain experts and may not be able to detect more subtle abnormalities of the FHR baseline. Moreover, human monitors may have other tasks to perform during the conduct of fetal testing. As indicated earlier, the linkage between raw FHR data and current/projected fetal condition is not consistent or readily understood. These issues present appropriate problems for computerized and progressively automated solutions.

Automated perinatal evaluation should lead to fewer errors of interpretation or prognosis. At the most basic level (see Figure 1), elements of automation are applied primarily to the signal processing which occurs within the devices used to examine the fetus. The clinician obtains the raw data, usually obtained from input–output devices (e.g., electronic fetal monitor, ultrasound imaging system) to pregnancy database, makes an overall assessment of fetal condition, and then applies this knowledge to further clinical management. This level characterizes most current obstetric assessment methods.

At the next level (2) of automated perinatal evaluation, the data-generating device uses analytic programs either onboard or through a link to a computer system. The new "monitor" system can simulate the experienced clinician's attempts to analyze the acquired fetal data. Its apparent advantages are the more rapid, accurate, and reproducible processing of a complex set of signals. The clinician must still generate the next step in formulating prognosis and therapy.

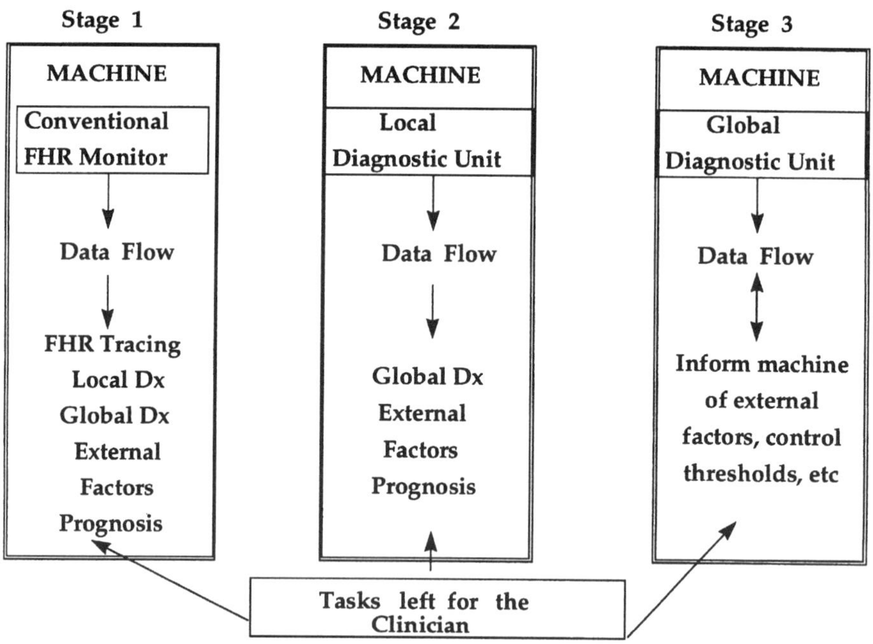

Figure 1. Scheme for automated perinatal assessment. Level I represents current status of conventional fetal monitoring systems. Level II is that afforded by algorithmic analytic systems for FHR, usually incorporating a fetal monitor interfaced with a computer. Level III represents the use of "intelligent" or expert systems for interpretation and management counselling.

The final level (3) of automated perinatal assessment adds an intelligent program which weights test data in the context of the current pregnancy, renders a prognosis, and offers management options for the clinician. The assessment program requires an extensively validated clinical knowledge base and offers reasonable explanations for its decisions.

The data requirements for computerization of FHR are well-defined and include:

1. Discrete, processible raw signals accessible to PC acquisition. The frequencies of FHR events can be handled through oversampling repetition in ranges which are easily addressed with current desktop computing systems—that is, 10 msec to 100 msec (16 times to 4 times).
2. Events which can be quantitated for digitization. FHR baseline can be characterized by quantitative features—for example, rate, variation, and the frequency of episodic events (accelerations, decelerations).
3. Normal ranges of FHR parameters can be established for comparison and classification of test outcomes.
4. FHR data can be discriminated, in most cases, from background noise or maternal signal and, therefore, is relatively unambiguous.
5. FHR signal can be compressed for easy, minimal lossy mass storage and can be reconstructed rapidly with high fidelity to original sources.

All of the systems studied and described below take advantage of these properties to assist the process of analysis and interpretation.

COMPUTERIZATION AND FETAL ASSESSMENT: CLINICAL APPLICATIONS

Systems Developed for Computerization of FHR Signals

Current operating systems for computerized analysis of continuous FHR recordings have been summarized in two recent reviews (16,17). These systems obtain the processed FHR signal online and, through different software routines, determine the basal FHR from which FHR accelerations and decelerations can be detected, signal quality can be assessed, and some measure of FHR variability can be calculated.

Table 1. Oxford Sonicaid System 8000 analysis criteria (14)

1. High FHR variation (> 32 msec) occurs in at least 5 of 6 consecutive minutes.
2. No large decelerations are present.
3. At least one fetal movement or three FHR accelerations occur.
4. Overall (long-term) variation >22 msec; short-term variation > 3 msec.
5. Basal heart rate > 115 bpm, < 160 bpm.
6. Short-term variation is within three standard deviations of value expected from the the mean range.

The only commercially available system in the United States and Europe is the Oxford Sonicaid System 8000 (Chichester, UK), based on the Dawes–Redman FHR analysis system referenced earlier (14). It is configured as either a dedicated single-computer–FHR-monitor system or as a self-contained portable FHR monitor with an EPROM chip containing the FHR analytic routine (Oxford Sonicaid TEAM™ monitor). Table 1 summarizes the system criteria for "analyzing" the FHR recording. An example of the System 8000 analytic report is shown in Figure 2. This system is weighted most heavily toward complex analysis of "long-term" and "short-term" variability, expressed in milliseconds. The thresholds for abnormal FHR variability were derived from a large set of infants who had had antepartum monitoring and subsequent

MEDICAL COLLEGE OF GEORGIA/FHR TESTING

Oxford Sonicaid - System 8000 - Objective CTG Analysis System - Rev GB2.12
Printed on 26-Apr-93 at 13:36:15

Reprint for	Reference No.
Date of recording 26-Apr-1993	Time of recording 12:57
Record Number A 972	Gestation 34 weeks 0 days

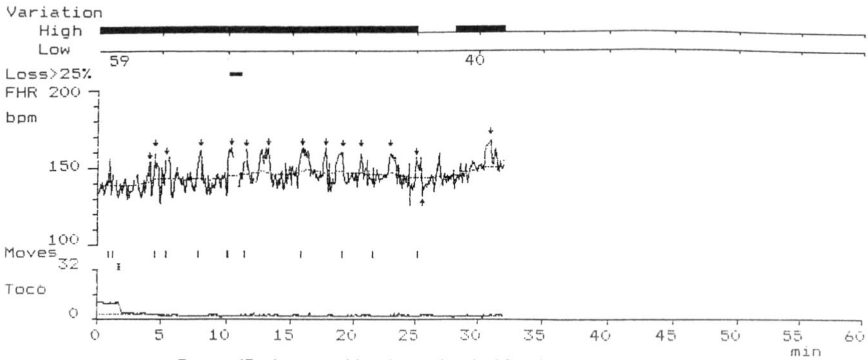

Dawes/Redman criteria met at 10 min

ANALYSIS at 32 min.

Normal Values		
(0)	1. SIGNAL LOSS (%)	3.3
	2. CONTRACTION PEAKS	1
(>12)	3. FETAL MOVEMENTS (per hour)...............	24
	per min in High 0.41	
(<160)	4. BASAL HEART RATE (bpm).....................	139
(>8/hr)	5. ACCELERATIONS >10 bpm & 15 sec.............	14
	>15 bpm & 15 sec.............	7
(0)	6. DECELERATIONS > 20 lost beats	0
(>4)	7. HIGH EPISODES (min) : Threshold 32 msec....	29
	LOW EPISODES (min)........................	0
	8. VARIATION OVERALL (Mean range : msec)......	55.9
	(Mean range : bpm)......	20.6
	SHORT TERM VARIATION (ms)	11.5

INTERPRETATION OF VARIATION		
	Normal	> 30 msec
	Questionable	20 - 30 msec
	Abnormal	< 20 msec

ADVICE ONLY. THIS IS NOT INTENDED AS A DIAGNOSIS

Figure 2. Standard computerized printout for the Oxford Sonicaid System 8000.

delivery. The mean minute range of 22 msec (long-term) and 3 msec (short-term) were chosen as those values with the best correlation to neonatal hypoxia and acidemia. The System 8000 renders an "ADVICE" notification when sufficient time has elapsed to reach the reassuring criteria (minimum = 10 minutes) or pathologic features exist, such as a flat (low variability tracing with or without FHR decelerations.

Normative FHR Data in Third Trimester Pregnancy

Over the past decade, we have archived more than 7000 normal pregnancies that have undergone serial antepartum testing using our computerized FHR analysis system at the Medical College of Georgia. Typical system output is shown in Figure 3. These data have enabled us to develop normograms for the major FHR baseline features as they evolve with increasing length of gestation. Figure 4 shows a bar graph for acceleration frequency per 30-min window using 10 bpm and 15 bpm acceleration peak thresholds. Similar graphs have been established for all measures of the baseline FHR, including rate, variation, and deceleration frequency. Using a threshold value of

```
FETMON(1.10) Copyright (c) 1992 by the Medical College of Georgia, all rights reserved.
PATIENT#                 TEST# 1   NAME:

TEST DATE:                 4/18/97
AGE:                      33
PREGNANCIES (GTPAL):      1 0 0 0 0
RACE:                     W
EDC:                       5/22/97
EGA:                      35
TIME OF STUDY:            14:30
DIAGNOSIS:                Decreased amniotic fluid volume
LAST MEAL:                12:30
LAST SMOKED:              00:00
MEDICATION & TIME:        :
AMNIOTIC FLUID:            0.0 x  0.0
SD:                        0.00
PI:                        0.00
RI:                        0.00
TEST TIME:                30 MINUTES
```

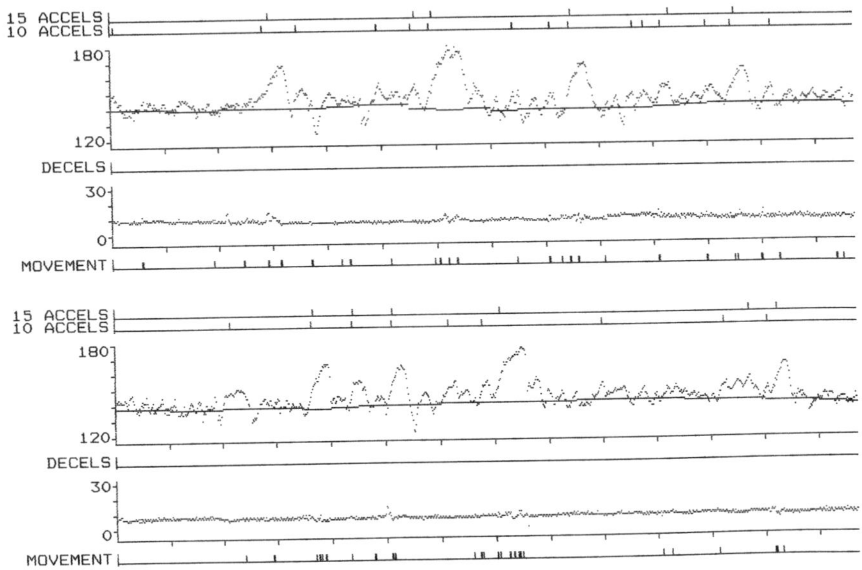

FETMON(1.10) Copyright (c) 1992 by the Medical College of Georgia, all rights reserved.
PATIENT# TEST# 1 NAME:

NONSTRESS TEST: NORMAL VALUES

PARAMETER	MEAN	ABNORMAL
BASELINE FETAL HEART RATE (BPM)	140	<120 or >155
STANDARD DEVIATION	5.6	< 2.3
COEFFICIENT OF VARIATION (LONG TERM VARIABILITY)	0.04	< 0.02
ACCELERATION COUNT (>15 BPM)	7.4	< 3
ACCELERATION AMPLITUDE (BPM)	22	< 15
ACCELERATION DURATION (MIN)	0.67	< 0.25
PERCENT ACCELERATION TIME	15	< 5
DECELERATION COUNT	0	> 0
DECELERATION AMPLITUDE (BPM)	0	> 0
DECELERATION DURATION (MIN)	0	> 0
PERCENT DECELERATION TIME	0	> 0

NONSTRESS TEST: TEST RESULTS

MEAN BASELINE FHR		139
STANDARD DEVIATION		9.912
MEAN BASELINE VARIABILITY (COV)		0.071
PERCENT SIGNAL LOSS		0.1
ACCELERATIONS:	10 BEAT	15 BEAT
NUMBER	26	13
AMPLITUDE	17.9	24.3
DURATION	0.48	0.63
PERCENT ACCELERATION TIME	41.33	27.39
DECELERATIONS:		
NUMBER		0
AMPLITUDE		0.0
DURATION		0.00
PERCENT DECELERATION TIME		0.00

CLASSIFICATION:
NORMAL: ALL PARAMETERS ARE WITHIN NORMAL LIMITS
ABNORMAL: AT LEAST ONE PARAMETER IS OUTSIDE NORMAL LIMITS *)

Interpretation: [ ] Abnormal, Normal, Unsatisfactory
Recommendation: Retest [ ] hours
Retest [ ] days
BPP [ ]
CST [ ]
Aminocentesis [ ]
Deliver [ ]

Comment:

Signature MD: ____________

Signature RN: ____________

Figure 3. Standard computerized printout for the Medical College of Georgia NST-ANALYST.

5th percentile for these objective FHR parameters resulted in a misclassification ("abnormal" for "normal") of less than 1% of this population, which is far better than achieved using the standardized visual criteria of 2 or 3 accelerations/20- or 30-min windows (false-positive rates typically range from 10% to 20%) (18).

Computerized Versus Visual FHR Analysis

Visual interpretation of the FHR record has been a long-standing source of problems in the detection of compromised fetuses (19), because disagreement often results when different observers analyze the same FHR records. Computerized FHR analysis could

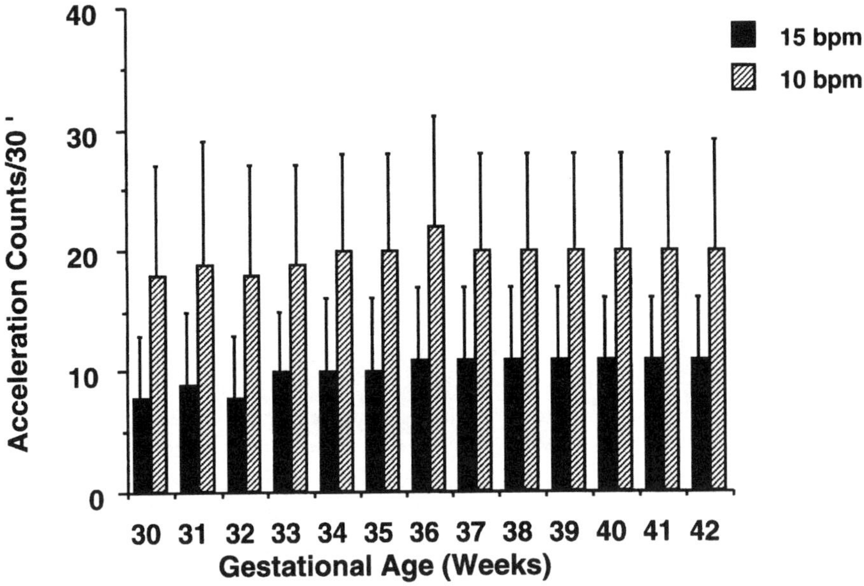

Figure 4. Computer-derived normogram for FHR acceleration counts/30 min obtained throughout the last trimester from a population of 7255 normal fetuses at the Medical College of Georgia.

virtually eliminate both intra- and interobserver variability. Hiett et al. (20) compared visual versus computerized (Oxford Sonicaid System 8000) antepartum FHR analysis in more than 500 cases in which two clinicians had achieved a priori agreement for FHR interpretation. Computer–clinician agreement was good for normal tracings (94%) but relatively poor for abnormal tracings (30–40%). Either source would have yielded similar sensitivity, specificity, and predictive values. Use of the System 8000 would have reduced the need for further testing (from 50% to 9%) and might have promoted delivery in nine cases, six of which had confirmed abnormal outcomes.

Visual analysis, even among experts, can yield frank interpretative errors when arrayed against objective computer analysis of the same records. Gagnon et al. (21) compared the readings of 100 antepartum records by five experts with computerized FHR analyses of the same records. While the experts could identify baseline rate with high accuracy and reproducibility, they missed more than 90% of potentially abnormal tracings, failed to agree on baseline variability, and tended to consider most tests as normal.

In summary, these reports suggest that, at the minimum, computerization of antepartum FHR records could improve accuracy and consistency of test analysis, reduce the frequency of follow-up tests, and lead to more appropriate obstetric interventions. Because no published national consensus exists on the interpretation of FHR baseline parameters, objective, consistent FHR interpretation might be readily achieved by adoption of any of the algorithmic software routines which have been published and subjected to extensive trials in clinical care settings.

Computerized FHR Systems applied to Fetal Assessment

Predictive thresholds for computerized FHR analysis have been established for the Oxford Sonicaid System 8000 (22,23): long-term FHR variation < 20 msec associated with a high probability of fetal hypoxemia; short-term variability < 2.6 msec associated with a high probability for antepartum fetal death and metabolic acidemia. Relatively few studies have approached specific high-risk conditions and computerized testing, prospectively.

Reliance on measures of FHR variation alone may be less than ideal in predicting outcome for growth-restricted fetuses. Snijders et al. (24) conducted a longitudinal study of such pregnancies and noted that, as a group, while reduced FHR variation often preceded delivery of the most compromised infants, considerable individual variations in FHR patterns occurred. Larger studies would certainly be needed to extend these observations before recommending their routine use in such cases. Weiner et al. (25) examined computerized FHR assessment in 310 pregnancies > 41 weeks' gestational age. This group found that a threshold of <30 msec as reduced long-term FHR variability yielded a 60% detection of neonatal acidosis and 90% detection of intrapartum fetal distress. These sensitivity figures bettered those produced by either Doppler velocimetry or amniotic fluid volume assessment.

Expert Systems Developed for FHR Analysis

The experience summarized above relates to the application of algorithmic solutions to FHR "analysis" and "interpretation." However, this type of software is limited in its ability to handle unfamiliar or eccentric cases, as illustrated by Gagnon et al. (26). They reported on two cases in which signal loss or change in fetal behavioral state misled the Sonicaid System 8000 to classify a normal fetus as pathologic. The next step in automating perinatal assessment systems (see Figure 1) is expert system software using either rule-based routines, neural networks, or hybrids of both approaches.

Rule-based expert systems have been applied to the clinical management of antepartum FHR records. Our collaborative group has accumulated nearly a decade of experience with such system development (27). The "NST-EXPERT" project has resulted in a comprehensive system which incorporates knowledge modules that include past maternal history, current pregnancy risk factors, and the actual FHR record data. A series of queries leads the user to a probable prognosis and set of therapeutic recommendations. This system can be asked to justify or explain its decision-making process. Initial validation, using a set of clinical cases and four clinical experts, resulted in a high-level of agreement in interpretation and management recommendation (28). Where NST-EXPERT excelled was in rendering the prognosis in cases complicated by fetal hypoxia/acidemia, generating an accuracy of 88%. In contrast, the most experienced clinician generated a prognostic accuracy of only 50% for the same set of cases. Such systems can offer very potent solutions to complex clinical scenarios provided that their knowledge base is extensive and the rule structure enables coverage of all likely contingencies.

Neural networks, unlike rule-based expert systems, are "intelligent" software routines that solve problems by achieving pattern recognition of outcomes derived from programmed sets of known inputs (e.g., FHR elements) and outputs (e.g., FHR classifications). So-called hidden layers of neurons link these input and output neuronal layers. Network development employs a repetitive training process in which input–output pairs are presented to the network. Over time, the network develops associations which lead to more accurate identification of known outcomes and, thereby, becomes able to handle unknown cases. Neural networks, unlike traditional expert systems, do not require rules and can "learn" or improve with additional data to handle increasingly difficult cases. However, networks cannot explain how they arrived at their solutions; training may be very difficult if highly sophisticated answers beyond "normal" or "abnormal" are sought.

Kol et al. (29) constructed a neural network for classifying nonstress tests (NSTs) as normal or abnormal. Their network addressed 3600 raw data inputs (FHR and uterine activity data noted each second for 30 minutes) and combined these with 17 classificatory inputs of the FHR recording. This network's hidden layer contained 50 hidden neurons and there were two outputs ("normal" or "abnormal"). The clinical experts evaluated 950 tracings; the network arrived at an 89% correct identification of normal and 87% correct identification of abnormal tracings, when experts agreed a priori on test interpretation. Unfortunately, network performance suffered when there was expert disagreement or uncertainty.

Devoe et al. (30) used a series of neural networks to test the stability of NST parameters derived from System 8000 analyses and conducted over time intervals, ranging from 1 to 4 days in normal third-trimester pregnancies. No networks could be developed to project future NST appearance for testing intervals that exceeded

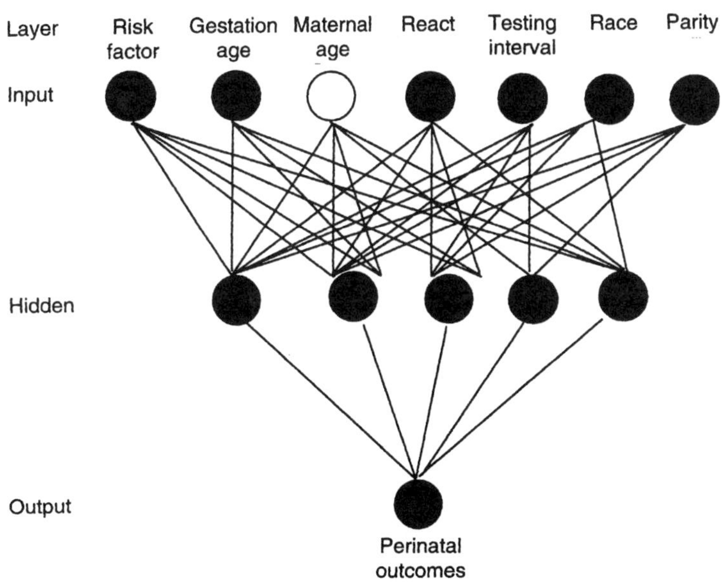

Figure 5. Schematic structure of neural network for evaluating perinatal condition based on the nonstress test and other pregnancy data, including maternal characteristics and risk factors.

Table 2. Prediction of perinatal outcome using a neural network

A. Conventional Prediction Using NST Alone

	Nonreactive	Reactive	Total
Bad Outcome	41	245	286
Good Outcome	127	2084	2211
Total	168	2329	2497

Sensitivity:	24%	Positive Predictive Value:	14%
Specificity:	90%	Negative Predictive Value:	94%
Prevalence:	11.4%	Test Accuracy:	85%

B. Prediction Using a Trained Neural Network

250 test cases:	249 correctly predicted			Test Accuracy:	99.6%
Sensitivity:	100%	Specificity:	99%	Prevalence:	10%

2 days. The most stable single FHR baseline parameter was long-term variability (mean-minute range of heart period over 30 minutes). More recently, we addressed the issue of network development for fetal prognosis based on contextual risk factors and NST outcome (31). The structure of this network, shown in Figure 5, incorporated (a) input data readily available to clinicians and (b) objective evaluation of NST results based on computerized analysis, and it was trained on a set of 2500 high-risk pregnancies. Compared to standard prediction, based on NST alone, the trained network shows a nearly perfect prediction of both compromised and normal fetal outcomes (see Table 2).

CONCLUSIONS

Where do we stand with computerized approaches to FHR analysis, interpretation, and integration into schemes for predicting fetal hypoxia and asphyxia? There is little question that the hardware and software tools for accomplishing this task are already with us. A number of investigative centers have accumulated more than a decade's experience with computerized FHR analysis in the antepartum setting and have implemented these systems in their daily practice. The minimum virtues of currently available systems are their ability to provide reproducible, consistent, and objective analysis of the FHR baseline. Their potential value resides in the ability to extend prediction of outcome by incorporating the FHR analysis into a contextual appraisal of the current pregnancy, as illustrated by the expert system approaches.

The obstacles that remain in the pathway of progress towards realizing improved assessment of fetal condition using these tools are as follows:

1. The lack of a national consensus on standard definitions and criteria for FHR baseline properties and events.

2. Imperfect interpretation of *all* FHR tracings which might occur, however infrequently, in clinical practice.
3. Requirement for large-scale clinical trials of current or future automated systems.
4. Need to clarify the legal status of archived records and interpretations (although precedents exist for cardiology and radiology).

It is to be hoped that such overviews as those presented in this monograph will both stimulate curiosity and demand that these systems be introduced to wider clinical settings. It is also accepted that the holy grail of fetal testing, which is the precise and early identification of the fetus at risk for asphyxia, will be more closely approached in this new era of perinatal assessment.

REFERENCES

1. Low JA, McGrath MJ, Marshall SJ, et al. The relationship between antepartum fetal heart rate, intrapartum fetal heart rate, and fetal acid–base status. *Am J Obstet Gynecol* 1986; 154:769–776.
2. Rosen MG, Dickinson JC. The paradox of electronic fetal monitoring: more data may not enable us to predict or prevent infant neurologic morbidity. *Am J Obstet Gynecol* 1993;168:745–751.
3. Evidence-based medicine working group. Evidence-based medicine: a new approach to the teaching of the practice of medicine. *JAMA* 1992;268:2420–2425.
4. Thacker SB, Berkelman RL. Assessing the accuracy and efficacy of selected antepartum fetal surveillance techniques. *Obstet Gynecol Survey* 1986;41:121–141.
5. Devoe LD, Cardner P, Dear C, et al. The diagnostic values of concurrent nonstress testing, amniotic fluid measurement, and Doppler velocimetry in screening a general high risk population. *Am J Obstet Gynecol* 1990;163:1040–1048.
6. Visser GHA, Sadovsky G, Nicolaides KH. Antepartum heart rate patterns in small-for-gestational age third-trimester fetuses: correlation with blood gas values obtained at cordocentesis. *Am J Obstet Gynecol* 1990;162:698–702.
7. Vintzileos AM, Gaffney SE, Salinger LM, et al. The relationship among the fetal biophysical profile, umbilical cord pH and Apgar scores. *Am J Obstet Gynecol* 1987;157:627–631.
8. Manning FA, Snijders RL, Nikolaides KH, et al. Fetal biophysical profile score. VI. Correlations with antepartum umbilical venous fetal pH. *Am J Obstet Gynecol* 1993;169:755–760.
9. Devoe LD, Castillo RA, Searle N, Searle J. Prognostic components of computerized fetal biophysical testing. *Am J Obstet Gynecol* 1988;158:1148–1152.
10. Nicolaides KH, Bilardo CM, Soothill PW, Campbell S. Absence of end-diastolic frequencies in the umbilical artery: a sign of fetal hypoxia and acidosis. *Br Med J* 1988;297:1026–1027.
11. Devoe LD, Castillo RA, McKenzie J, et al. Sequential nonstress testing with use of each fetus as its own control. *Am J Obstet Gynecol* 1986;154:931–936.
12. Yeh S-Y, Betyar L, Hon EH. Computer diagnosis of fetal heart rate patterns. *Am J Obstet Gynecol* 1972;114:890–896.

13. Wickham PJD, Dawes GS, Belcher R. Development of methods for quantitative analysis of the fetal heart rate. *J Biomed Eng* 1983;5:302–310.
14. Dawes GS, Redman CWG. Antenatal heart rate analysis at the bedside using a microprocessor. In Kunzel W (ed). *Fetal heart rate monitoring.* Berlin: Springer-Verlag, 1985:63–65.
15. Searle JR, Devoe LD, Phillips MC, Searle NS. Computerized analysis of resting fetal heart rate tracings. *Obstet Gynecol* 1988;71:407–412.
16. Devoe LD. Automated methods of fetal assessment: the future of antenatal testing. *Clin Perinatol* 1994;21:863–878.
17. Farmakides G, Weiner Z. Computerized analysis of the fetal heart rate. *Clin Obstet Gynecol* 1995;38:112–120.
18. Devoe LD, Castillo RA, Sherline DM. The nonstress test as a diagnostic test: a critical reappraisal. *Am J Obstet Gynecol* 1985;152:1047–1053.
19. Lotgering FK, Wallenburg HCS, Schouten HJA. Interobserver and intraobserver variation in the assessment of antepartum cardiotocograms. *Am J Obstet Gynecol* 1982;144:701–705.
20. Hiett AK, Devoe LD, Youssef A, et al. A comparison of visual and automated methods of analyzing fetal heart rate tests. *Am J Obstet Gynecol* 1993:168:1517–1521.
21. Gagnon R, Campbell MK, Hunse C. A comparison between visual and computer analysis of antepartum fetal heart rate tracings. *Am J Obstet Gynecol* 1993;168:842–847.
22. Smith JH, Dawes GS, Redman CWG. Low human heart rate variation in normal pregnancy. *Br J Obstet Gynecol* 1987;94:656–664.
23. Street P, Dawes GS, Moulden M, Redman CWG. Short-term variation in abnormal antenatal fetal heart rate records. *Am J Obstet Gynecol* 1991;165:515–523.
24. Snijders RJM, Ribber LSM, Visser GHA, Mulder EJH. Numeric analysis of heart rate variation in intrauterine growth-retarded fetuses: a longitudinal study. *Am J Obstet Gynecol* 1992;166:22–27.
25. Weiner Z, Farmakides G, Schulman H, Kellner L, Plancher S, Maulik D. Computerized analysis of fetal heart rate variation in postterm pregnancy: prediction of intrapartum fetal distress and fetal acidosis. *Am J Obstet Gynecol* 1994;171:1132–1138.
26. Gagnon R. Bocking AD, Richardson BS, Maclean P. A flat decelerative fetal heart rate tracing with normal fetal heart rate variability. *Am J Obstet Gynecol* 1994;1717:1379–1381.
27. Alonso-Betanzos A, Guijarro-Berdinas B, Moret-Bonillo V, Castro-Martinez A, Devoe LD. An expert system approach to antenatal assessment. *New Rev Appl Expert Sys* 1996;2:139–153.
28. Alonso-Betanzos A, Moret-Bonillo V, Devoe LD, Searle JR, Banias B, Ramos E. Computerized antenatal assessment. *Automedica* 1992;14:3–22.
29. Kol S, Thaler I, Paz N, Shmueli O. Interpretation of nonstress tests by an artificial neural network. *Am J Obstet Gynecol* 1995;172:1372–1379.
30. Devoe LD, Carlton E, Prescott P. Neural network prediction of nonstress test results: how often should we perform nonstress tests? *Am J Obstet Gynecol* 1995;173:1128–1131.
31. Devoe LD, Nezhat A, Prescott P. Enhanced prediction of perinatal outcome using a neural network based on nonstress testing, obstetric characteristics, and pregnancy risk factors. *J Soc Gynecol Invest* 1995;3:238.

15

COMPUTERIZED ANALYSIS OF FETAL HEART RATE FOR RECOGNIZING ANTEPARTUM FETAL COMPROMISE

Domenico Arduini, M.D., Francesco Giacomello, M.D., Flavio Giannini, M.D., and Herbert Valensise, M.D.

Department of Obstetrics and Gynecology, University of Rome "Tor Vergata," Policlinico Nuovo "S. Eugenio," Rome, Italy

INTRODUCTION

The recent history of fetal heart rate (FHR) monitoring is characterized by two major advances. The first consists of the possibility to explain many suspicious or pathological FHR patterns with sonographic observation of fetal structure, behavior, environment and circulation. The second is represented by computerized analysis of FHR.

The aim of this chapter is to examine the possibilities of computerized analysis of FHR for recognizing antepartum fetal brain damage since, despite striking advances in prenatal diagnosis, it continues to be an important social and medicolegal problem.

Asphyxia and Fetal Brain Damage, Edited by Dev Maulik, M.D., Ph.D.
ISBN 0-471-18427-6

ELECTRONIC FETAL HEART MONITORING AND BRAIN DAMAGE

Electronic fetal heart rate (FHR) monitoring has been widely available for about 30 years, and the benefits derived from its use in the prevention and/or diagnosis of fetal brain damage are still being discussed (1,2). The lack of correlation between FHR monitoring results and prenatal brain damage can be explained, at least in part, by the following observations.

The plasticity of the developing human brain is capable of overcoming much of the prenatal injury. A correlation was observed between ominous FHR patterns and abnormal neurological performance at 1 year (3) but follow-up of the same infants at 6–9 years demonstrated normal children (4) even if FHR patterns consisted of long-lasting periods of decelerations (5). In addition, lesions of cerebral areas uninvolved in the control of FHR will not result in any prenatal FHR abnormality (6).

Prenatal brain damage has often already occurred before labor. In a retrospective study, 25 of 75 infants with cerebral palsy had chronic fetal distress and acid–base studies, when available, did not reveal acidosis (7). Persistent nonreactive FHR in two-thirds of neurologically impaired infants at the time of the admission indicated that injury occurred prior to arrival at the hospital, the mechanism being static rather than progressive, probably related to oligohydramnios with episodes of cord compression, since compensatory tachycardia was frequently absent (8). In a recent retrospective study of 209 brain-damaged infants, 46% were persistently nonreactive at the time of admission, confirming that damage occurred before admission (9).

The FHR pattern associated with brain damage can differ according to gestational age and site of the lesion. A FHR pattern characteristic of abnormal neurologic development was described in close proximity to a reactive nonstress test (NST), and it consisted of a normal baseline, persistently absent variability, and mild variable decelerations with overshoot (7). This pattern, frequently associated with postmaturity, meconium staining, intrauterine growth retardation (IUGR), and neonatal seizures, was related to chronic, intermittent cord compression resulting in repetitive antepartum central nervous system (CNS) ischemia and was unrelated to the presence of acidosis. On the other hand, in preterm fetuses, an oscillatory tracing pattern (10) or moderate variable decelerations (11), always related to cord compression, were associated with the occurrence of periventricular leukomalacia. In other studies there was no specific FHR abnormality or pattern associated with fetal neurologic injury (1,9). On the contrary, mildly elevated baseline heart rate, low variability, and the absence of accelerations and decelerations were the specific findings of fetal brain death (12).

The relationship between particular FHR patterns and damage to specific areas of the CNS was studied, correlating the site of the anatomic defect with traces in autopsy material from 20 anencephalic infants (13). The following concluding hypotheses about the neurologic control of FHR patterns were drawn: The baseline FHR is controlled by the medulla oblongata and vagus nerve; the sleep–awake pattern is controlled by the cerebral cortex; accelerations are controlled by the midbrain; long-term variability is controlled by medulla oblongata and midbrain amplified by the cortex; U-shaped decelerations are controlled by medulla oblongata; and V-shaped decelerations are controlled by intracardiac reflexes and myocardial stretch.

One study of anencephalic fetuses, using probability distribution matrices, led to the hypothesis that at 27–28 weeks' gestation the medulla oblongata appears to play a primary role in the regulation of fetal heart rate variation (FHRV), whereas at 29–30 weeks the brain cephalad to the medulla oblongata probably participates (14). In addition, since the site of neuronal necrosis following asphyxia was demonstrated to vary in degree and distribution in preterm and term infants (15), this may explain why FHR patterns associated with brain damage may differ (1,9) according to the time and characteristics of the asphyxial insult.

Prenatal brain damage is often associated with cerebral ischemia and multiorgan dysfunction, occurring before labor. In animal experiments, only long periods of asphyxia with consequent FHR abnormalities were demonstrated to induce brain damage (16), whereas lesions resembling those of infants with cerebral palsy can be easily produced by intermittent cord occlusion in the absence of systemic acidosis or continuing asphyxia (17). Therefore, besides a severe hypoxic insult, some associated cardiocirculatory failure or collapse is required to produce brain damage (18), and ischemia of the brain is the critical factor in the etiology of fetal neurological injury (19). The "brain sparing" vasodilation of the mean cerebral artery (MCA) in IUGR fetuses does not seem to be associated with neonatal neurologic problems up to the age of 2 years (20,21).

In the human fetus, hematological and pathological findings indicate that between 43% and 66% of cases of brain damage occur in the antepartum period (15,22,23). Profound metabolic acidemia is often not sufficient to cause brain damage or cerebral dysfunction (24,25), except in the case of preterm fetuses (26,27).

The American College of Obstetricians and Gynecologists has proposed that before a plausible link between FHR abnormalities and brain damage can be made, besides severe acidemia (pH less than 7.00), persistent (more than 5 min) low Apgar score (0–3), and neurological sequelae (e.g., seizures, coma, or hypotonia), multiorgan system dysfunction (e.g., cardiovascular, gastrointestinal, hematological, pulmonary, or renal) must be demonstrated (28). If this assessment is true, with few exceptions (29), then by hypothesizing an efficient brain-sparing mechanism in all fetuses, postasphyxial antepartum brain damage should always be associated with or follow multiorgan system dysfunction secondary to the redistribution of cardiac output. In this case, antepartum FHR monitoring and/or Doppler ultrasonography detecting low FHRV and abnormal fetal waveforms (30) could be sensitive enough in the prevention of asphyxial brain damage. On other occasions the intrauterine environment can suddenly change, and, as in the case of stroke, the ischemic injury may develop rapidly (e.g., cord accidents), precluding benefit from any intervention.

Several factors may indeed explain the difficulty in the diagnosis of fetal asphyxia at a stage that could permit the prevention of brain damage: (1) the wide period of its antenatal occurrence, and its sudden and ischemic character, (2) the absence of specific risk factors in 50% of the cases, (3) the failure of periodic assessment, in complicated pregnancies, to identify the asphyxial episodes, and (4) the late cardiotocographic evidence of CNS damage (31).

Computer analysis may improve the predictive value of FHR monitoring, allowing an objective evaluation of FHR patterns and calculation of FHRV that appears persistently reduced in the case of fetal brain damage. Besides all these difficulties, antepartum FHR monitoring is criticized because the interpretation arising from visual analysis could vary according to different observers and even for the same observer on different occasions. Computerized systems allow an objective numerical analysis of all FHR traces, eliminating the observer bias (32). In addition, the quantitative evaluation of FHRV is possible, being, at least in the case of normal values, the best single assessment of fetal health (33,34). Persistently reduced FHRV appears to be the most common FHR pattern encountered in the case of fetal brain damage (1,34); since its quantitative determination by visual evaluation is impossible, computerized FHR monitoring could have a more efficient role in progressive cerebral damage prevention by recognizing FHRV reduction at an early stage.

The computer analysis of FHR will be the topic of this chapter, and we will focus our attention on fetal neurological aspects.

SYSTEMS FOR COMPUTERIZATION OF FHR SIGNALS

The conversion of FHR signals to digital data by a personal computer allows its acquisition, storage (archival), transmission (telemetry), and analysis (on-line and off-line). With computerized analysis all the information included in FHR, even if hidden to the naked eye, can be assessed in a precise quantitative way and compared to normal values. In addition, the objective assessment of the effects of physiological and pathological factors on FHR is possible.

FHR interpretation algorithms may be constructed according to different models. In a computerized interpretation each heart beat is sampled at regular intervals, the frequency of sampling being different according to the system adopted (35–37).

All systems receive the FHR signal online and should first determine the basal FHR defined as the reciprocal of the modal FHR period over time.

The baseline should be calculated in the absence of fetal movements and uterine contractions rather than in the absence of accelerations and decelerations, because it is necessary to know the baseline before the identification of an acceleration or a deceleration is possible (38). This calculation is most important when the goal of a computerized system is to mimic the clinician's visual interpretation since the recognition of the accelerations and decelerations depends on the baseline. If the baseline is overestimated, the number of accelerations decreases dramatically and the number of decelerations can increase (Figure 1). Examples of ambiguous records due to a misleading baseline calculation may correspond to the physiological type D trace recorded in the awake fetus (39,40). The systems also recognize the signal quality (artifacts and signal loss), discriminating between true and false decelerations or ac-

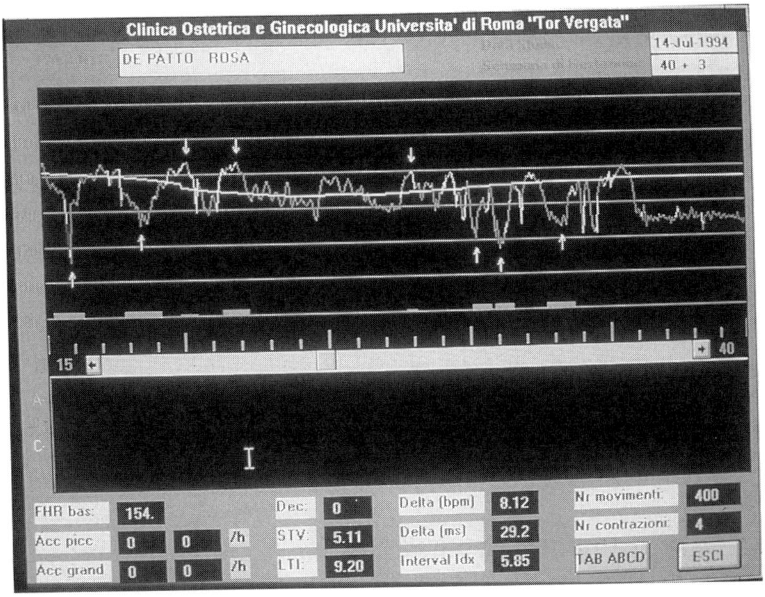

Figure 1. Error in baseline determination in the case of pattern D.

celerations (41). The evaluation of signal loss is of particular importance in younger fetuses, especially before 30 weeks' gestation, since at this time the incidence of errors is greater and the decision to deliver the fetus more relevant because of prematurity (42). Although most systems consider the traditional parameters of visual cardiotocography comparing quantitative obtained results to normal data, the complex analysis of long- and short-term variability (43) expressed in milliseconds (msec) is given particular importance since it represents the advantage of the system over the experts and their irreducibly different definitions of FHR patterns (44). Variability is a mathematical approximation of true variability since the source of antepartum signals is Doppler rather than ECG. The thresholds for reduced FHR variability are set at different values depending on the system adopted, but it is very important for each center to establish cutoff limits since persistently decreased FHRV with or without decelerations is described in over half the cases of cerebral palsy in several series (8,22,24).

HEART RATE VARIABILITY

Heart rate variability is the spontaneous fluctuation in sinus rate. The source of FHRV is a healthy well-working feedback between the autonomic system and the sinoatrial node. The sinoatrial node is innervated by sympathetic and parasympathetic (vagus) systems. The vagus nerve stimulation hyperpolarizes the node decreasing both the rate of spontaneous firing and the cardiac rate, whereas the sympathetic system releasing cathecolamines has the opposite effect. Due to the high turnover of acetylcholine the node response to vagal stimulation is faster, allowing beat-to-beat regulation.

Physiological Factors Affecting FHRV

Fetal respiratory movements, by changing blood pressure during each movement, stimulate and inhibit baroreceptors, thereby causing reflex changes in FHR (Bainbridge reflex) and increasing variability (45). The ultimate shape of the FHRV spectrum may result from the interaction of respiratory influences (vagally mediated) and behavioral influences (sympathetically mediated) (46). During breathing time (24.8%) there is an increase of beat-to-beat variability and of the baseline FHR, while during moving time (16.4%) there is an increase of baseline FHR but a decrease in beat-to-beat variability (47). Variability increases with gestational age as does the time spent in high heart rate variation and the number of accelerations (48). Such an increase, together with accelerations and episodes of high variation, primarily occurs during fetal activity (49,50). Every 3-min epoch of the FHR trace is classified in four different patterns (A, B, C, D) with the following definitions (51):

FHR Pattern A: Absence of accelerations and delta value < 10 bpm or presence of one acceleration and delta value < 5 bpm.

FHR Pattern B: Presence of accelerations or of one acceleration with delta value > 10 bpm.

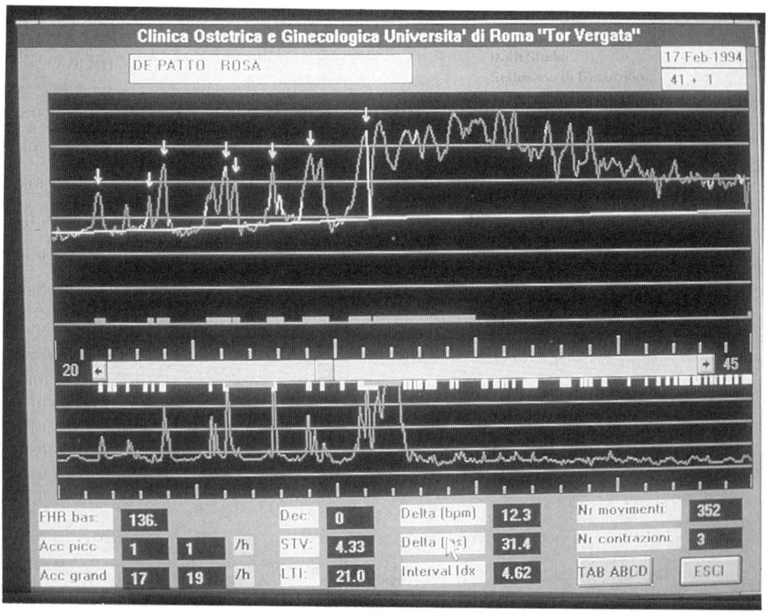

Figure 2. Example of 2 CTG System recording: FHR pattern B is followed by pattern D.

FHR Pattern C: Absence of accelerations and delta value ≥ 10 bpm.
FHR Pattern D: Presence of accelerations lasting more than 60 sec (Figures 1 and 2).

Significantly lower values of all FHRV indices were found during pattern A when compared with pattern B by using 2CTG system (52). In addition, with increasing gestational age, long-term variability increases in type B trace and decreases in type A (49) and the detection of behavioral state change becomes easy by visual evaluation (Figure 3).

Heart Rate Variability, Acute and Chronic Hypoxia, Acidemia

While acute experimental hypoxia is associated with an increase in variability (53,54) with a decrease in heart rate, the disappearance of FHRV is most often considered a sign of chronic hypoxia and may represent decompensation of the autonomic system undergoing prolonged and increasing stress with disruption of the equilibrium between sympathetic and parasympathetic systems. Basal FHR and long- and short-term variability increased with acidemia in ewes similar to the increase reported with acute hypoxia, suggesting that the decrease in FHRV in the case of chronic asphyxia is not the result of acidemia alone (55). Interestingly enough, when the hypoxemia of IUGR fetuses with antenatal reduced variability, is corrected after birth, FHRV is not restored immediately to normal levels (56), indicating that metabolic factors could be involved in variability regulation or that a transient or permanent damage has already occurred to the cardiac autonomic system.

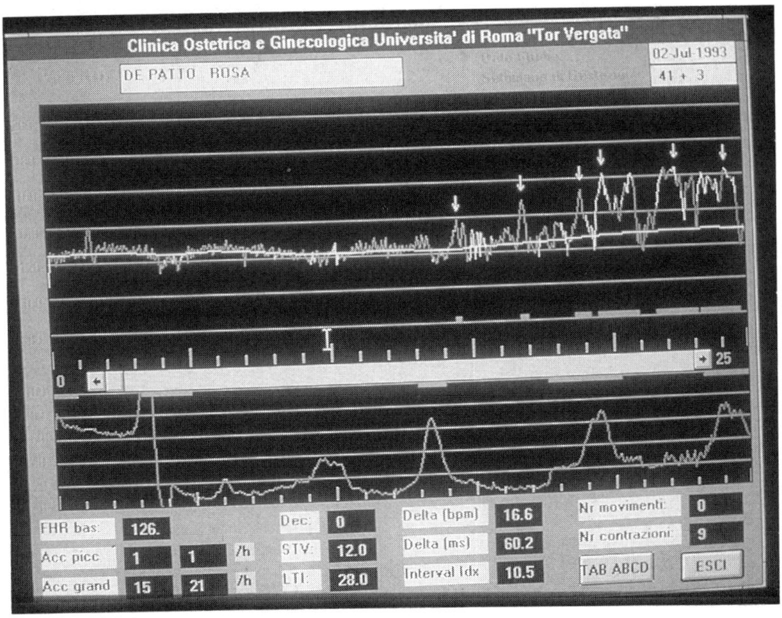

Figure 3. Example of 2 CTG System recording: FHR pattern A is followed by pattern B.

COMPUTERIZED SYSTEMS

Quantification of FHRV was first described (47,53,57–60) and reviewed (44); then autocorrelation was introduced (61), and in the same period the first computerized system originated from the work of Dawes and Redman (35). The FHR pulse interval is averaged every 3.75 sec in System 8000-8002 (Oxford Sonicaid Ltd., Oxford, UK) but is averaged every 2.5 sec in the 2CTG System (Hewlett Packard, Italy), and sampling intervals of 1 msec of the ECG signal that allows the computer to analyze and associate parameters of the fetal behavior are also used (36).

PARAMETERS

System 8000-8002 considers variability among the most important measures of fetal normality with a cutoff level of 22 msec (long-term variation) and 3 msec (short-term variation).

Normative data on FHR variation, accelerations, and time spent in high variation from 20 to 41 weeks' gestation are available for System 8000-8002, and abnormal patterns have been reported (41,62–64). Long-term variation greater than 30 msec is associated with normal outcome, whereas when it decreases to less than 20 msec it is associated with hypoxemia and metabolic changes (65,66). Short-term variability of less than 2.6 msec is linked to a high probability of fetal death or metabolic acidemia (63). Besides System 8000 (Figure 4), other analogous computerized systems have been introduced in the United States and Europe. In particular we gave our

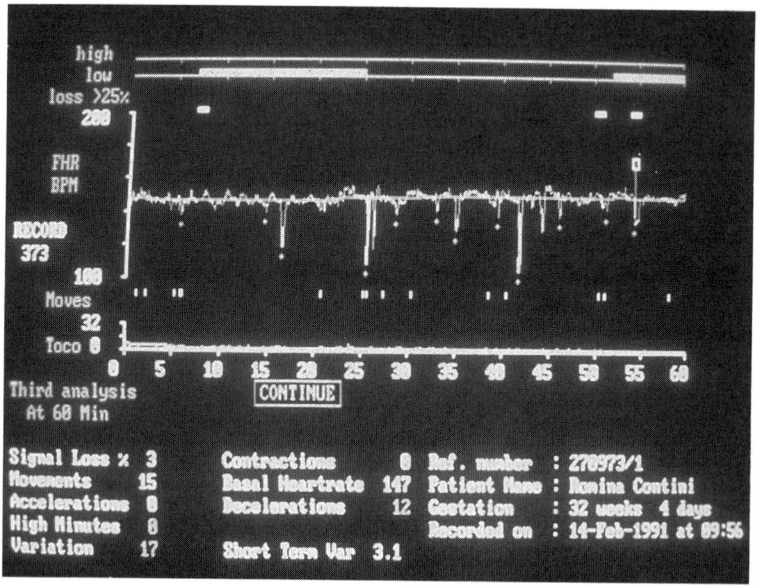

Figure 4. Example of System 8000 recording.

contribution to the development of the 2 CTG system (37,52) which will be briefly presented (Figures 1–3).

DESCRIPTION OF THE 2 CTG SYSTEM

Hardware

FHR, uterine contractions, and fetal movements are recorded by means of a commercially available fetal monitor (Hewlett Packard 8040A). The system of analysis is based on a 386 Personal Computer with Intel 80386X processor running at 20 MHz (Hewlett Packard Vectra 386/20N). The configuration includes 3 Mb of RAM and 50 Mb of hard disk. The operating system is MS-DOS 5.0 with MS-Windows 3.1. The system employs priority interrupts every 100 msec from the central processor unit to address the fetal monitor via its RS232 port to acquire the pulse interval of FHR, the quality of signal (autocorrelation function), the tocodynamometer value, and fetal movements. The signals captured are displayed graphically in a dedicated window of the computer screen and stored on the hard disk. The quality of the signal is continuously evaluated and the percentage of signal loss of FHR, as determined by the autocorrelation function, is continuously provided on the computer screen.

Software

After the first 10 minutes of recording, the FHR baseline is fitted and accelerations, decelerations, and variability indices are calculated. Uterine contractions are identified and analyzed. These parameters are reanalyzed every 5 minutes thereafter until the end of recording. The procedure of analysis is as follows:

Baseline Determination. A real-time version of the procedure described by Mantel et al. (67) is used. After 10 min of recording, the fetal heart pulse interval is averaged over 2.5-sec epochs. A frequency distribution is obtained and the starting point is calculated on the basis of the first prominent peak near the high end of the frequency distribution using a previously described algorithm (68). The value of the starting point is then used as a guide for baseline calculation based on a low-pass filter with a time constant of 0.1 min^{-1} and a trim function interacting in a five-run iterative process (67). Only the first 5 min of the resulting baseline are considered valid, while the remaining portions are discarded. This selection is made in an attempt to minimize the border effect errors that may result with the procedure of filtering used. After an additional 5 min (15 from the beginning of the acquisition) the computation window is shifted 5 min forward and the baseline is recalculated on the next 10 min using as a starting point the last valid value of the previously calculated baseline and similarly discarding at the end of the calculation the last 5 min. The procedure is repeated every 5 min until recording stops. The selection of the 10-min window shifted every 5 min is the result of a compromise between theoretical considerations on the time constant of the low-pass filter requiring a sufficiently long period of acquisition to have negligible border errors and the clinical usefulness of frequent reanalysis of the data acquired.

Acceleration and Deceleration Identification

Accelerations and decelerations are defined as deviations from the baseline with a certain amplitude and duration. Large accelerations are longer than 15 sec with an amplitude of > 15 bpm, whereas the amplitude of small accelerations is between 10 and 15 bpm. Decelerations are periods of >20 bpm below the baseline lasting >30 sec or periods with an amplitude >10 bpm lasting >60 sec. For each deceleration the nadir, duration, and area under the baseline is calculated as well as the temporal association between the onset of contractions and the deceleration.

Variability

Variability is calculated excluding accelerations and decelerations. For each minute the amplitude bandwidth around the baseline (delta) is then calculated as the difference between the maximum and minimum value of FHR and expressed in bpm and msec. Long-term variability is evaluated by means of the long-term irregularity index (LTI) as described by de Haan et al. (57). Short-term variability is calculated every 60 sec with two different indices. The short-term variation (STV) is the average of successive 2.5-sec pulse interval epochal differences (epoch to epoch variation) (53), and the interval index is the coefficient of variations (SD/mean) of the difference between averaged pulse interval of consecutive 2.5-sec epochs (58).

Uterine Contractions

Resting tone is calculated by the same method used for FHR baseline. A contraction is an increase from the resting tone lasting >30 sec exceeding a value of 25% from basal value.

FHR Patterns

At the end of recording (off-line) the system reanalyzes the data using a 3-min moving window shifted every 1 min. According to Nijhuis et al. (51), every 3-min epoch is classified in different patterns (A–D) (37).

THE OBSERVER COMPARED TO THE COMPUTER

Disagreement may occur when different observers are faced with the same FHR trace (69). Computerized FHR analysis eliminates the problem of intra/interobserver variability (32) and the high false-negative rate of visual evaluation (39). Poor agreement between visual and computer evaluation of abnormal tracings was recorded (70) with fewer follow-up tests and more appropriate obstetric interventions in the case of computer evaluation. A consistent amount of the interobserver variation may be caused by the different definitions of FHR patterns among experts and institutions (44), but also in this case the computer may help to form a general agreement. Computerized analysis of FHR can identify and measure abnormal characteristics of the FHR before the appearance of nonreactive FHR at visual analysis (71). Computer analysis of FHR may also occur without the intervention of human observers since the computer itself can be trained to recognize normal and abnormal patterns. This can be achieved by using neural networks.

NEURAL NETWORKS

Neural networks are a group of intelligent software mimicking the function of the human brain that can recognize patterns through a programmed set of known inputs (FHR elements) and outputs (FHR classifications) linked by associative elements (neurons). Through repetitive training the final accurate identification of unknown cases is possible, since these systems can learn or improve by themselves. Nevertheless, networks cannot indicate how they arrived at their solutions, and training may be very difficult whenever high levels of sophistication are required.

NST results are classified as normal or abnormal by a neural network. When expert agreement on test interpretation is high, the network works well, whereas it is in difficulties in the case of expert disagreement or uncertainty (72). This phenomenon can be explained by the rarity of adverse outcome and by the ambiguity of some patterns that can belong to normal or abnormal outcomes. In such instances, training of the neural network becomes difficult (73). In network training it would be ideal to have an equal number of pathological and nonpathological cases. Since fetal cerebral damage is very rare in clinical practice, it would be very difficult to train the system to recognize typical FHR patterns indicative of cerebral palsy when its existence is still in doubt. Networks were employed to assess test stability in normal pregnancies from 1 to 4 days demonstrating that NST is unstable when intervals exceeded 2 days, the only parameter relatively stable over 2 days being long-term variability (74). Neural networks can also be trained to read power spectra of FHRV.

STUDYING THE EFFECTS OF MATERNAL DRUG ADMINISTRATION ON FHR

The use of corticosteroids to accelerate fetal pulmonary maturation causes inhibition of fetal movements and a significant reduction of FHR variation in the case of betamethasone (75), but an increase in the case of dexamethasone administration is no longer evident in the case of low biophysical score (76). The use of dexamethasone instead of betamethasone is suggested to accelerate fetal pulmonary maturation and could represent a test of fetal assessment since the lack of increased variability can be interpreted as a sign of fetal jeopardy.

No changes in FHR patterns occurs in preeclamptic patients receiving methyldopa or isradipine (77), while magnesium decreases both long- and short-term variability and accelerations (78–80).

Phenytoin reduces only the short-term variation (79).

Maternal hyperoxia produces a greater increase in accelerations and variability in the case of IUGR (81).

STUDYING THE EFFECTS OF FETAL STIMULATION

The effects of vibroacoustic stimulation in a sleeping near-term fetus are fetal movements with a variability shift of indices toward that recorded in the previous spontaneous active period (82,83).

THE CLINICAL USE

The clinical use of computerized FHR monitoring concerns the threshold values of long-term variability to predict fetal hypoxemia (63,66,84), death, or metabolic acidemia. Reduced FHRV was reported in fetal anemia caused by Rhesus alloimmunization (85).

Short-term and long-term FHRV are strongly correlated with the exception of sinusoidal FHR pattern. Sinusoidal rhythm can sometimes result in high long-term and low short-term FHRV (63), but the low ratio of short-term/long-term FHRV warns the clinician of the presence of this ominous rhythm. In the case of IUGR fetuses, no uniform behavior was noted with respect to FHRV alone (86), most fetuses having low values before delivery. Using each fetus as its own control in longitudinal studies is therefore warranted. FHRV proved more reliable in measuring fetal deterioration than umbilical artery (UA) velocimetry (87), whereas its value was recently challenged in comparison with venous Doppler in IUGR fetuses (30,88). When FHRV is reduced, the presence or absence of decelerations is not helpful in assessing outcome, in comparison with the measurement of FHRV (63,87). Computerized FHR monitoring was studied in the case of absent end-diastolic velocities (AEDVs) in UA Doppler waveforms, and reduced FHRV was shown to select the most compromised fetuses requiring immediate delivery since it was associated with decreased left cardiac output, followed by loss of MCA dilation and by the appearance of FHR decelerations (89,90). FHRV was significantly reduced when the MCA reached its maximal dilation, but it was only with the rise of cerebral impedance that all fetuses had a further reduction of FHRV and decelerations. Therefore, at least in IUGR fetuses with AEDV in UA, the fetal brain loses autonomic reactivity first and the heart responds to the cerebral impedance increase. Only later, worsening hypoxia causes a loss of autonomic reactivity in the heart. In a recent paper (88), venous Doppler was demonstrated to be a more accurate method of determining the optimum time of delivery in

IUGR fetuses than computerized cardiotocography. An abrupt increase in pulsatility of the ductus venous waveforms with loss of forward flow velocity during atrial contraction preceded abnormally low short-term FHRV. In contrast with a previous study (89), the authors found neither a further decrease in pulsatility index (PI) nor a loss of MCA vasodilation with an increase in PI before a decrease in FHRV occurred. This confirms the results of a longitudinal study of IUGR fetuses in which no changes in PI of MCA were found preceding the onset of late FHR decelerations (91).

Pregnancies exceeding 41 weeks were followed by computerized FHR monitoring, and its better diagnostic efficiency was demonstrated over other measures of fetal condition such as amniotic fluid index or Doppler waveforms (92,93). Not only decreased interval index, but also increased basal FHR, seems to predict intrapartum fetal distress (93). In addition, in post-term pregnancy a reduction of both left and right cardiac output was noticed in association with decreased long-term FHRV (<30 msec) while MCA impedance was normal, indicating a cardiogenic origin of decreased FHRV (90). Decreased FHRV may be related not only to a number of physiological and pathological factors, but also to a dysfunction of the autonomic control of the cardiocirculatory system, since it occurs in the case of myocardial ischemia, infarction, or impaired left ventricular function in adults (45). Further longitudinal studies are necessary in high-risk pregnancies (IUGR, postdate, diabetes) to assess the correlation between reduced FHRV, cardiac dysfunction (abnormal fetal venous circulation), and cerebral dysfunction (circulatory or behavioral alterations). Actually, abnormal hemodynamics have been described in fetuses of insulin-dependent diabetic mothers, and IUGR and post-date fetuses may have an abnormal cardiac function (90,94,95). Nevertheless, low human FHRV can occur in normal pregnancy, indicating that the intrauterine environment could have a role in some cases (65). The role of antepartum computerized FHR analysis was evaluated in the antenatal prediction of fetal distress during labor in 577 healthy term pregnancies. The multivariate analysis showed that FHR baseline and the percentage of small accelerations were independently and significantly related to the labor outcome (96). In other studies, prediction of morbidity in normally grown fetuses by FHRV, biophysical profile score, and umbilical Doppler studies performed within 7 days of delivery failed all these tests of fetal well-being (97), as in the case of unexplained antepartum hemorrhage (98).

Since approximate entropy and fractal analysis correlate with variability, they have been recently studied in the evaluation of fetal well-being (99,100).

FRACTAL ANALYSIS

The FHR is a "chaotic" signal and may contain diagnostic information that is hidden to visual evaluation. The mathematical theory of deterministic chaos used to describe nonlinear and nonrandom (borderline) phenomena was successfully applied to the study of FHR. A brief terminology glossary is reported in the appendix of a recent article (99). The normal traces at term show a large central attractor with lots of random projection of energy and a fractal dimension index ranging from 4.22 to 5.22. Questionable traces show smaller attractors with fewer emissions. Highly pathological traces show very small attractors without random projections and a fractal dimension index ranging from 2.0 to 3.09 (99). In the case of chaos, the expert's interpretation is not necessary because the dimension value is a qualitative measure for interpretation.

APPROXIMATE ENTROPY (ApEn)

FHR variability was studied in fetuses by incorporating the nonlinear analytic techniques of phase-space reconstruction and next-dimensional analysis to the raw FHR signals (100–102). Approximate entropy is a statistical measure of complexity or regularity of signals derived from non-linear dynamic analysis that is proportional to the degree of regularity in a signal (103). This system may pose difficulties in case of noise in the detection of periodic pathological patterns that power spectrum can easily identify (104). It offers no advantage over measurement of short-term FHR variation antepartum (100), at least in the case of averaged FHR signal. The normogram of ApEn is reported in Figure 5.

SPECTRAL ANALYSIS OF FHRV

Power spectral analysis is widely used to study the dysfunctions of the autonomic nervous system in cardiology, neurology, and neonatology where heart rate traces are not considered for well-being evaluation (45). It identifies rhythmic variations by decomposing the variations of heart rate period into their underlying frequency components

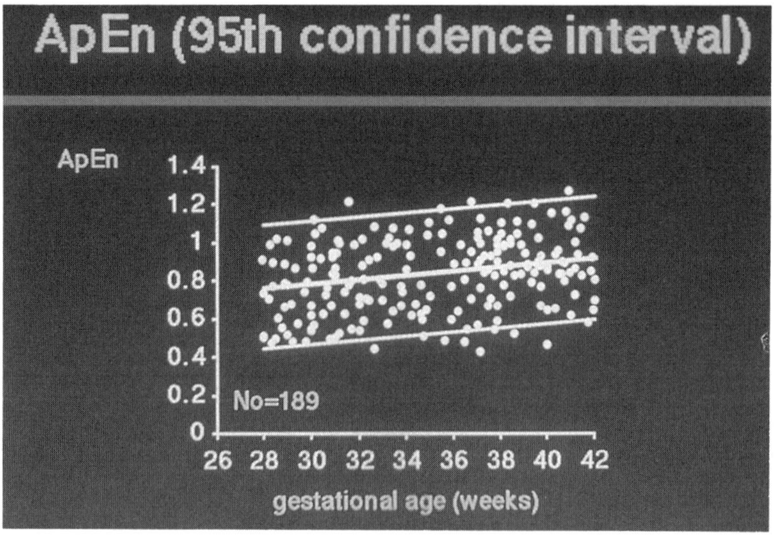

Figure 5. Normogram of ApEn.

(105). There are three major identifiable peaks in normal adults (106). The high-frequency peak (0.15–0.30 Hz), representing respiratory sinus arrhythmia, is parasympathetic since it can be abolished by muscarinic antagonist and vagotomy (107). The midfrequency band (0.05–0.15 Hz) is most likely linked to baroreceptor feedback activity related to blood pressure oscillations, whereas the low-frequency peak (0.01–0.05 Hz) is linked to peripheral vasomotor control (108). The area under the curve of an individual peak represents the power or the amount of variance in the data within that frequency range. Spectral analysis of FHRV obtained by Doppler ultrasound signals was comparable to that obtained from fetal scalp electrocardiogram (109).

Most authors have found similarities between adult and FHR spectra (110,111), with differences concerning the high-frequency component of the fetal power spectrum. This component seems particularly important in the fetus, being apparent in the third trimester during fetal breathing movements (109,110,112,113). Since a reduced respiratory sinus arrhythmia was demonstrated in asphyxiated term infants by using spectral analysis (114), it can be hypothesized that the same finding can account for the smooth FHR pattern commonly associated with perinatal asphyxia.

Peaks of 0.30 Hz may identify fetuses with chronic distress (115) and may reflect the presence of movements of unchanged amplitude but higher frequency such as mouthing or thoracic movements. Real-time spectral estimation of FHRV (116) could be useful in the near future to establish a correlation between new spectral components and fetal behavioral patterns, breathing, or hypoxic stimuli such as uterine contractions. Both visual and computerized cardiotocography reduce FHRV to a single number that represents an average value between different fetal behavioral states. Therefore, the same value may correspond to thousands of traces while a considerable amount of information can be extracted by means of spectral analysis.

The biological relevance of spectral analysis of FHRV is very limited in the case of artifacts and/or restricted variance as in tachycardia. Nevertheless, in flat FHR recordings a shift of the position of the maximum energy peak from 0.20 Hz to 0.30 Hz may signify a chronic distress condition (117). Periodic low-frequency fluctuations in the vicinity of 0.05 Hz have been found in various abnormal conditions and are considered a sign of malfunctioning autonomic control of the cardiovascular system (sinusoidal pattern).

Vibroacoustic stimulation increases the power and shifts the spectrum toward the very low frequency band (0–0.05 Hz) representing sympathetic activity (118). Power spectral analysis has been used to study the development of the autonomous nervous system in monkey fetuses. The frequency bands were classified into low frequency (LF = 0.05–0.2 Hz) and high frequency (HF = 0.4–1.0 Hz), mediated by the sympathetic and parasympathetic systems respectively. Both LF and HF showed significant increase with gestational age, but the rate of the increase in HF was three times more than that in LF. The LF/HF ratio showed a positive correlation both to LF and to LF/HF ratio (sympathetic activity). Short-term variability increased only during fetal breathing movements, and showed a positive correlation to HF (parasympathetic activity) and an inverse correlation to LF/HF ratio (119). Examples of spectral analysis are reported in Figure 6.

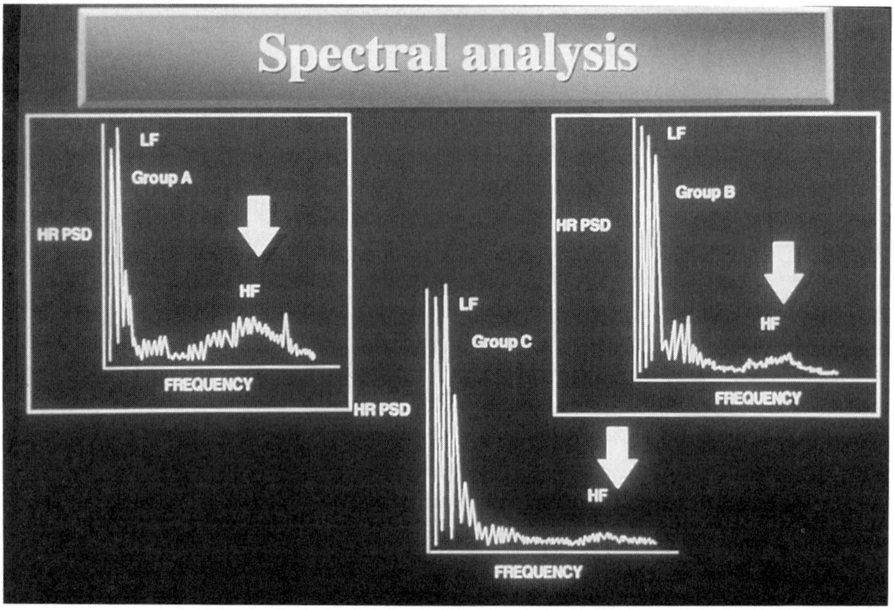

Figure 6. Patterns of spectral analysis. Group A: healthy preterm fetus. Group B: healthy near-term fetus. Group C: IUGR fetus. LF, low frequency; HF, high frequency.

CONCLUSIONS

Computerized FHR monitoring allows a reproducible and objective analysis of FHR tracings, a quantitative evaluation of FHR variability, and the possibility to archive or transmit all the traces. It remains to be seen in the near future whether technical advances will improve, and to what extent, the predictive value of cardiotocography in the evaluation of fetal well-being by extracting the neurological and cardiac information hidden in the sequence of fetal heart beats. Many open questions still remain such as: Which comes first, myocardial or neurological dysfunction? Does FHR reflect better neurological or myocardial function? Can myocardial dysfunction be considered a first step in prenatal brain damage? Actually, the time sequence of fetal deterioration is still discussed in the IUGR fetus and is almost unknown in other pregnancy complications like postdatism, diabetes, and alloimmunization. Computerized analysis could be helpful in finding an answer to all these questions. However, because of the low prevalence of cerebral damage in high-risk pregnancy, the predictive value of computerized cardiotocography will never be high, with a large proportion of false-positive findings. For the general population the predictive value will be even lower since decreased FHRV could be related to a great number of factors other than cerebral damage. Nevertheless, the treatment paradox will lead to thinking that a positive test with a satisfactory newborn condition is the result of appropriate obstetrical intervention and not a false-positive finding. On the other hand, computerized cardiotocography will produce emergency obstetrical intervention in a number of cases where nonprogressive prenatal cerebral damage has already occurred (31) during the spontaneous recovery period. The awareness of all these difficulties and of the possibility that fetal brain damage can occur very rapidly at home in the case of cerebral ischemia will avoid the replacement of FHR monitoring utopia with that of other contemporary methods of fetal well-being evaluation such as venous Doppler.

REFERENCES

1. Rosen GM, Dickinson JC. The paradox of electronic fetal monitoring: more data may not enable us to predict or prevent infant neurologic morbidity. *Am J Obstet Gynecol* 1993; 168:745–751.
2. Nelson KB, Dambrosia JM, Ting TY, Grether JK. Uncertain value of electronic fetal monitoring in predicting cerebral palsy. *N Engl J Med* 1996;334:613–618.
3. Painter MJ, Depp R, O'Donoghue PD. Fetal heart rate patterns and development in the first year of life. *Am J Obstet Gynecol* 1978;132:271–277.
4. Painter MJ, Scott M, Hirsch R, O'Donoghue PD, Depp R. Fetal heart rate pattern during labor: neurologic and cognitive development at six to nine years of age. *Am J Obstet Gynecol* 1988;159:854–858.
5. Painter MJ. Fetal heart rate patterns, perinatal asphyxia, and brain injury. *Pediatr Neurol* 1989;5:137–144.
6. Horimoto N, Koyanagi T, Maeda H, Takashima T, Minami T, Nakano H. Can brain impairment be detected by in utero behavioural patterns? *Arch Dis Child* 1993;69:3–8.
7. Shields JR, Schifrin BS. Perinatal antecedents of cerebral palsy. *Obstet Gynecol* 1988;71: 899–905.
8. Phelan JP, Ahn MO. Perinatal observations in forty-eight neurologically impaired term infants. *Am J Obstet Gynecol* 1994;171:424–431.
9. Ahn MO, Korst L, Phelan JP. Intrapartum fetal heart rate patterns in 209 brain damaged infants. *Am J Obstet Gynecol* 1996;174:492.
10. Okamura M, Itakura A, Kurauchi O, Mizutani S, Tomoda Y. Fetal heart rate patterns associated with periventricular leukomalacia. *Int J Obstet Gynecol* 1997;56:13–18.
11. Ito T, Kadowaki K, Takahashi H, Nagata N, Makio A, Terakawa N. Clinical features of cardiotocographic findings for premature infants with antenatal periventricular leukomalacia. *Early Hum Dev* 1997;47:195–201.
12. Nijhuis JG, Kruyt N, Van Wijck JAM. Fetal brain death. Two case reports. *Br J Obstet Gynaecol* 1988;95:197–200.
13. Terao T, Kawashima Y, Noto H, Inamoto Y, Lin TY, Sumimoto K, Maeda M. Neurological control of fetal heart rate in 20 cases of anencephalic fetuses. *Am J Obstet Gynecol* 1984;149:201–208.
14. Yoshizato T, Koyanagi T, Takashima T, Satoh S, Akazawa K, Nakano H. The relationship between age-related heart changes and developing brain function: a model of anencephalic human fetus in utero. *Early Hum Dev* 1994;36:101–112.
15. Low JA, Robertson DR, Simpson LL. Temporal relationships of neuropathologic conditions caused by perinatal asphyxia. *Am J Obstet Gynecol* 1989;160:608–614.
16. Adamsons K, Myers RE. Late decelerations and brain tolerance of the fetal monkey to intrapartum asphyxia. *Am J Obstet Gynecol* 1977;128:893–900.

17. Mann LI. Pregnancy events and brain damage. *Am J Obstet Gynecol* 1986;155:6–9.
18. de Courten-Myers GM, Folgeson HM, Kleinholtz M, Myers RE. Hypoxic brain and heart injury thresholds in piglets. *Biomed Biochem Acta* 1989;48:S143–S148.
19. Vannucci RC. Mechanisms of perinatal hypoxic-ischemic brain damage. *Semin Perinatol* 1993;17:330–337.
20. Scherjon SA, Smolders-de Haas H, Kok JH, Zondervan HA. The "brain sparing" effect: antenatal cerebral Doppler findings in relation to neurologic outcome in very preterm infants. *Am J Obstet Gynecol* 1993;169:169–175.
21. Chan FY, Pun TC, Lam P, Lam C, Lee CP, Lam YH. Fetal cerebral Doppler studies as a predictor of perinatal outcome and subsequent neurologic handicap. *Obstet Gynecol* 1996;87:981–988.
22. Paul RH, Yonekura ML, Cantrell CJ, Turkel S, Pavolova Z, Sipos L. Fetal injury prior to labor: does it happen? *Am J Obstet Gynecol* 1986;154:1187–1193.
23. Naeye RL. Can meconium in the amniotic fluid injure the fetal brain? *Obstet Gynecol* 1995;86:720.
24. Ruth VJ, Raivio KO. Perinatal brain damage: predictive value of metabolic acidosis and the Apgar score. *Br Med J* 1988;297:24–27.
25. Dennis J, Johnson A, Mutch L, Yudkin P, Johnson P. Acid–base status at birth and neurodevelopmental outcome at four and one-half years. *Am J Obstet Gynecol* 1989;161:213–220.
26. Soothill PW, Ajayi RA, Campbell S, Ross EM, Candy DLA, Snijders RM, Nicolaides KH. Relationship between fetal acidemia at cordocentesis and subsequent neurodevelopment. *Ultrasound Obstet Gynecol* 1992;2:80–83.
27. Low JA, Panagiotolous C, Derrick EJ. Newborn complications after intrapartum asphyxia with metabolic acidosis in the preterm fetus. *Am J Obstet Gynecol* 1995;172:805–810.
28. American College of Obstetricians and Gynecologists. *Fetal and neonatal neurologic injury.* Washington, DC: American College of Obstetricians and Gynecologists, 1992 Jan; ACOG technical bulletin no 163.
29. Goodlin RC. Do concepts of causes and prevention of cerebral palsy require revision. *Am J Obstet Gynecol* 1995;172:1830–1836.
30. Black RS, Campbell S. Cardiotocograph versus Doppler. *Ultrasound Obstet Gynecol* 1997;9:148–151.
31. Low JA, Simpson LL, Ramsey DA. The clinical diagnosis of asphyxia responsible for brain damage in the human fetus. *Am J Obstet Gynecol* 1992;167:11–15.
32. Arduini D, Rizzo G, Giannini F, Garzetti GG, Romanini C. Computerized analysis of fetal heart rate. II. Comparison with the interpretation of experts. *J Matern Fetal Med* 1993B;3:165–168.
33. Martin C Jr. Physiology and clinical use of fetal heart rate variability. *Clin Perinatol* 1982;9:339–342.
34. Schifrin BS. Antenatal fetal assessment: overview and implications for neurologic injury and routine testing. *Clin Obstet Gynecol* 1995;38:132–141.
35. Dawes GS, Redman CWG. Antenatal heart rate analysis at the bedside using a microprocessor. In Kunzel W (ed). *Fetal heart rate monitoring.* Berlin: Springer, 1985:63–65.
36. Divon MY. Microcomputer-assisted evaluation of fetal wellbeing. In Geisow MJ and Barrett AN (eds). *Microcomputers in medicine.* New York: Elsevier Science Publishers, 1987:207–222.

37. Arduini D, Rizzo G. Quantitative analysis of the fetal rate: its application in antepartum clinical monitoring and behavioural pattern recognition. *Int J Biomed Comput* 1990;25: 247–252.

38. Bernades J, Costa-Pereira A, van Geijn H, Pereira-Leite L. A more objective fetal heart rate baseline estimation. *Br J Obstet Gynecol* 1996;103:714–715.

39. Gagnon R, Campbell MK, Hunse C. A comparison between visual and computer analysis of antepartum fetal heart rate tracings. *Am J Obstet Gynecol* 1993;168:842–847.

40. Gagnon R, Bocking AD, Richardson BS, McLean P. A flat decelerative fetal heart rate tracing with normal fetal heart rate variability. *Am J Obstet Gynecol* 1994;171:1379–1381.

41. Dawes GS, Lobb M, Moulden M, Redman CWG, Wheeler T. Antenatal cardiotocogram quality and interpretation using computers. *Br J Obstet Gynaecol* 1992A;99:791–797.

42. Dawes GS, Moulden M, Redman CWG. Limitations of antenatal fetal heart rate monitors. *Am J Obstet Gynecol* 1990;162:170–173.

43. Parer WJ, Parer JT, Holbrook RH, Block BSB. Validity of mathematical methods of quantitating fetal heart rate variability. *Am J Obstet Gynecol* 1985;153:402–409.

44. Parer JT, Quilligan EJ. Lack of consistency in definitions of fetal heart rate (FHR) patterns. *Am J Obstet Gynecol* 1996;174:492.

45. Kristal-Boneh E, Raifel M, Froom P, Ribak J. Heart rate variability in health and disease. *Scand J Work Environ Health* 1995;21:85–95.

46. Davidson SR, Rankin JHG, Martin CB, Reid DL. Fetal heart rate variability and behavioral state: analysis by power spectrum. *Am J Obstet Gynecol* 1992;167:717–722.

47. Divon MY, Zimmer EZ, Yeh SY, Vilensky A, Sarna EZ, Paldi E, Platt LD. Modulation of foetal heart rate patterns by foetal breathing: the effect of maternal intravenous glucose administration. *Am J Perinatol* 1985A;2:292–295.

48. Dawes GS, Houghton CRS, Redman CWG, Visser GHA. Pattern of normal fetal heart rate. *Br J Obstet Gynaecol* 1982A;89:276–284.

49. Dawes GS, Moulden M, Redman CWG. Improvements in computerized fetal heart rate analysis antepartum. *J Perinat Med* 1996;24:25–36.

50. Mantel R, Van Geijn HP, Ververs IAP, Colenbrander GJ, Kostense PJ. Automated analysis of antepartum fetal heart rate in relation to fetal rest–activity states: a longitudinal study of uncomplicated pregnancies using the Sonicaid System 8000. *Eur J Obstet Gynecol* 1996;71:41–51.

51. Nijhuis JG, Prechtl HFR, Martin CB Jr, Bots RSGM. Are there behavioural states in the human fetus? *Early Hum Dev* 1982;6:177–195.

52. Arduini D, Rizzo G, Piana G, Bonalumi A, Brambilla P, Romanini C. Computerized analysis of fetal heart rate. I. Description of the system 2CTG. *J Matern Fetal Med* 1993A;3:159–163.

53. Dalton KJ, Dawes GS, Patrick JE. Diurnal respiratory and other rhythms of fetal heart rate in lambs. *Am J Obstet Gynecol* 1977;127:414–424.

54. Ikenoue T, Martin CB, Murata Y, Ettinger BS, Lu PS. Effects of acute hypoxemia and respiratory acidosis on the fetal heart rate in monkeys. *Am J Obstet Gynecol* 1981;141:797–806.

55. Chaffin D, Barnard J, Phemetton T, Newman A, Reed K. The effect of acidemia on fetal heart rate variability. *Am J Obstet Gynecol* 1996;174:380.

56. Smith JH. Low human fetal heart rate variation. Thesis. Cambridge, England: University of Cambridge, 1989:167pp.

57. de Haan JV, Bemmel JHV, Vesteeg B, Veth AFL, Stolte FL, Janssens LAM, Eskes TKAB. Quantitative evaluation of fetal heart rate patterns. I. Processing methods. *Eur J Obstet Gynecol* 1971;3:95–102.
58. Yeh SY, Forsythe A, Hon EA. Quantitation of fetal heart rate beat-to-beat interval differences. *Obstet Gynecol* 1973;41:355–363.
59. Saini VD, Maulik D. Computation of short term fetal heart rate variability from heart-rate waveforms. *Comput Biol Med* 1982;12:81–86.
60. Maulik D, Saini V, Zigrossi ST. Clinical significance of short-term variability computer from heart-rate waveforms. *J Perinat Med* 1983;11:243–248.
61. Divon MY, Torres FP, Yeh S, Paul RH. Autocorrelation techniques in fetal monitoring. *Am J Obstet Gynecol* 1985B;151:2–6.
62. Snijders RJM, Mc Laren R, Nicolaides KH. Computer-assisted analysis of fetal heart rate patterns at 20–41 weeks' gestation. *Fetal Diagn Ther* 1990;5:79–83.
63. Street P, Dawes GS, Moulden M, Redman CWG. Short-term variation in abnormal antenatal fetal heart rate records. *Am J Obstet Gynecol* 1991;165:515–523.
64. Dawes G, Meir YS, Mandruzzato GP. Computerized evaluation of fetal heart-rate patterns. *J Perinat Med* 1994;22;491–499.
65. Smith JH, Dawes GS, Redman CWG. Low human fetal heart rate variation in normal pregnancy. *Br J Obstet Gynaecol* 1987;94:656–664.
66. Smith JH, Anand KJS, Cotes PM, Dawes GS, Harkness RA, Howlett TA, Rees LH, Redman CWG. Antenatal fetal heart rate variation in relation to the respiratory and metabolic status of the compromised human fetus. *Br J Obstet Gynaecol* 1988;95:980–989.
67. Mantel R, Van Geijn HP, Caron FJM, Swartijes JM, van Worden EE, Jongsma HW. Computer analysis of antepartum fetal heart rate. 1. Baseline determination. *Int J Biomed Comput* 1990;25:261–272.
68. Dawes GS, Houghton CRS, Redman CWG. Baseline in human fetal heart-rate records. *Br J Obstet Gynaecol* 1982B;89:270–275.
69. Todros T, Preve CU, Plazzotta C, Biolcati M, Lombardo P. Fetal heart rate tracings: observers versus computer assessment. *Eur J Obstet Gynecol Reprod Biol* 1996;68:83–86.
70. Hiett AK, Devoe LD, Youssef A, Gardner P, Black M. A comparison of visual and automated methods of analyzing fetal heart rate tests. *Am J Obstet Gynecol* 1993;168: 1517–1521.
71. Ferrazzi E, Rigano S, Mezzopane R, Bellotti M, Barbera A, Pardi G. Computerized heart rate monitoring of growth restricted fetuses. *Am J Obstet Gynecol* 1996;174:337.
72. Kol S, Thaler I, Paz N, Shmueli O. Interpretation of nonstress test by an artificial neural network. *Am J Obstet Gynecol* 1995;172:1372–1379.
73. Stock A, Rogers MS, Li A, Chang AMZ. Use of the neural network for hypothesis generation in fetal surveillance. *Baillière's Clin Obstet Gynecol* 1994;8(3):533–548.
74. Devoe LD, Carlton E, Prescott P. Neuronal network prediction of nonstress test results: how often should we perform nonstress test? *Am J Obstet Gynecol* 1995;173:1128–1131.
75. Mulder EJH, Zonneveld MF, Derks JB, Bruinse HW, Visser GHA. Transient reduction in fetal activity after maternal betamethasone administration. *Proc Soc Study Fetal Physiol* 1993;19:B27.
76. Dawes GS, Serra-Serra V, Moulden M, Redman CWG. Dexamethasone and fetal heart rate variation. *Proc Soc Study Fetal Physiol* 1993;20:30.

77. Wilde-Swensson D, Montan S, Arukumaran S, Ingemarsson I, Ramam S. Effect of methyldopa and isradipine on fetal heart rate pattern assessed by computerized cardiotocography in human pregnancy. *Am J Obstet Gynecol* 1993;169:1581–1585.

78. Hiett AK, Devoe LD, Brown HL, Watson J. Effect of magnesium on fetal heart rate variability using computer analysis. *Am J Perinatol* 1995;12:259–261.

79. Guzman E, Conley M, Stewart R, Ivan J, Pitter M, Kappy K. A comparison of the effects of phenytoin and Mg_2SO_4 on fetal heart rate tracings using computer analysis. *Am J Obstet Gynecol* 1992;166:299–304.

80. Atkinson MW, Belfort MA, Saade G, Moise KJ. The relationship between magnesium sulfate therapy and fetal heart rate variability. *Obstet Gynecol* 1994;83:967–970.

81. Bartnicki J, Sailing E. Influence of maternal oxygen administration on the computer-analyzed fetal heart rate patterns in small-for-gestational-age fetuses. *Gynecol Obstet Invest* 1994;37:172–175.

82. Bartnicki J, Dudenhausen JW. Antepartum vibroacoustic stimulation in patients with low fetal heart rate variability. *Int J Obstet Gynecol* 1995;48:173–177.

83. Giacomello F, Rizzo G, Sonnino A, Capponi A, Arduini D, Romanini C. Are there any changes in the computer-measured fetal heart rate variation after vibroacoustic stimulation in near-term uneventful pregnancies? *J Matern Fetal Invest* 1995;5:148–151.

84. Ribbert LSM, Snijders RJM, Nicolaides KH, Visser GHA. Relation of fetal blood gases and data from computer-assisted analysis of fetal heart rate patterns in small for gestation fetuses. *Br J Obstet Gynaecol* 1991;98:820–823.

85. Economides DL, Selinger M, Ferguson J, Bowell PJ, Dawes GS, Mackenzie IZ. Computerized measurement of heart variation in fetal anemia caused by rhesus alloimmunization. *Am J Obstet Gynecol* 1992;167:689–693.

86. Snijders RJM, Ribbert LSM, Visser GHA, Mulder EJH. Numeric analysis of heart rate variation in intrauterine growth-retarded fetuses: a longitudinal study. *Am J Obstet Gynecol* 1992;166:22–27.

87. Dawes GS, Moulden M, Redman CWG. Short-term fetal heart rate variation, decelerations, and umbilical flow velocity waveforms before labor. *Obstet Gynecol* 1992B;80: 637–678.

88. Hecher K, Hackeloer B-J. Cardiotocogram compared to Doppler investigation of fetal circulation in the premature growth-retarded fetuses: longitudinal observations. *Ultrasound Obstet Gynecol* 1997;9:152–161.

89. Weiner Z, Farmakides G, Schulman H, Penny B. Central and peripheral hemodynamic changes in fetuses with AEDV in umbilical artery: correlation with computerized FHR pattern. *Am J Obstet Gynecol* 1994;170:509–515.

90. Weiner Z, Farmakides G, Schulman H, Casale A, Itskovitz-Eldor J. Central and peripheral haemodynamic changes in post-term fetuses: correlation with oligohydramnios and abnormal fetal heart rate pattern. *Br J Obstet Gynaecol* 1996;103:541–546.

91. Arduini D, Rizzo G, Romanini C. Changes of pulsatility index from fetal vessels preceding the onset of late decelerations in growth-retarded fetuses. *Obstet Gynecol* 1992; 79:605–610.

92. Weiner Z, Farmakides G, Schulman H, Lopresti S, Schneider E. Surveillance of growth-retarded fetuses with computerized fetal heart rate monitoring combined with Doppler velocimetry of the umbilical and the uterine arteries. *J Reprod Med* 1996;41:112–118.

93. Valensise H, Dell'Anna D, Menghini S, Rizzo G, Arduini D, Romanini C. Computerized analysis of fetal heart rate in postterm pregnancy. *J Matern Fetal Invest* 1994;4:251–256.
94. Rizzo G, Arduini D, Romanini C. Accelerated cardiac growth and abnormal cardiac flow in fetuses of type I diabetic mothers. *Obstet Gynecol* 1992;80:369–376.
95. Rizzo G, Arduini D. Fetal Cardiac function in intrauterine growth retardation. *Am J Obstet Gynecol* 1991;165:876–882.
96. Valensise H, Arduini D, Giannini F, Conforti R, Giacomello F, Romanini C. Role of antepartum computerized fetal heart rate analysis in the prediction of fetal distress during labor. *Eur J Obstet Gynecol Reprod Biol* 1997;73:129–134.
97. Soothill PW, Ajayi RA, Campbell S, Nicolaides KH. Prediction of morbidity in small and normally grown fetuses by fetal heart rate variability, biophysical profile score and umbilical Doppler studies. *Br J Obstet Gynaecol* 1993;100:742–745.
98. Ajayi A, Soothill PW, Campbell S, Nicholaides KH. Antenatal testing to predict outcome in pregnancies with unexplained antepartum haemorrhage. *Br J Obset Gynaecol* 1992; 99:122–125.
99. Di Renzo GC, Montani M, Fioriti V, Clerici G, Branconi F, Pardini A, Indraccolo R, Cosmi EV. Fractal analysis: a new method for evaluating fetal heart rate variability. *J Perinat Med* 1996;24(3):261–269.
100. Dawes GS, Moulden M, Sheil O, Redman CWG. Approximate entropy, a statistic of regularity, applied to fetal heart rate data before and during labor. *Obstet Gynecol* 1992C; 80:763–768.
101. Chaffin DG, Goldberg CC, Reed KL. The dimension of chaos in the fetal heart rate. *Am J Obstet Gynecol* 1991;165:1425–1429.
102. Gough N. Fractals, chaos and fetal heart rate. *Lancet* 1992;339:182–183.
103. Pincus SM, Viscariello RR. Approximate entropy: a regularity measure for fetal heart rate analysis. *Obstet Gynecol* 1992;79:249–255.
104. Sapoznikov D, Luria MH, Gotsman S. Detection of regularities in heart rate variations by linear and non-linear analysis: power spectrum versus approximate entropy. *Comput Methods Programs Biomed* 1995;48:201–209.
105. Marple L. *Digital spectral analysis with applications.* Englewood Cliffs, NJ: Prentice-Hall, 1987:264–265.
106. MacDonald AH. Mechanisms affecting heart-rate. *Int J Biomed Comput* 1990;25:3–13.
107. Pomeranz B, Macualay RJB, Caudill MA, Kutz I, Adam D, Gordon D, Kilborn KM, Barger AC, Shannon DC, Cohen RJ, Benson H. Assessment of autonomic function in humans by heart rate spectral analysis. *Am J Physiol* 1985;248H:151–153.
108. Akselrod S, Gordon D, Ubel FA, Shannon DC, Barger AC, Cohen RJ. Power spectrum analysis of heart rate fluctuation: a quantitative probe of beat-to-beat cardiovascular control. *Science* 1981;213:220–222.
109. Kimura Y, Okamura K, Yajima A. Spectral analysis of beat-to-beat intervals of the fetal heart obtained by Doppler ultrasound. *Gynecol Obstet Invest* 1996;41:5–9.
110. Cerruti S, Civardi S, Bianchi A, Signorini MG, Ferrazzi E, Pardi G. Spectral analysis of antepartum heart rate variability. *Clin Phys Physiol Meas* 1989;10:27–31.
111. Breborowicz G, Moczko J, Gadzinowski J. Quantification of the fetal heart rate variability by spectral analysis in growth-retarded fetuses. *Gynecol Obstet Invest* 1988;25: 186–191.

112. Ferrazzi E, Pardi G, Setti PL, Rodolfi M, Civardi S, Cerutti S. Power spectral analysis of the heart rate of the human fetus at 26 and 36 weeks of gestation. *Clin Phys Physiol Meas* 1989:10(Suppl B):57–60.

113. Karin J, Hirsch M, Akselrod S. An estimate of fetal autonomic state by spectral analysis of fetal heart rate fluctuations. *Pediatr Res* 1993;34:134–138.

114. Divon MY, Winkler H, Yeh SY, Platt LD, Langer O, Merkatz IR. Diminished respiratory arrhythmia in asphyxiated term infants. *Am J Obstet Gynecol* 1986;155:1263–1266.

115. Sibony O, Fouillot J-P, Benaoudia M, Benhalla A, Oury J-F, Sureau C, Blot P. Quantification of fetal heart rate variability by spectral analysis of fetal well-being and fetal distress. *Eur J Obstet Gynecol Reprod Biol* 1994;54:103–108.

116. Basano L, Ottonello P, Poggi A, Adezati L, Semino S, Ubaldi P, Viviana GL. An instrument for real-time spectral estimation of heart rate variability signals. *Comput Methods Programs Biomed* 1995;47:229–236.

117. Sibony O, Fouillot J-P, Bennaoudia M, Luton D, Blot P, Sureau C. Spectral analysis of fetal heart rate in flat recordings. *Early Hum Dev* 1995;41:215–220.

118. Lewinsky RM, Degani S. Spectral analysis of fetal heart rate variability gives new insight into fetal autonomic response to vibroacoustic stimulation. *Am J Obstet Gynecol* 1996;174:380.

119. Matsuura M, Murata Y, Hirano T, Nagata N, Doi S, Suda K. The effects of developing autonomous nervous system on FHR variabilities determined by the power spectral analysis in rhesus monkey features. *Am J Obstet Gynecol* 1996;174:380.

16

FETAL BIOPHYSICAL VARIABLES AND FETAL STATUS

Christopher R. Harman, M.D., Savas M. Menticoglou, M.D.,
Frank A. Manning, M.D., and Ian Morrison, M.B., Ch.B.

Department of Obstetrics, Gynecology, and Reproductive Sciences, University of Maryland Medical Center, Baltimore, Maryland (C.R.H.); and Department of Obstetrics, Gynecology and Reproductive Sciences, University of Manitoba, Winnipeg, Canada (S.M.M.); and Sloane Hospital for Women, Columbia-Presbyterian Medical Center, New York, New York (F.A.M.); and St. Boniface General Hospital, University of Manitoba, Winnipeg, Canada (I.M.)

Systematic observation of fetal behavior by real-time ultrasound surveillance can provide important information about fetal well-being. Motives for antenatal monitoring are many, and they range from individual disease-specific fetal concerns to general population goals of enhanced health care in pregnancy. Circumstances and gestational timing are varied: Each fetus–placenta–mother unit presents unique features throughout pregnancy, all of these potentially acute, chronic, or superimposed. Thus, many demands are placed on any system used to detect fetal compromise. Monitoring systems continue to evolve as technology, fetal data, and experience provide new insight. With new information about cerebral palsy added to our large database, it is an appropriate time to review one such approach to detailed fetal monitoring: the Biophysical Profile Score (BPS).

Asphyxia and Fetal Brain Damage, Edited by Dev Maulik, M.D., Ph.D.
ISBN 0-471-18427-6

PREMISES OF BPS

Biophysical profile scoring was developed to detect chronic fetal compromise (1). Its application assumes several things about normal fetal behavior and about adaptive responses to hypoxemia and acidemia.

Cyclicity of Fetal Behaviors

Near term, the human fetus has progressed to a complicated pattern of interrelated activities. These can be grouped into defined behavioral states analogous to the behavioral states (states 1–5) of the newborn infant (2), termed 1F-4F for the fetus (3). During "active sleep" (Stage 2F), many behaviors (body movement, limb movement, swallowing, fetal breathing movements, frequent fetal heart rate (FHR) accelerations, high FHR variability, and many more) are clustered. In "quiet sleep" (Stage 1F), movements are infrequent, except for rapid eye movements and mouthing movements, which are associated with reduced FHR variability, and so on (4). Fetal breathing movements mirror blood glucose levels, thus following a pattern related to maternal meals (5). Fetal urine production, fetal corticosteroid production, and probably a number of fetal metabolic functions follow diurnal patterns (6–8).

Many behaviors change as the fetus grows older. Respiratory activity at early gestation is dominated by hiccups, while episodes of rhythmic fetal breathing assume the majority in the third trimester (9). The total-body "startles" of the first half of pregnancy give way to recognizable kicks, and even these diminish, often dramatically over a few days at 34–38 weeks, and sophisticated, small-amplitude "baby movements" take their place. FHR variation increases weekly, as do the amplitude of FHR accelerations and the discrete boundaries between periods of high and low variation (10).

This is a sampling of the interwoven patterns which must be considered in the use of fetal observations to describe fetal status. Clearly, a system based on the presence or absence of a *single* factor might be confounded if that factor appeared only part of the time.

Multiple Parameters of Well-Being

The original development of biophysical profile scoring showed that the combination of variables produced a more accurate representation of fetal status than did any single variable (1). While intermediate results were obtained using pairs or triads of behaviors the most precise definition of fetal status came from a combination of all five variables which form the biophysical profile score. This premise was validated with a number of endpoints, with an example shown in Figure 1 for variable analysis when low 5-min Apgar was the endpoint (1,11–12).

The original variables have undergone some modification, but the principle has withstood evaluation in over 100,000 high-risk pregnancies. The choice of these variables was not entirely accidental. The time period of BPS variables (Table 1) allows for significant overlap, addressing the possibility that one or other variable may be

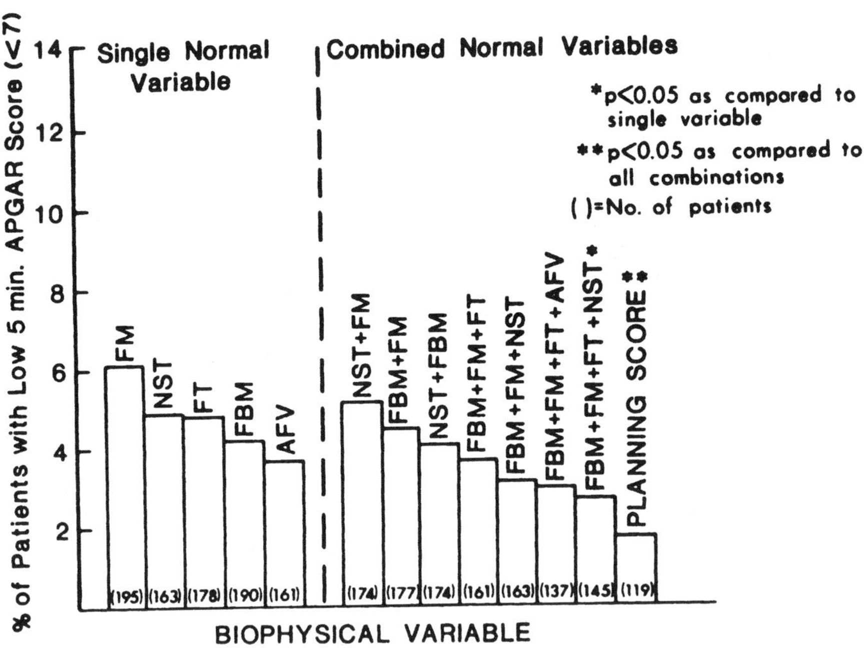

Figure 1. Analysis of individual BPS variables, and combinations of variables, in predicting low 5-min Apgar score. Sensitivity of single variables improved in combinations, and the most reliable relationship was derived when all five variables were combined (1). (The "planning score" was originally named for Platt and Manning.)

Table 1. The time period of BPS variables

Fetal tone	FT	Continuous/minutes ?
Fetal movement	FM	Minutes
Fetal breathing movement	FBM	20–30 min
Cardiotocogram	CTG	30–60 min
Amniotic fluid volume	AFV	Days

absent at a given moment. On many occasions, many of these variables occur at the same time, so the normal fetus very often demonstrates its normal status in only a few minutes.

The principle of multiple variable assessment does not mean that the original five variables are inviolable. Similar results may be obtained when substituting the contraction stress test for the CTG (13), doing just amniotic fluid volume and/or breathing movements under ultrasound, inferring fetal movements from the CTG (14,15), and so on. The principle remains that the most accurate depiction of the complex process of fetal adaptation to abnormal intrauterine environment will use *multiple* parameters.

Fetal Responses to Asphyxia

This discussion is complex beyond the scope of this chapter. For example, previous exposure to hypoxemia, chronic respiratory status of the placenta, previous placental damage, actual gestational age, maturational effects (if any) of factors such as IUGR, maternal diabetes, and so on, rate of onset and depth of the hypoxemic challenge, the opportunity to recover even partially between hypoxemic episodes, the ambient pO_2 and placental bed blood flow, and more, interact in determining fetal responses. Those responses, likewise, are multiple and of varying significance.

Biophysical profile scoring addresses three facets of fetal adaptation to hypoxemia:

1. *Get More Oxygen.* These maneuvers may be sufficient to deal with most of the decreases in oxygen supply experienced by most fetuses throughout pregnancy and delivery. Much has been inferred from the fetal sheep model and other experimental situations; but with advancing information from human fetuses, the following seem to be important: mild to moderate increase in basal heart rate, minor increases in cardiac size and therefore mechanical advantage, and significant increases in oxygen extraction (16). The last of these may be most significant, contributing up to 14% additional oxygen, and is a ready explanation for the ability of the term fetus to tolerate repetitive severe variable decelerations without any long-term debt (17).
2. *Use Oxygen Differently.* Redistribution of cardiac outflow seems designed to preserve or even increase oxygen delivery to brain, heart and adrenals, while restricting distal aortic outflows such that only placental perfusion is maintained (18–20). Even within "favored" organs, differences may exist between regions. For example, in fetuses with increased total brain perfusion, the cortex may remain relatively under-perfused, while the brain stem experiences an absolute increase (21). Redistribution is probably not an all or none phenomenon, with increments and short-term readjustment as circumstances warrant. For example, the linear correlation of hourly fetal urine output with severity of fetal hypoxemia, implies that minor changes in fetal pO_2 produce equally minor adjustments in renal blood flow, as central perfusion is maintained (22). This second tier of responses accounts for the majority of situations not addressed by increased oxygen supply. The majority of asymmetrically growth-retarded infants are delivered intact with reasonable pH, although with generally lower pO_2's, evidence of the effectiveness of their compensatory mechanisms.
3. *Use Less Oxygen.* Sudden acute hypoxemia, or chronic descent into absolute cerebral hypoxemia, can trigger loss of fetal variables (23). The fetal sheep promptly abolishes almost all activity with relatively minor drops in umbilical venous pO_2 (16). In this artificial situation, fetal oxygen consumption falls dramatically when movements cease (up to 17%, for example, when the fetus is paralyzed) (24). Again, this mechanism of homeostasis is not binary: total fetal activity (the sum of fetal breathing, gross body movement, and heart rate variation) documented in normal fetuses, and the striking diminution in growth-retarded fetuses, probably represent two points on a continuum (25,26). Thus, a gradual reduction in activity, with larger spaces between active intervals along with blurring of the circadium rhythm, may be among the first fetal responses to diminished oxygenation. Vintzileos et al. (27) observed that individual vari-

ables were lost progressively as fetal pO_2 fell. Fetal heart rate reactivity was lost before fetal breathing movements; and then fetal movements, and ultimately fetal tone, were lost with further declines in cord artery pO_2 in unlaboring fetuses delivered by cesarean section. (Sampling interval may suggest a more absolute change in activity than really exists: Perhaps FBM episodes become so far apart, and are so short when they do occur, as to be statistically absent. The use of minimum criteria to count the BPS variable as normal is of obvious importance here.)

These responses are likely not mutually exclusive. They can be triggered by different degrees of hypoxemia, appearing in the above order in the instrumented fetal lamb (16,28,29). The impact of the previous hypoxemic status, the duration, and the gestational age of that individual fetus probably means that, in humans, these responses are overlapping and on a continuous sliding scale. Successful adaptation (e.g., combining decreased splanchnic perfusion, increased O_2 extraction, increased FHR, and increased duration of quiet sleep) may stabilize the situation, allowing the growth-retarded fetus to resume normal activity and remain safely in utero for a number of weeks, despite patently abnormal placental circulation (Figure 2). The impact

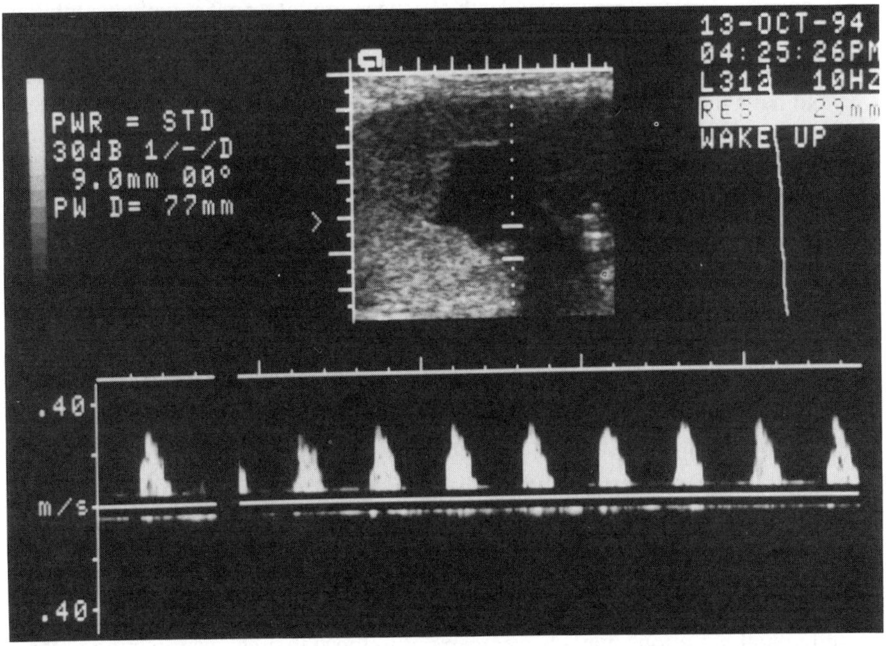

Figure 2. At 22 weeks 6 days' gestation, this fetus had absent end-diastolic velocities. At the time of the first visit (4 weeks previously), for elevated maternal serum AFP, diastolic velocities were present. Frequent monitoring, using biophysical profile scoring and mandatory NST ("score out of 10"), showed normal growth along the 10th to 15th percentile, maintenance of normal amniotic fluid, and other parameters of fetal well-being. Elective delivery was at 36 weeks 5 days for a male infant just < 10th centile, whose cord vein pH was 7.28. Statistically, Doppler correctly predicted the IUGR. BPS determined that intervention was not required for about 14 weeks.

of these multiple mechanisms of fetal adaptation on fetal monitoring, is obvious: Solitary observations of single variables may be misleading. Serial observations of multiple parameters on multiple time scales are more likely to give an accurate status report.

BPS FORMAT

Evolution of Individual Variables

Biophysical profile scoring has been modified through ongoing analysis of results and outcome, so its *current* format is shown in Table 2 (30). The evolution of BPS in this regard is a process which makes a clear statement about the method: It is flexible, subject to question, and subject to modification, and it should not be applied as a rigid formula. A detailed evaluation of the application of BPS is available for the interested reader (30).

A few comments illustrate some principles of our BPS application:

1. Amniotic fluid volume (AFV) (30–34)—criteria are now 2.0 cm minimum, 3.0 cm normal, using maximum depth of a clear amniotic pocket without umbilical cord present.
2. Amniotic fluid index has been analyzed versus pocket depth and has been found to have no particular advantage, probably because AFV is a binary (normal/abnormal) variable rather than a continuous one.
3. Impressions of "Subjectively decreased" AFV suggest that fluid is significantly less than average. These include restricted extension on limb movement, uterus or placenta conforming to contours of the fetus (e.g., the uterus follows the curve of the fetal neck), no cord-free pocket > 3.0 cm, FHR decelerations with transducer pressure, spontaneous FHR decelerations on CTG with fetal movement, maternal impression of decreased FM, and/or a sharp drop in maximum pocket depth between serial visits. These call for increased frequency of BPS (30).
4. Cord-free pocket of fluid is verified with pulsed and/or color Doppler.
5. Numerical FHR analysis (System 8000) (35) is adjusted for gestational age.
6. Fetal movement periodicity is utilized in timing repeat BPS. For example, if a 26-week fetus does move three or four times in a 30-min scan, then it meets minimum criteria but would not satisfy expectations for the continual movement pattern usually seen, so the BPS interval would be shortened.

Individual variations may be averaged out in the statistical examination of large populations, but when BPS is evaluated in small populations of extremely compromised infants, there may be variations in technique which would not be accepted in our Unit. For example, in a recent review of BPS versus umbilical artery Doppler velocimetry in detecting fetal acidemia, fetal tone was scored in the complete absence of movements, an impossibility with orthodox BPS (36). One problem with wide use of any method is that rote application may cloud the underlying principles.

Table 2. Interpretation of BPS variables

Fetal Variable	Normal Behavior (score = 2)	Abnormal Behavior (score = 0)
Fetal breathing movements	Intermittent, multiple episodes of more than 30-sec duration, within 30-min BPS time frame. Hiccups count. Continuous FBM for 30 min = R/O fetal acidosis.	Continuous breathing without cessation. Completely absent breathing or no sustained episodes.
Body or limb movements	At least four discrete body movements in 30 min. Continuous active movement episodes = single movement. Includes fine motor movements, rolling movements, and so on, but not REM or mouthing movements.	Three or fewer body/limb movements in a 30-min observation period.
Fetal tone/posture	Demonstration of active extension with rapid return to flexion of fetal limbs and brisk repositioning/trunk rotation. Opening and closing of hand, mouth, kicking, and so on.	Low-velocity movement only. Incomplete flexion, flaccid extremity positions, abnormal fetal posture. Must score = 0 when FM completely absent.
Cardiotogram	Normal mean variation (computerized FHR interpretation), accelerations associated with maternal palpation FM (accelerations graded for gestation), 20-min CTG.	Fetal movement and accelerations not coupled. Insufficient accelerations, absent accelerations, or decelerative trace. Mean variation < 20 on numerical analysis of CTG.
Amniotic fluid evaluation	At least one pocket > 3 cm with no umbilical cord. See text regarding subjectively decreased fluid.	No cord-free pocket > 2 cm, or elements of subjectively reduced amniotic fluid volume definite.

Binary Interpretation: Minimum Normal Criteria

The initial biophysical profile score was designed to permit finer gradations, allowing a 0–1–2 format, but time has shown that those original criteria are a minimum for normal, rather than an expression of average, behavior (11,37,38). For example, better ultrasound technology allows discernment of smaller FM, better detection of FBM, more accurate depiction of AFV, and so on. Although the minimum criteria outlined in Table 2 still apply, an experienced group using BPS will integrate some fine-tuning: subjectively decreased fluid (see discussion above), range and vigor of FM relative to gestation, fine motor movements of hand and face as substitutes for gross body and limb movements, the subjectivity of fetal tone, and so on.

Vintzileos et al. (39) introduced a 0–1–2 system, which includes placental grading, so the total score ranges in single points from 0 to 12. This system validates the multiple variable approach, but does not appear to offer improved precision and does automatically increase with gestation (i.e., placental grade advances), so we have not moved in that direction. We have also resisted the temptation to "weight" variables (11,30). Although some variables are missing more frequently and may have a statistically stronger connection with fetal hypoxemia, all do contribute, and all combinations of variables missing do occur, when the population is large enough. Thus, score analysis (normal = 2, missing/abnormal = 0) remains consistent. The binary system is easy to apply, easy to teach, and less subjective than fine grades of distinction, and we believe that the coarse gradations of classical BPS have the correct connotation of an *approximate* description of fetal behavior and status.

Systematic Responses

Since its inception, biophysical profile scoring has been evaluated "under fire." Following the original blinded trial (1), estimation of fetal status by BPS has always been attached to a defined management protocol (Table 3) (30,40). Like BPS format, the management has changed somewhat. The gestational ages for intervention have shifted downward with advances in neonatal care. Confidence in the correlations of poor scores with adverse outcome facilitates intervention earlier than may have been the case in the past, thus improving the condition of neonates. Application of these management principles is not by rote but, instead, depends on the clinical situation of both mother and fetus and is integrated with critical short-term measures such as maternal transport, dexamethasone administration, maternal stabilization, and ancillary fetal testing. When delivery is prohibited, we consider intrauterine therapy (amnioinfusion, chronic maternal oxygen administration, uterine relaxation, antihypertensive therapy, etc.). In addressing fetal compromise, our primary option is safe delivery, so the analysis may be decided on the probabilities of death inside the uterus versus inside the intensive care nursery (Table 4).

Gestational age has the biggest impact in varying the responses to non-normal scores. Beyond the gestational age of viability (24–25 weeks), the definitely abnormal score (2/10 or 0/10) is a mandatory indication for delivery (11,41). At early ges-

Table 3. Biophysical profile score indicates clinical management

BPS	Interpretation	Predicted PNM/1000[a]	Recommended Management
10/10 8/8 8/10 (AFV-normal)	No evidence of fetal asphyxia present.	Less than 1/1000	No acute intervention on fetal basis. Serial testing indicated by disorder-specific protocols.
8/10-OLIGO	Chronic fetal compromise likely.	89/1000	For absolute oligohydramnios, prove normal urinary tract, disprove asymptomatic rupture of membranes, then deliver at any viable gestation.
6/10 (AFV-normal)	Equivocal test, fetal asphyxia is not excluded.	Depends on progression (61:1000 on average)	Repeat testing immediately, before assigning final value. If score is 6/10, then 10/10, in two continuous 30-min periods, manage as 10/10. For persistent 6/10, deliver the mature fetus, repeat within 24 hours in the immature fetus, then deliver if less than 6/10.
4/10	Acute fetal asphyxia likely. If AFV-OLIGO, acute on chronic asphyxia very likely.	91/1000	Deliver by obstetrically appropriate method, with continuous monitoring.
2/10	Acute fetal asphyxia, most likely with chronic decompensation.	125/1000	Deliver for fetal indications (cesarean section).
0/10	Severe, acute asphyxia virtually certain.	600/1000	Deliver *immediately* by cesarean section.

[a]Per 1000 live births, within 1 week of the test result shown, if no intervention. For scores of 0, 2, or 4, intervention should commence virtually immediately, provided the fetus is viable.

Table 4. Risks of asphyxial death in utero versus premature death in the NICU

BPS	Stillbirth Rate[a]	Equivalent Neonatal Death Rate (Weeks)
0	560	25.4
2	153	28.3
4	91	29.1
6	61	30.0
8	0.5	Full term
10	0.5	Full term

[a]When no intervention is used, survival statistics in our NICU improve yearly, so these figures change and will differ between centers. This table illustrates one step in the decision to intervene. Risk of intrauterine death (at any gestation) with a score of zero, for example, is about 560/1000, equivalent to the risk of neonatal death of an intact infant, as early as 25.5 weeks. At any viable gestation therefore, the fetus with 0/10 has a better (although no "good") chance in the nursery. With a normal BPS, on the other hand, the argument that the fetus is "better off delivered" is a difficult one to make before term.

tation, however, neonatal consultation and a clear depiction to the parents of our expectations is imperative.

The equivocal or abnormal BPS should generate a differential diagnosis which should be resolved prior to intervention. So, especially in the situation where the fetus is being assessed for the first time, consideration must be given to *external factors* (e.g., maternal condition, drug ingestion), *intrinsic factors* (e.g., aneuploidy, syndromic problems), *acquired fetal problems* (e.g., viral infection, previous asphyxial insult), and the significant likelihood that the fetus is *completely normal,* with an unusual coincidence of the absence of many variables at the same time. For this final reason, prolonged testing, retesting after a short interval, or adding tests (contraction stress test or oxytocin challenge test, and/or fetal blood gas and pH measurement by cordocentesis) are primary steps in finalizing the differential diagnosis when intensive care of the neonate carries any liability (30,42). With the fetal and neonatal correlates illustrated below, family counseling in the face of abnormal or equivocal scores can be reasonably confident. It is emphasized, however, that statistics do not tell the entire story about a given fetus.

In every case, serial testing, a consistent set of observers, and additional information (e.g., karyotype, maternal antiphospholipid antibody status, history of superimposed preeclampsia, serial fetal growth estimations, etc.) can aid in determining action. The contributions of an abnormal Doppler in this scenario are many, including explaining etiology, narrowing the differential diagnosis, mandating more frequent BPS, providing early warning of placenta-based maternal complications, and indicating a need for routine performance of CTG. The principle of accepting information from all possible sources, upon which BPS is based, obliges flexibility.

BPS—TECHNICAL ASPECTS

The Manitoba Context

In Manitoba, where BPS application has been practiced for more than 17 years, some features exist which may favor both application and effect. Referral is centralized, and there are only two tertiary-care perinatal units; both of these are university teaching hospitals with Fetal Assessment Units under our direction. Universal access is by publicly funded medical insurance. The team is an experienced one, and most of the nurse-ultrasonographers have been in the Unit for more than a decade, so their fetal sensing may be as important as the BPS format in depicting fetal status. There is centralized intake through a single AFP screening program, a single genetics program, an Rh program, and an obstetrical ultrasound outreach program, all of which facilitate selection of cases and early referral in complicated pregnancy. We have virtually complete follow-up: Information is available on 98.8% of newborns. Perinatal mortality has fallen progressively in our jurisdiction (Figure 3) (43). (This means that perinatal mortality rates are of declining potential in outcome evaluation, making newborn follow-up data even more critical.)

There seems little doubt that these "environmental" factors influence BPS results and impact. This does not render the method insignificant; it does emphasize the necessity for flexibility and integration.

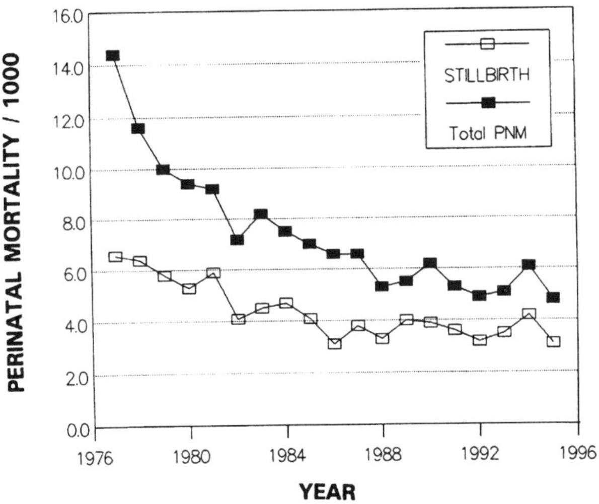

Figure 3. Perinatal mortality (■) and stillbirth rate (□) in the Province of Manitoba over the last 20 years. This ongoing improvement in perinatal results needs to be considered when evaluating the impact of testing programs.

BPS Performance

Many details of our practice of BPS have been mentioned already. Performance characteristics and distribution of test results are shown in Table 5. A few items of clarification deserve emphasis:

1. *False-Negative Rate 0.54/1000 tests* (44). This rate describes the number of fetuses who have died within 7 days of their last BPS, which was normal. It does not include a substantial number of fetuses with lethal congenital anomalies who die following normal tests, nor does it include cases where the fetus, found to be normal and discharged from surveillance, died at a time remote from referral. It is imperative to note that this false-negative rate does not apply to non-normal scores: In the face of an equivocal or abnormal score, BPS testing may be repeated as often as every 6 hours.

2. *BPS = 6/8 Does Not Exist.* In the case of a single missing ultrasound variable, two points having been awarded for the other three variables on the scan, the cardiotocogram is always completed, yielding a score based on 10 (30,45). Our experience is that in the compromised fetus, there may be bursts of activity which would achieve three normal ultrasound behavior variables, even in the face of absent amniotic fluid and a nonreactive CTG. If the surveillance was truncated at the ultrasound variables and the score of 6/8 was reported, the impression of near-normality would

Table 5. BPS performance statistics

Normal score 8/8	Completion mean 11 min	
Abnormal score	*Requires* 30-min scan to meet definition of abnormal.	
Test score distribution		
Normal score	10/10 8/8	97.84%
Equivocal score	6/10	1.0%
Abnormal scores	4/10	0.56
	2/10	0.19
	0/10	0.07
Negative predictive value (BPS normal, 7-day duration)		99.946%
Positive predictive values (Change with test score, endpoint)		
Examples:		

BPS	Endpoint	PPV
0/10	Perinatal mortality	100% (no intervention)
0/10	Neonatal mortality	43% (despite intervention)
0/10	Perinatal morbidity	100%
4/10	Perinatal morbidity	63%
6/10	Perinatal morbidity	35%

be erroneous. An equivocal score (6/10) may well represent the maximum range of behavior of a compromised fetus, who oscillates between virtual hibernation (2/10, only fluid normal) and moderate activity at 6/10, emphasizing again the importance of obtaining information from multiple sources.

3. *BPS Applied in Midtrimester.* We have evaluated data subsets examining fetuses at 24–26 weeks. These data confirm the impression that compartments of fetal quiet and active sleep are less well demarcated, and the CTG contains lower-amplitude variation and lower-amplitude accelerations; but when parameters are modified with regard to gestational age, the BPS concept remains valid (30,42).

4. *Roles of Cardiotocography.* BPS is performed most efficiently in sequential fashion (45). If not all ultrasound variables are normal, a CTG is always done. In the context of an ultimately normal score (8/10), FBM is the variable most frequently absent, which is understandable based on its long period of variation. (This sequential use of cardiotocography accounts for fetal heart rate monitoring in about 10% of our referred population.) This approach was validated by a randomized, blinded trial, in which BPS was compared to the nonstress test alone in predicting fetal compromise (46). That study has often been misquoted, as giving evidence that the nonstress test should not be done, far from our actual position. The use of the word "cardiotocography" emphasizes that we are not simply watching FHR accelerations, but attending FHR variation and/or decelerations, especially "minimal variables" (connoting decreased amniotic fluid) (Figure 4A) and "desaturation variables" (connoting transient drop in fetal pO_2, unrelated to labor) (Figure 4B). Numerical analysis is used to interpret the CTG; normal variation (mean variation > 30 msec) (35) can be substituted for

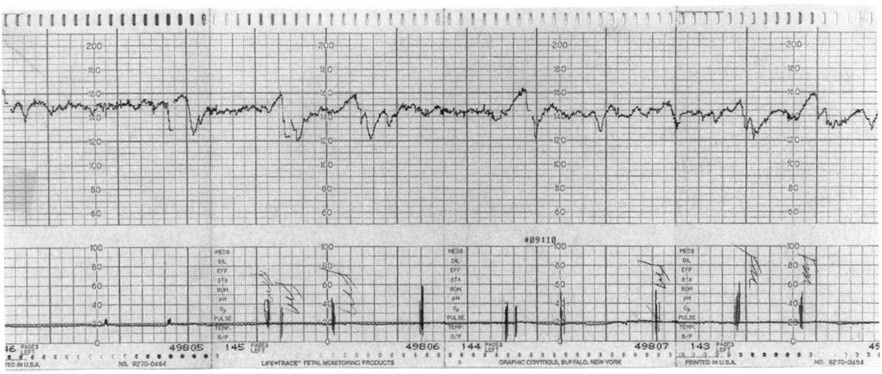

A

Figure 4. A: "Minimal variable" decels. This CTG demonstrates small decelerations simultaneous with fetal movements, indirect evidence of oligohydramnios. Ultrasound examination and full BPS should follow. **B:** "Desaturation" FHR deceleration, mother not in labor. Although normal variation may follow such an episode, the tracing would be regarded as equivocal, score as 0. Not infrequently, this tracing would be typical of the IUGR fetus with abnormal Dopplers and would also be typical of maternal problems such as renal impairment with superimposed preeclampsia (all true in this particular case), and BPS monitoring would be as often as daily, depending on the precise condition.

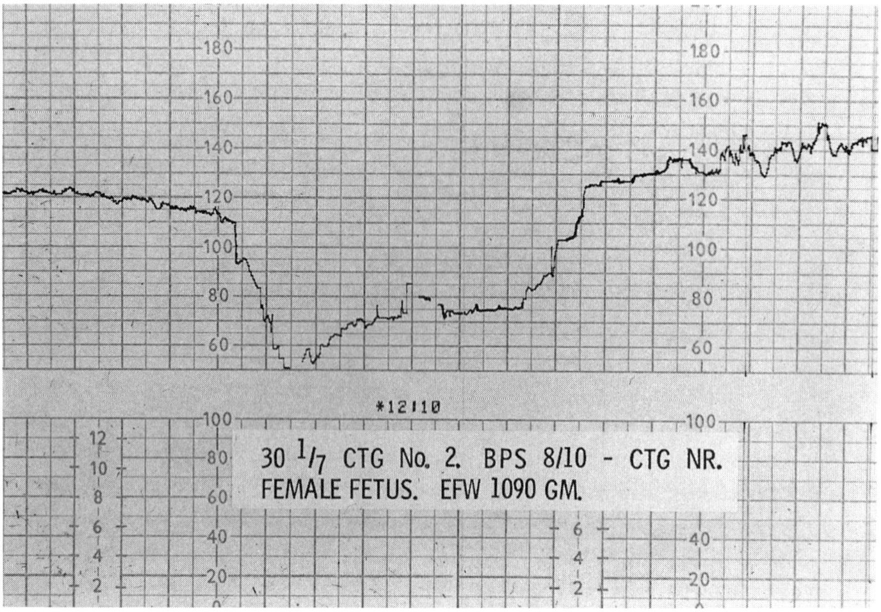

Figure 4. B. *continued*

accelerations, in determining normal CTG (score = 2). If the FHR shows abnormally decreased variation, even in the presence of some accelerations, the interval of BPS is shortened.

In addition to the detailed analysis of the CTG, used sequentially, mandatory "score out of 10" situations exist. These reflect severity or instability of maternal or fetal condition and would include proteinuric preeclampsia, severe intrauterine growth retardation, absent or reverse end-diastolic velocities on Doppler investigation, borderline AFV, or the accelerating macrosomic fetus in the out-of-control diabetic mother (30,47–49).

In summary, there are many technical aspects of BPS which may not be recognizable in a statistical analysis of the method. The Manitoba context may be critical to BPS application. BPS performance is attractive, because it involves the family, nurse-ultrasonographers, and the resources of a health care team, rather than pivoting on a few selected high-risk pregnancy obstetricians. The roles of cardiotocography are sequenced, selective, and objective, not in competition with the ultrasound variables. The high uptake of fetal assessment services in the context of universal access to health care, high compliance of referring obstetricians with recommendations, and ease of application, in a supportive university academic atmosphere, substantiated by a very large database, gives confidence to the analyses and recommendations about BPS. It is recognized, however, that these concepts need to be challenged and evaluated in other less ideal environments.

VALIDATION OF BIOPHYSICAL PROFILE SCORING

Intratest Comparisons

In all normal, equivocal, and abnormal scores, we have evaluated the impact of the individual variables. Stepwise logistic regression to determine the best predictors, produces hierarchies of variables which change with the endpoint (Table 6) (11). The dissection of all possible combinations is complicated: There are 10 different ways to achieve a score of 6/10 and there are 10 ways to achieve a score of 4/10, a total of 32 different potential score combinations within the method. Almost all combinations of variables have occurred, although some very infrequently.

There has been much discussion about ranking or weighting variables and about the sequenced disappearance of individual behaviors as the fetus becomes more compromised. This is discussed in some detail in the section below on correlations with absolute fetal parameters, but in summary the *combination of all variables into an overall score always produces the best predictive accuracy, regardless of the endpoint.*

Intertest Comparisons with Biophysical Profile Scoring

Biophysical profile scoring has been compared with several other methods of fetal assessment. Versus the NST (46), versus the NST/CST protocol (50), versus the contraction stress test (13), or versus the oxytocin challenge test (51,52), the relatively straightforward comparison of two testing regimes favors biophysical profile scoring.

Morrison et al. (53) have compared sequential testing in a highly selected group of fetuses. All fetuses underwent all tests, following referral because of intrauterine growth restriction, decreased AFV, or both. Biophysical profile scoring (scored out of 10), umbilical artery Doppler velocimetry, and contraction stress test or oxytocin challenge test were compared. Two important conclusions arise from these data. First, there is incomplete concordance between tests. If a fetus produced one or more abnormal test results, sensitivities of the individual tests for this situation were: BPS 42%, Doppler 34%, CST/OCT 17%. This suggests there is not a close relationship between these different tests: They may well examine different facets of fetal compensation/compromise.

Table 6. Test comparisons of BPS variables

Endpoint	BPS Variable Ranking[a]
Low Apgar: 5	NST/AFV FBM FT FM
Fetal distress	NST AFV/FBM/FM/FT
NICU admission	NST/AFV FBM FM/FT
pH <7.20	FBM NST AFV FM/FT
PN mortality	AFV NST FM/FT FBM

[a]Rank order by logistic regression, slashes denote equivalence of variables.

The second conclusion of this study was emphatic: *Combining* tests improves performance. A single abnormal test conferred a risk of perinatal morbidity of 10%, while multiple abnormal tests were associated with significant morbidity in 39%; sequenced testing in the highly compromised infant seems to be the best approach. Different investigators start with a different test and progress if test results are abnormal, accepting that normal results usually mean that further tests will not add further information. Several groups have published results using cardiotocography as the primary tool, with backup from biophysical profile scoring, umbilical Doppler velocimetry, or both, when the CTG was abnormal. Although outcome differences between cardiotocography and BPS always favor BPS, the differences may be modest. Ultrasound detection of fetal anomalies and other serendipitous factors independent of fetal asphyxia contribute to the BPS superiority, and the distinction in our practice is moot: Cardiotocography is an integral and important part of BPS.

A number of teams have evaluated experience with different formats of multiple-parameter fetal testing. We do not have direct experience with these methods, termed variously "modified biophysical profile score" (13–15), "fetal assessment score" (54), "fetal biophysical assessment" (39), or "duplex BPS" (55), but believe that all these methods embrace the principles of noninvasive determination of fetal status by observation of various fetal behaviors. In some cases the original BPS has been validated, in some cases the efficacy of a shortened exam (amniotic fluid assessment and CTG without ultrasound observation of fetal activity) (56) improves economies but without significantly detracting from results, and in other cases (as one would expect from such multiple comparisons) some endpoints are better illustrated by some combinations of antenatal variables than others (15). As emphasized in the review by Morrison (53), in the severely compromised IUGR infant, sequences of tests may provide the only path to *absolute* documentation of fetal status.

Miller et al. (14) evaluated the modified biophysical profile (classical nonstress test (NST), plus ultrasound-derived amniotic fluid index) in 15,482 high-risk pregnancies, totaling 54,617 modified BPS. The "full" biophysical profile score was used as the backup for equivocal or abnormal results of either of the test components, and ultimately it was performed in 15,075 (27%) antepartum tests. The authors compared the false-negative rate (0.6/1000 women for full BPS versus 0.8/1000 for modified BPS) and the false-positive rate (40% for complete BPS, 60% for modified BPS) and found that either method produced results superior to heart rate monitoring alone. Performance of a complete biophysical profile score could be more time-consuming and requires enhanced ultrasound experience, they noted. These authors were content with the iatrogenic prematurity rate of approximately 1.5% of women tested before term. We have focused on the details of this study because it is perhaps the largest study in which the biophysical profile scoring model has been analyzed in comparison with a simpler method, and secondly because their population of high-risk women represents a profile of the perinatal experience and is not confined simply to growth-retarded infants with abnormal placentation.

Studies which compared BPS with various Doppler protocols are reviewed later. An interesting offshoot of this comparison was the "fetal Apgar score," a more or less literal attempt to define fetal aspects as they are defined for the neonate (heart rate, skin color, respiratory quality, tone, and reflexes) (54). The study substituted FHR patterns for heart rate, Doppler assessment of blood flow redistribution for skin color, uteroplacental (maternal) perfusion for respiratory quality, fetal tone examined by real-time ultrasound, and reflex response to vibroacoustic stimulation. Receiver–operator curves comparing BPS and the "fetal assessment score" showed that the fetal assessment score appears to have advantages in the prediction of fetal distress in both small-for-dates and postdates categories, and it appears to be similar in the prediction of pH and low 1-min Apgar score in both categories. With a study population of only 213 pregnancies, statistical analysis produces many theoretical arguments and leaves some fundamental questions unanswered. Linear regression of categorical variables such as in the BPS is arguable; cases with low 5-min Apgar (taken as a more reliable index of neonatal compromise) were too few to allow comparison; with the most objective measure, umbilical artery pH, the ROCs are virtually identical. This trial has appeal because it portrays the functional relationships of Doppler velocimetry measurements in terms of their likely impact on fetal characteristics.

Direct Fetal Parameters

Fetal Apgar score notwithstanding, standards for fetal well-being broadly accepted in perinatal research are focused on fetal blood gases and pH. This does not deny the importance of neonatal review, incorporating information about catchup growth, lactic acidosis, hypoglycemia, delayed metabolites of asphyxia, long-term follow-up, and correlation with neurologic function in childhood (57–59). In fact, a major emphasis of this chapter is information about cerebral palsy in our database. However, the close chronology of biophysical profile scoring and fetal blood results does allow for detailed analysis.

Delivery Cord Gases (see Table 7) (12,30,36,54,59–62). Three reports are helpful here. Manning et al. (64) first reported their prevalence of low umbilical vein cord blood pH (pH <7.20) associated with poor biophysical profile scores in 1990. This population has been expanded to 557 high-risk fetuses delivered by elective cesarean section without labor, showing correlation of last BPS before delivery with fetal cord gases (12). The significant inverse linear correlation between BPS and venous pH is shown in Figure 5. Fetuses with normal scores had a mean cord venous pH of 7.35 ± 0.13 ($N = 495$). Among fetuses with an equivocal score of 6/10 the pH averaged 7.21 ± 0.23 ($N = 39$), and in 23 fetuses with an abnormal score of 4/10 or less the mean pH was 7.13 ± 0.16.

Vintzileos et al. (27) detailed the relationship between fetal biophysical variables (not including AFV) and umbilical cord blood gas and pH measurements at delivery. Fetuses with a variable absent always had lower pH than those with that particular variable present. While the demarcation between fetuses with reactive versus nonreactive NSTs was fairly narrow (umbilical artery pH 7.29 versus pH 7.21, $p < 0.0007$, respectively), the difference in fetuses with and without tone was striking (umbilical artery pH 7.27 versus pH 7.03, $p < 0.0001$). Their analysis suggested that different variables might be lost at different levels of acidosis, the NST becoming nonreactive

Table 7. BPS versus umbilical venous pH at delivery

Authors	Year	*N*	Comment	Correlation[a]
Harman et al. (30)	1985	24	All had repetitive FHR decels	BPS positive[a], BPS > CTG
Vintzileos et al. (60,61)	1987	124	All high risk	BPS positive[a], BPS > Apgar
Vintzileos et al. (62)	1991	62	All high risk	BPS positive[a], BPS > NST > Doppler
Yoon et al. (36)	1992	105	Pre-C/S nonfetal reasons	BPS positive[a], Doppler ≥ BPS
Soothill et al. (59)	1993	191	161 normal / 30 IUGR	No, Doppler ≥ BPS (weak)
Arabin et al. (54)	1993	213	IUGR/postdates	BPS positive[a], FAS[b] ≥ BPS
Ribbert et al. (63)	1993	19	Severe IUGR	BPS positive[a], TFA ≥ BPS
Manning (12)	1995	557	All high risk	BPS positive[a], BPS > CTG

[a]Statistically significant correlations in predicting pH<7.20 and/or pH on a continuum.
[b]Fetal assessment score.

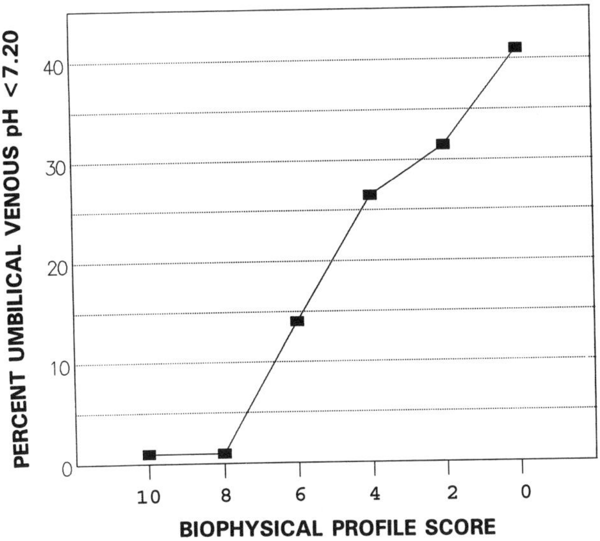

Figure 5. Relationship between last biophysical profile score prior to delivery and umbilical venous pH collected at delivery. There is a graded relationship, with strong statistical correlation, between the incidence of acidosis and poor biophysical performance.

at pH 7.21 ± 0.10, FBM lost at pH of 7.21 ± 0.12, FM lost at pH 7.08 ± 0.10, and tone lost at pH 7.03 ± 0.04, on average. With falling pO_2, rising pCO_2, and decreasing bicarbonate, parameters were lost in consistent order.

In a separate study, they further examined the relationship between fetal acidosis and overall score composition, FHR reactivity, and umbilical artery velocimetry (62). Normal BPS (8 or greater, Vintzileos criteria, $N = 49$) had mean pH 7.27 arterial, while 13 fetuses with abnormal BPS had mean pH 7.15. The difference in pH between NST results was also statistically significant: pH 7.29 with a reactive test, and pH 7.21 with a nonreactive test. With Doppler velocimetry, there was no statistically significant difference between groups: 25 with normal systolic:diastolic ratio; 30 with elevated ratios but present diastolic velocity; and seven fetuses with absent end-diastolic velocities, who had, respectively, pH values of 7.26, 7.23, and 7.24. These two papers should be read together, and the detail of the analysis should be appreciated. Our data support the conclusion that different biophysical variables are susceptible to abolition in association with different pH and pO_2 levels (Figure 6) (64) on a population basis, but our experience with individual cases is that there can be variation in this pattern (30).

The third study of interest with correlations between biophysical profile scoring and cord gases at delivery concerns a subsection of acutely compromised fetuses with repetitive decelerations immediately prior to emergency cesarean section (30). Since the cardiotocogram was decelerative, the maximum score obtainable by any fetus was 8/10. Figure 7 demonstrates the distribution of umbilical venous pH values, corresponding to the truncated scores in these compromised fetuses. All mothers had

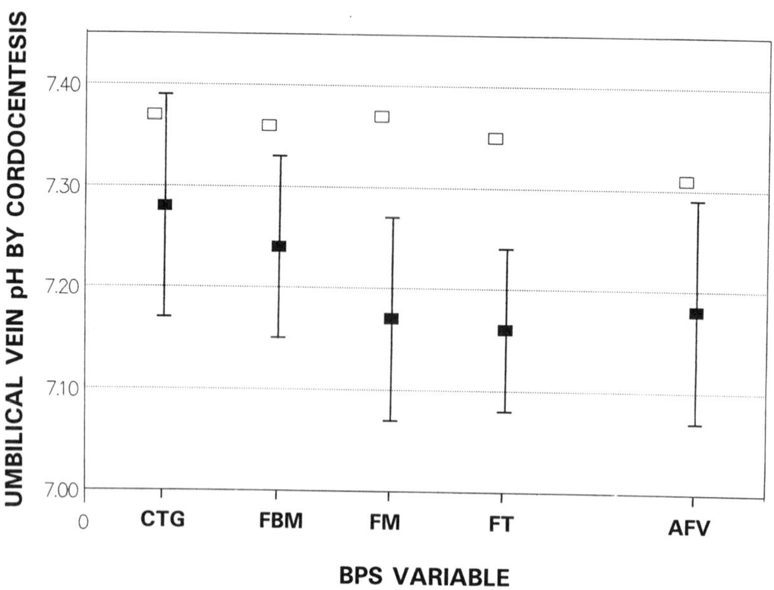

Figure 6. Biophysical variables: progressive loss with increasing acidosis. As the pH falls in the umbilical vein, there may be sequential loss of specific individual behaviors. This figure displays the mean pH plus one standard deviation for fetuses in whom the BPS variable was abnormal/missing. Amniotic fluid volume, which does not necessarily follow in this sequence, is shown separately on the right. Mean pH for fetuses with the given variable *present* are shown in open boxes across the top of the graph. These data suggest, but do not prove, that behaviors can be lost in sequential fashion. Serial observation of fetuses losing one behavior at a time is rare: Persistent loss of two variables would mandate delivery (repeated BPS = 6/10) at any age beyond viability. However, the sequence is the same in a limited number of fetuses followed serially: CTG becomes unreactive, fetal breathing movements cease, and fetal movement and tone become abnormal sometime later, sensitive to virtually the same level of acidemia (27).

proteinuric preeclampsia, and 18 of 24 were <10th percentile for gestational age. As judged by the remaining BPS parameters, fetal behavior in this group still reflected fetal status, despite the clearly unstable condition. In many cases, BPS gave a more accurate impression (in this circumstance, a normal BPS suggested normal pH in the face of an ominous CTG).

Antenatal Blood Gases and pH by Cordocentesis (Figure 8) (65–70). A number of studies have documented the relationship between antenatal fetal umbilical (usually venous) blood pH/pO_2 and BPS obtained immediately prior to the test. Table 8 summarizes relationships between antenatal cordocentesis results and the noninvasive techniques being assessed, including biophysical profile scoring, modified BPS, cardiotocography, and various forms of Doppler analysis (maternal and/or fetal).

Overall, the trials in Tables 7 and 8, totaling more than 2000 patients, show a reliable correlation between final BPS and fetal blood pH by either method. There are two

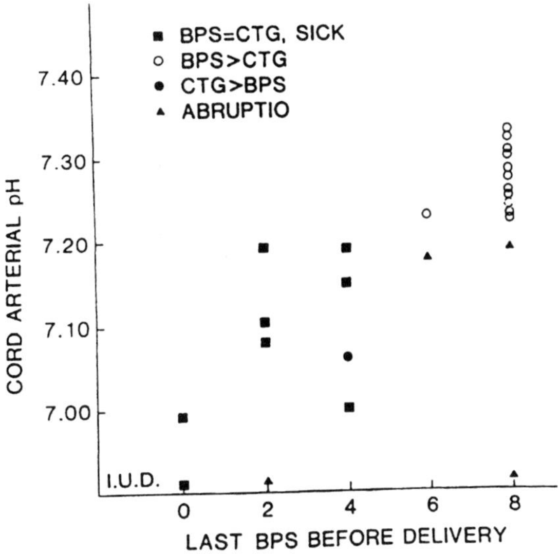

Figure 7. Biophysical profile scoring under unstable conditions. These fetuses had repetitive decelerations, not in labor. Mothers all had proteinuric preeclampsia at premature gestations, and the majority were growth-retarded fetuses. Even with repetitive large decelerations, the remaining behavior reflected umbilical cord pH. Three exceptions along the bottom of the graph had acute abruption and fetal demise. In all but one case (●), BPS equaled or outperformed CTG in indicating fetal pH status. The *combination* of CTG and BPS (in other words, the complete BPS) correctly predicted fetal acidemia in all cases.

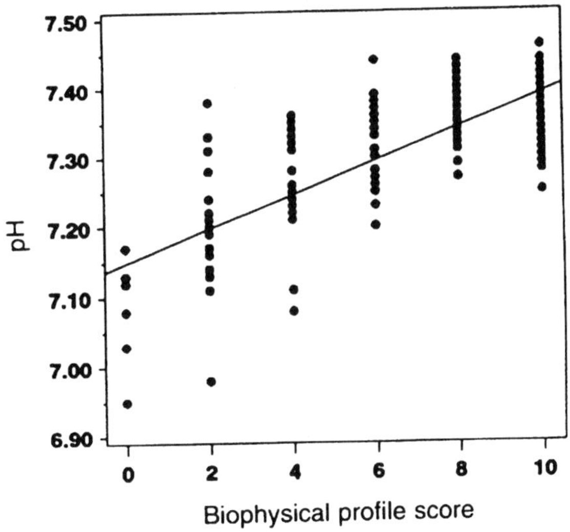

Figure 8. Biophysical profile score versus umbilical vein pH at antenatal cordocentesis. Paired observations of biophysical profile score and umbilical vein pH, $N = 493$. BPS of 0/10 was always associated with a pH <7.20; and when BPS equals 10/10, pH was always >7.20.

Table 8. Correlation of biophysical profile score with umbilical venous pH at cordocentesis

Author	Year	*N*	Comment	Correlation[a]
Ribbert et al. (66)	1990	14	Severe IUGR	BPS positive
Okamuar et al. (67)	1991	150	53% anomalous fetuses	BPS no correlation
Montenegro et al. (68)	1992	57	IUGR	BPS positive Doppler > BPS
Manning et al. (65)	1993	493	IUGR/Rh	BPS positive
Shalev et al. (69)	1993	23	IUGR	BPS positive
Yoon et al. (70)	1993	24	IUGR	BPS,OCT,NST > > Doppler BPS positive Doppler = BPS
Salvesen et al. (71)	1993	41	Diabetes	BPS positive but limited value

[a]Positive, statistically significant correlation with pH.

exceptions. Okamura et al. (67) (with cordocentesis) failed to show a correlation between BPS and fetal pH, but over half of the fetuses were being assessed for structural congenital anomalies, trisomies, and so on; there are no separate data for normal fetuses. Soothill et al. (59) (with delivery cord blood) studied 191 fetuses longitudinally to determine the best indicators of hypoxic morbidity, but only seven of 161 normal-sized infants and five of 30 IUGR infants had abnormal pH values, so the comparison was difficult. BPS was a poor predictor, while abnormal Doppler indices were statistically important in indicating which of the 30 small fetuses might have morbidity. For all tests (umbilical artery Doppler, FHR pattern, BPS), morbidity occurred more often in the groups with normal results than in those with abnormal results.

With these exceptions, biophysical profile scores have shown excellent correlation with fetal pH and blood gases: A normal BPS is a highly reliable indicator of normal pH, while progressive deterioration in BPS reliably predicts progressively worse pH values.

In the acutely changing situation, BPS may be an excellent guide as to the success of fetal intervention (72). In a group of 19 acidotic moribund alloimmune hydrops,

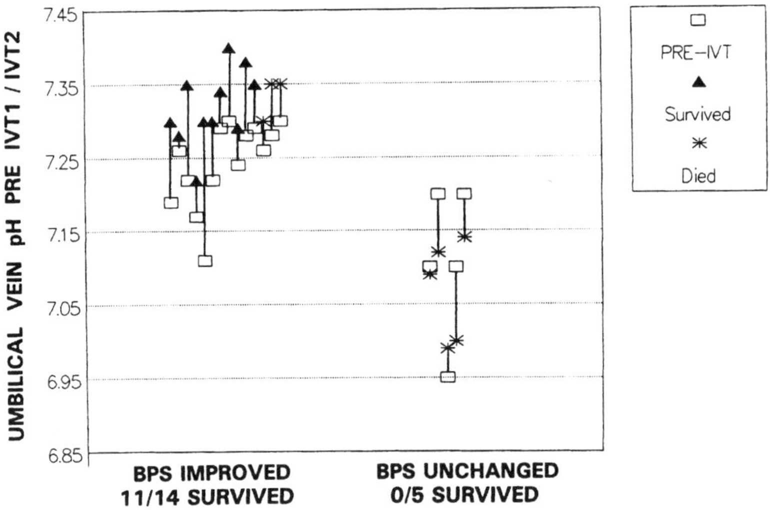

Figure 9. Biophysical profile score and response to intravascular transfusion. In 19 moribund fetuses (Class 4 hydrops, BPS ≤4/10, flat/decelerative CTG, gross physical hydrops), the biophysical profile score was used to monitor between transfusions. In those fetuses with improved BPS after the first or second transfusion (N = 14, group on left), 11 survived, with their pH at the time of the next procedure shown by the filled triangles. In eight fetuses (indicated by the asterisk, signifying pH at the time of the subsequent procedure), the fetus died. In three fetuses, in the left-hand group, BPS had improved, pH was somewhat improved, but traumatic complications led to fetal demise. In the right-hand group, with no improvement in BPS, mean pH fell among this group between first and second procedures, there was no resumption of normal fetal behavior, and all fetuses died. Fetuses in the right-hand group had more severe disease: lower pre-IVT pH and lower pre-IVT hemoglobin level. BPS reflected the success/failure of IVT to return pH towards normal. This study demonstrates the sensitivity of BPS behaviors to pH, not only in worsening acidosis but in improving fetal acidemia. This suggests that the success of efforts at intrauterine resuscitation for fetal asphyxia can be monitored successfully by BPS.

BPS was ≤4/10 in all, prior to first transfusion. Within minutes of transfusion, BPS improved in 14, 11 of whom survived. Mean umbilical venous pH improved from 7.27 to 7.34 as the BPS was restored. In the five with no improvement in BPS, pH fell after the first transfusion, and *none* survived. In this situation, restoration of an improved BPS is emphatic evidence of successful therapy, and it reliably demonstrates return towards normal pH (Figure 9).

With regard to BPS validation, then, consensus is broad on several issues:

1. For all variables and all endpoints, multiple variable fetal assessment is superior to single variable testing.
2. Many modifications have been evaluated. Superiority of any one approach over standard BPS has not been demonstrated, but multiple tests may be complementary.
3. BPS accurately reflects fetal pH and pO_2. With progressive change the acute BPS variables may disappear, or reappear, sequentially.

PERINATAL MORTALITY

Relationship to Test Score

BPS directly predicts perinatal mortality (Figure 10). Score/mortality figures are variable (obstetric intervention and neonatal care produce consistent improvements), but the exponential relationships (low scores confer high risk of mortality) have remained constant (42,73). For individual components, there is a hierarchy (AFV = 0, NST-NR, FM/FT-ABS, FBM-ABS by logistic regression), but performing the classic 10-point BPS produces the highest order of prediction. The low risk of stillbirth within 7 days of a normal score, 0.545 per 1000 tests, is a reliable clinical standard (stable over 17 years) which allows successful, safe extension of pregnancy in many high-risk perinatal situations (44). Intermediate scores provide surveillance alerts. Abnormal BPS justifies intervention across the gestational range of viability.

Population Impacts of BPS Programs

When BPS is incorporated into a centralized high-risk perinatal program, perinatal mortality falls (Table 9) (12,14,74,75). Enhanced management has been demonstrated in centers in Europe, North America, South America, Japan, and, recently, China, where 1066 tests in 649 high-risk pregnancies accurately predicted fetal hypoxemia at an early stage, "so that the perinatal mortality rate declined remarkably" to 3.00/1000 (76). These impacts are seen in both stillbirth and neonatal statistics: Prompt intervention can prevent intrauterine death from asphyxial causes while reducing neonatal mortality and morbidity when the intervention is able to prevent the intrauterine deterioration, which led to compromised neonates. These are the results of clinical *implementation* of the biophysical profile scoring management scheme. This is *not* "prediction" or "extrapolation"; that is, the relationships have

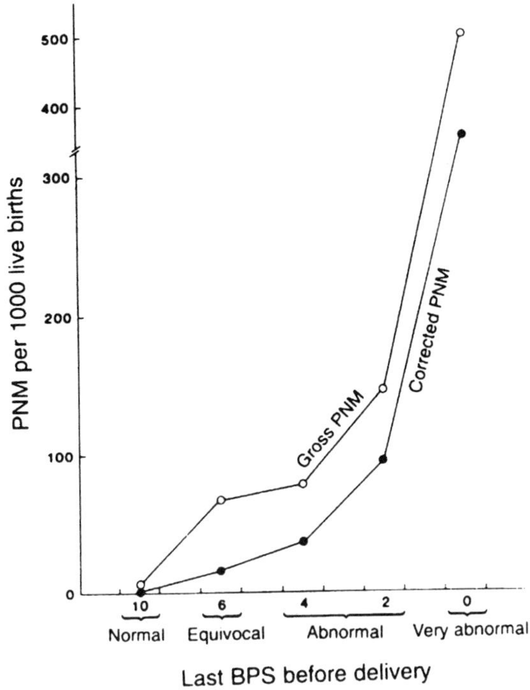

Figure 10. Biophysical profile score versus perinatal mortality. There is a progressive, exponential relationship between perinatal mortality and declining biophysical behavior. There is an important contribution to perinatal mortality by fetuses with congenital anomalies, as depicted in the gross PNM distribution.

Table 9. Perinatal mortality appears to change with BPS application

Author	N[a]	PNM[b] Tested	PNM Not Tested
Chamberlain (74)	3,200	4.1	10.7
Baskett et al. (75)	4,800	3.1	6.6
Manning (12)	56,000	1.9	7.7
Miller et al. (14)	16,000	1.3	8.8

[a]Number tested. In all trials, nontested population was much larger—for example, Manning 104,000 not tested, Miller et al. 53,000 not tested.
[b]PNM = Perinatal mortality/1000.

been demonstrated in clinical practice in all centers using BPS as primary antenatal surveillance.

The chronological connection is inescapable. This does not prove cause and effect. Perhaps at least as important in impact on perinatology are the centralization, expertise, and effects of formalizing the referral process for complicated pregnancies.

Perhaps BPS serves as a framework for regarding the fetus as a patient, with the obvious impacts that attitude would have on decision-making, transfers of mothers to high-risk centers antenatally, fetal therapy, and neonatal therapy.

Do We Need an RCT?

We believe the implementation of a biophysical profile scoring-based perinatal service lowers overall perinatal mortality:

1. BPS is strongly related to perinatal mortality, demonstrated in the original blinded study, in the original prospective application study, and in numerous clinical and ongoing studies.
2. Population comparisons show lower perinatal mortality between tested and non-tested groups with similar characteristics.
3. Application of the BPS management scheme to an existing population produces a drop in the overall perinatal mortality.
4. Construction of appropriate randomized controlled trials (obviously such a trial could not be blinded) seems very unlikely.
5. Problems with the current state of knowledge, from our point of view, do not seem to be lack of effect, but rather defining the effect and determining ways to allocate resources.

Construction of such a trial would be very difficult, because obstetric ultrasound is so entrenched: One would have to, somehow, exclude data about fetal behavior acquired during normal morphometrics, Doppler velocimetry, and so on. (While conducting the ultrasound scan to measure "amniotic fluid index only" in their modified BPS, Miller et al. (14) performed, *en passant,* thousands of complete BPS!) Finally, an RCT may not be necessary because the growing databases in many centers utilizing BPS will allow highly precise enquiry.

PERINATAL MORBIDITY

With the relationships between objective parameters, individual variables, and overall BPS, along with an accurate depiction of the risk of perinatal mortality with BPS, it would be surprising if there was not the same type of relationship to immediate neonatal *morbidity.* Figure 11 shows the same curvilinear, accelerating relationship between the biophysical profile score nearest delivery and a group of intrapartum and neonatal characteristics (63).

As suggested by Tables 7 and 8, several groups have confirmed the early suggestion that BPS was a good predictor of neonatal condition. BPS and other versions of multiple variable antenatal testing have proven superior to the Apgar score in predicting neonatal acidemia (61). Intervention now based on this level of prediction seems to be associated with improved condition of neonates in our service. However, it is hard to prove neonatal impacts of antenatal intervention. Specific studies have been com-

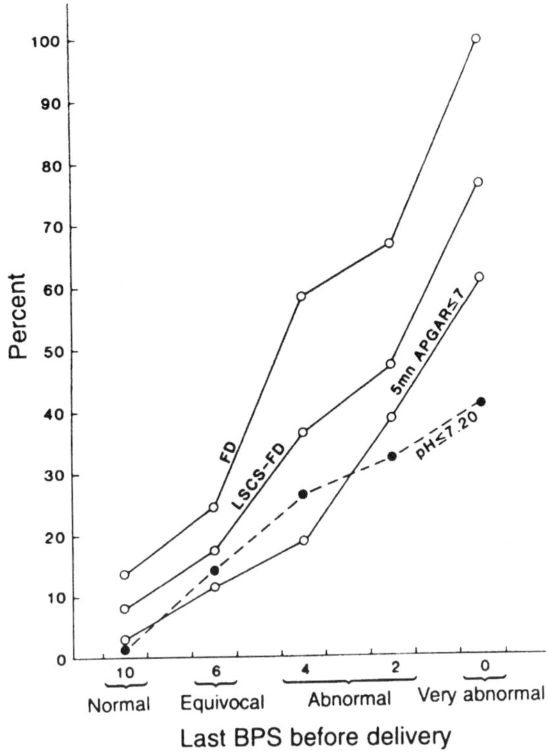

Figure 11. Biophysical profile score versus neonatal morbidity. Fetal distress (FD), emergency cesarean section in labor for fetal distress (LSCS-FD), 5-min Apgar scores <7, umbilical vein pH <7.20 at delivery, and admission to intensive care nursery (not shown) all show strong correlation with declining scores. This figure indicates the last biophysical profile score prior to delivery, plotted against the percentage of neonates who had one or more elements of perinatal morbidity.

pleted examining the role of BPS in postdate pregnancies (77,78), diabetic pregnancies (49,79), and multiple gestation (80,81), with favorable improvement in survival, neonatal condition, and iatrogenic complications. In complicated preterm pregnancy, where intervention previously was provoked by abnormal cardiotocography, continuation in utero by virtue of reassuring BPS was safe and effective, gaining up to 2 weeks (82). This policy in another situation reduced iatrogenic prematurity to 1.5% of high-risk pregnancies, from a previous standard of 2.5% (14). In our center, ancillary associations include a decline in antenatal admissions by 65%, intervention in postdate pregnancies reduced by 31%, and 28% fewer interventions in severe IUGR.

The role of BPS in preterm rupture of membranes, monitoring for intrauterine/fetal infection, is in dispute, with polarized viewpoints (83,84); and since asphyxia is often a very late step in the pathway of infections morbidity, this is not surprising. The critical role of Doppler in assigning fetal risk in intrauterine growth retardation will be stressed later; the equally critical role of BPS in determining the timing of delivery in such cases has seen sequenced testing adopted by many teams (14,82, 85,86). We are not so aggressive as some, and we favor the three-tiered approach described by James et al. (87) in many instances: IUGR is defined by size, risk is defined by Doppler, and intervention is determined by BPS.

Proving that neonatal benefits are attributable to antenatal testing is difficult. There is a background of steady improvement in neonatal care, due to antenatal steroids, better general maternal health, and great strides in neonatal care, all of which would tend to enhance a chronological association between BPS and neonatal survival rates. Specific interventions, such as cesarean section for fetuses with a score of 0/10, undoubtedly improve immediate survival (these fetuses usually died in the short term in utero), but may simply be generating asphyxiated newborns, who suffer severe consequences. Longer-term studies are needed to be certain about this.

BPS and Cerebral Palsy

Relation to Test Score. Study of the longer-term relationship mentioned above has begun. Such study, however, is even more complicated than the relationships to immediate neonatal morbidity. As observed by Pharoah (88), "it is inherently probable that different insults acting at different times have different effects on the developing brain," so relating evidence of a compromised intrauterine environment to longer-term evidence of central neurological impacts (in the form of cerebral palsy) is a daunting prospect. Although it is increasingly accepted that distant antenatal events contribute to the abnormal intrapartum performance and predetermine the long-term neurologic impacts in many cerebral palsy victims, documentation of the insult and antenatal *evidence* of its impact are unusual. (Murphy et al. (89), for example, found no cases of abnormal BPS associated with cerebral palsy in 59 extremely premature infants.) In our population, there is a >300-fold difference in the incidence of cerebral palsy for the extremes of BPS score (Figure 12). Fetuses who had a normal BPS had a rate of cerebral palsy of 0.82/1000 at 3 years of age, while fetuses with a score of 0/10 had a rate of 250/1000 (90).

We undertook a detailed review of cerebral palsy cases in the Province of Manitoba, our health care jurisdiction, to relate the last biophysical profile score result to subsequent cerebral palsy (90). The incidence of cerebral palsy in 22,336 high-risk pregnancies was determined by computer-assisted interrogation of two discrete databases. These were cross-referenced and were confirmed by a secondary audit of three additional user-group databases (extremely low-birthweight infant long-term follow-up, fetal assessment outcome database, Society of Manitobans with Disabilities database). The 27 children subsequently identified as having cerebral palsy, who had had biophysical profile scoring during pregnancy, had individual detailed chart review. These data were then analyzed in blinded fashion to classify the probable time of insult according to timing categories: antenatal, intrapartum, neonatal, (asphyxia, trauma, prematurity-specific complications, infection, combined etiology, and indeterminable), postnatal (remote in infancy, combined, or indeterminable) and genetic disorders.

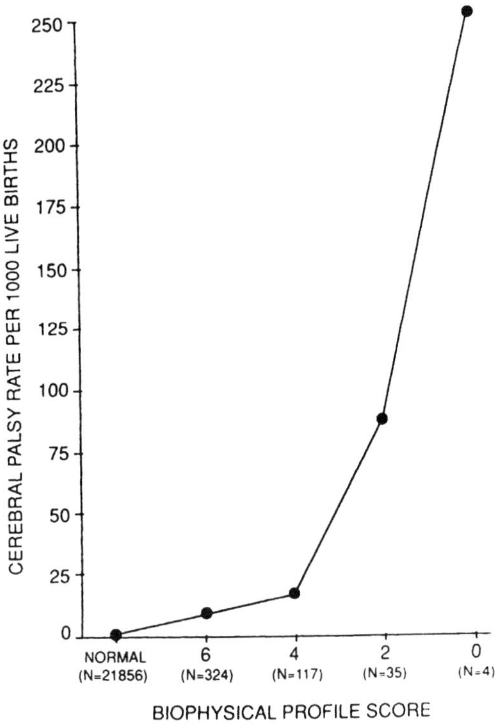

Figure 12. Biophysical profile score versus cerebral palsy rate. This figure depicts the relationship between the last biophysical profile score recorded prior to delivery and the frequency of cerebral palsy, in follow-up at 3 years of age, per 1000 live births. The issue is very complex (see text), but these data suggest that accelerated risk for cerebral palsy can be suspected in fetuses with overtly abnormal BPS.

Correlations seen between BPS and other adverse neonatal outcomes were duplicated in this population of infants with cerebral palsy: More fetal distress, more acidosis, and more frequent seizures were found in infants who had low BPS as fetuses (Table 10). The cerebral palsy group with abnormal BPS did not differ in gestational age, birthweight, incidence of IUGR, or frequency of normal-term vaginal delivery. Ultimate type of cerebral palsy did not differ with BPS score.

There *was* a significant difference in the timing of primary injury related to the cerebral palsy. (Classification of the timing of injury was done through detailed review of all available data, *blinded to BPS result.*) Overall, 29.6% of children who had cerebral palsy by age 3 had an antenatal origin (remember that *all* cases (e.g., child abuse, meningitis, congenital anomaly), were included). With normal BPS, only 5.5% of cerebral palsy cases were classified as antenatal in origin. This is significantly less than the 77.7% of fetuses with *abnormal* BPS prior to delivery, whose cerebral palsy insult occurred antenatally. Eighty-eight percent of cerebral palsy attributable solely to antenatal insult had abnormal BPS.

Table 10. Cerebral palsy cases in the BPS-tested population

Variable	BPS ≥8 Normal	BPS ≤6 Abnormal	Significance
Mean birthweight	2.1 kg ± 1.1	1.8 kg ± 0.77	NS
Mean gestational age weeks	34.0 ± 6.3	32.3 ± 4.4	NS
Gestational age ≤32 weeks	50%	66%	NS
% Fetal distress	16.1%	88.8%	p <0.01
% C/S fetal distress	5.5%	55.5%	p <0.01
% Cord pH <7.20	10%	77.7%	p <0.01
% NN seizures	27.7%	89%	p <0.05
% Antenatal insult	5.5%	78%	p <0.05[a]

[a]There were no significant differences in the frequencies of cerebral palsy caused by genetic/congenital, intrapartum, neonatal, or childhood factors.

The relationship of BPS to cerebral palsy is evident: A normal score is associated with a rate of cerebral palsy which is (a) very low and (b) caused by nonantenatal factors. In the group with abnormal BPS, the rate of cerebral palsy is higher; and while the number of cases caused by nonantenatal factors is similar, these are overshadowed by a large contribution from *antenatal* causes. Before the reader becomes impatient at this almost tautological argument ("Of course, sick fetuses have a higher rate of C.P.!"), be reminded that this is one of the first studies to relate handicap in a relatively large group of children to direct, prospective observations of their hampered intrauterine life.

Perhaps the most intriguing finding in this study was that the overall rate of cerebral palsy was only 1.21/1000. Since our referral practice concentrates infants with pregnancy complications, intrauterine growth retardation, premature labor and delivery—in fact, all of the suspected antecedents to cerebral palsy are indications for referral for BPS—it is quite surprising that the overall rate appears to be lower than many current published figures.

Impact of Biophysical Profile Scoring on the Incidence of Cerebral Palsy. Because the rate of cerebral palsy among tested children seemed so low, a further study was designed to determine the incidence of cerebral palsy in our high-risk referred population, evaluated and managed according to the BPS protocol, compared with a concurrent population of children delivered within our health care jurisdiction, who were not referred for BPS (91).

There are many reasons why the referred population might be expected to have a higher rate of cerebral palsy. The opposite, however, was found. The population assessed and managed according to BPS principles had a profoundly lower rate of cerebral palsy (Table 11). These results indicate a decreased rate of cerebral palsy in the BPS tested/managed population, which is so striking that one automatically turns for an explanation in definitions, treatment restrictions, data manipulations, and so on. A comparison of demographics of children in the two groups emphasizes the similarity

Table 11. Cerebral palsy rate in BPS-tested and nontested women delivered 1987–1991, cerebral palsy by age 3

Variable	Tested	Nontested	*p*
Deliveries	26,288	58,659	
Cerebral palsy cases	35	278	
Cerebral palsy rate	1.33/1000	4.74/1000	*p*<.001
Mean birthweight	2.09 kg ± ..99	2.28 kg ± .32	NS
< 1.0 kg	14%	6.7%	NS
Mean gestational age	33.4 ± 5.6 weeks	34.4 ± 2.1 weeks	NS
< 32 weeks	40.5%	37.8%	NS
< 28 weeks	13.5%	10.9%	NS
Type of cerebral palsy			
Quadriplegia	63%	56%	NS
Diplegia	22%	26%	NS
Hemiplegia	15%	18%	NS

of the populations: The different cerebral palsy rates exist despite a trend to earlier, lighter babies, among the tested group. (These differences were not statistically significant but would again suggest an increased liability in the BPS–managed group).

In this large population-based study of children born between 1987 and 1991, with detailed follow-up at age 3 years, management by the BPS protocol was associated with a *68% decline in the cerebral palsy rate.* The potential mechanisms for this association require further examination. It could be that intervention for an abnormal score interrupts the progression leading to cerebral injury. Among the tested population of 26,288 patients, intervention on the basis of an abnormal score was carried out 563 times (2.1%). The majority of such interventions, notably, were for intermediate scores of 4/10 and 6/10, which combined for a total of 91.9% of all low-score interventions. The incidence of cerebral palsy in these groups was low, suggesting that cerebral injury may have been prevented by delivery before the score declined further.

As noted at the beginning of this section, however, the contributors to cerebral palsy are very complex (92). Table 12 shows the distribution of timing of cerebral palsy, based on the blinded classification system explained earlier. Comparison between the tested and nontested population shows highly significant differences in *all* categories of insult timing, so there must be multiple explanations for the overall population differences—more than just obstetric factors at play. Population distribution, favoring socioeconomic classes, education levels, or other factors determining women's access to health care might be determinants. Examining pregnancy-related timing (the total of antenatal, intrapartum, and neonatal factors) shows a difference of more than threefold between the tested population (CP rate 1.14/1000) and the nontested population (3.73/1000, p <0.01). Early intervention, selection of fetuses for whom labor might not be safe, and delivery of neonates in better condition at tertiary-care neonatal units might collectively account for this large difference. Among those

Table 12. Cerebral palsy rate per 1000 live births according to presumed etiology of primary insult

Timing	Tested	Nontested
Antenatal	0.69	1.79
Intrapartum	0.08	0.41
Neonatal	0.38	1.55
Genetic/anomaly	0.16	0.51
Postnatal	0.12	0.48

with genetic anomalies related to their cerebral palsy, major components here are spina bifida and Down syndrome, in which case the tested population were quite likely to have undergone maternal serum screening and have had the birth frequency of neural tube defects/aneuploidy reduced by pregnancy termination. The postnatal category, which includes child abuse, infant and childhood infections, and accidental brain injury, as well as a few cases of delayed consequences of pregnancy-related asphyxia, could not be explained by perinatal interventions alone. Much work remains to be done to approach answers in this difficult area. Timing of intervention, based on multiple-parameter testing of the fetus, might be expected to contribute significantly in reducing the cerebral palsy rate, as BPS application continues to grow over time.

DOPPLER VELOCIMETRY AND THE BIOPHYSICAL PROFILE

Doppler Velocimetry Versus BPS

A large number of studies, both descriptive and more structured comparative trials, exist in which BPS and Doppler have been evaluated. Some of these include evaluation of BPS, Doppler, cardiotocography, and growth profiles, in varying combinations. Some of these studies confine their attention to diabetics, postdate pregnancies, or, most commonly, growth-restricted fetuses. The results are varied. They range from finding that the biophysical profile score is superior to CTG (62) and that Doppler velocimetry is a poor predictor of compromise among IUGR infants (69), to an equally reputable study where Doppler velocimetry was the only factor able to distinguish the sick IUGR infant from the healthy one (59)!

Since IUGR is inherently a complex disorder, it may be unreasonable to expect any method to cover all possibilities. Among the group with placental insufficiency as the most likely cause for IUGR (i.e., omitting aneuploidy, congenital abnormalities, infection, etc.), Doppler velocimetry has a highly significant diagnostic impact: These fetuses have a *vascular* disorder. Doppler performance in many trials of IUGR infants was superior to BPS in diagnostic timing, differentiation of severity, and likelihood of significant permanent compromise, especially when accompanied by, or in series with, fetal heart rate testing (93–95). However, in many of these studies and in our current practice, the biophysical profile score was the bottom line in determining management per se (96–99). The progression of events outlined by James et al. (87) in their detailed review of Doppler velocimetry, fetal growth prediction, and biophysical profile scoring offers a likely explanation: Placental limitation and/or injury is evidenced by abnormal Dopplers, which may progress as the placenta continues to deteriorate; third-trimester growth limitation is the first line of compensatory sacrifice made by the fetus; decline in biophysical variables marks the onset of decompensation and is the indicator for intervention. In their model, gestational age has a significant effect: After 34 weeks, in the growth-retarded fetus with abnormal Dopplers, intervention is suggested in the presence of a normal score, preventing the final stage of decline. From our perspective, the security of a normal BPS allows extension of the pregnancy into that zone when neonatal management can be expected to have the lowest possible rate of iatrogenic complications (12,14,30).

Similarly, in the diabetic population, there may be different routes to fetal compromise. In the subset of women with diabetic vasculopathy, Doppler velocimetry has a preeminent role (100). In many populations of diabetic women with lower rates of nephropathy, retinopathy, and so on, biophysical profile scoring offers detailed evaluation of the fetus at risk for metabolic compromise (in whom Doppler may be irrelevant) possibly supplemented by amniotic fluid insulin levels (49). One must have reservations about the efficacy of *any* method in the unstable diabetic (71,101).

The emergence of cardiac, cerebral, and cerebellar Doppler velocimetry as techniques capable of elucidating fetal compromise in the face of abnormal placental (umbilical) Dopplers (102,103) has recently been further enhanced by the evidence of cardiac failure in the late decompensation phase, as evidenced by umbilical venous pulsations (104). These refinements in Doppler technology undoubtedly will contribute to greater specificity of diagnosis in the subset of fetuses whose disorders are primarily vascular in nature. Nevertheless, even in these populations, biophysical profile scoring produces a reliable index of when to intervene, with many cautioning against the hasty overinterpretation of the Doppler waveform (97,98).

Doppler Velocimetry and Biophysical Profile Scoring

The discussion above is somewhat artificial from our point of view. Duplex scanning allows performance of all Doppler indices within the short time frame (11 min on average for the normal score, 30 min by protocol application for the abnormal score) of biophysical profile scoring. The precision afforded by Doppler in vessel-based fetal disease has enhanced BPS in our population (53). Doppler abnormalities of either the umbilical or cerebral vasculature are an indication to modify the usual timing of BPS performance. With absent end-diastolic velocities (AEDV), BPS is carried out biweekly, as long as fetal growth is demonstrated, regardless of centile. In this group, our record for prolongation of pregnancy from the time AEDV was first documented is 14 weeks! (See Figure 2.) In cases where serial monitoring has been possible (based on BPS 10/10 allowing the pregnancy to proceed further), the cardiotocogram is *always* performed ("score out of 10"), ancillary tests such as cordocentesis for fetal pH and pO_2 are used (86,105), and the oxygen uptake test (Figure 13) is utilized (106).

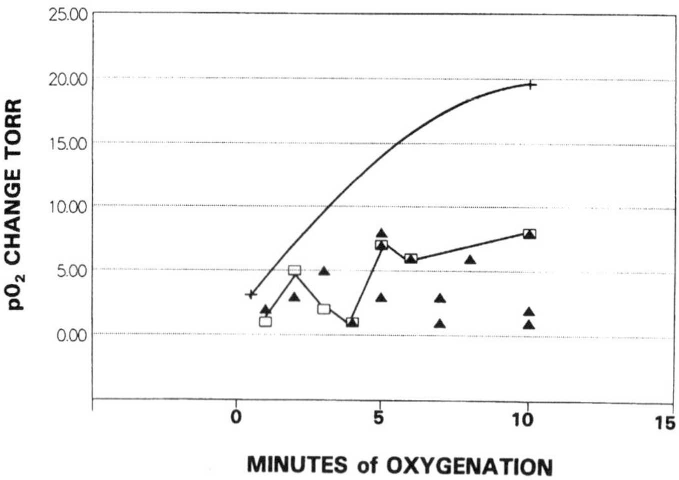

Figure 13. Oxygen uptake test. This figure illustrates response of fetuses to maternal hyperoxygenation, while cordocentesis is carried out. With the 22-gauge needle resident in the umbilical vein, the mother is placed on tightly sealed rebreathe oxygen by mask, to give FiO_2 of 45–55%. In healthy fetuses receiving top-up intrauterine transfusions, mean increase in pO_2 is shown by the curved line. In IUGR fetuses (usually undergoing combined sampling for karyotype, acid base status, pO_2, hemoglobin, and other metabolic indices), pO_2 levels do not rise, or rise only fractionally (▲). The pO_2 profile of a severely IUGR fetus with successive values is displayed by the open boxes. Lack of continuity of the line indicates a large variable deceleration which took place at approximately 3 min, blocking the increased transmission of oxygen. These data demonstrate the limited ability of the placenta to transmit improved maternal oxygen levels to the fetus.

In the severely affected group of IUGR fetuses with reverse end-diastolic velocities (REDV), BPS is done at least daily, often every 8–12 hours. Under these circumstances, fluid volume is often marginal, the CTG is borderline (registering mean variations in the 20–30 range), and decelerations with fetal movements are not uncommon. Intervention may be on the basis of the nurse ultrasonographer-perinatologist team illustrating changes in biophysical parameters at or near the threshold of the BPS variables. Sometimes this will be on the basis of decline in total activity, even though the BPS will not have fallen all the way to zero. We believe that the BPS in these severely compromised infants offers a framework, rather than an absolute guideline, for timing of the delivery and successful outcome.

SERENDIPITY

BPS Versus Ultrasound (Figure 14)

There may be significant impact on perinatal mortality as nonasphyxic events are modified or prevented under the guidance of the BPS protocol. Cord accidents,

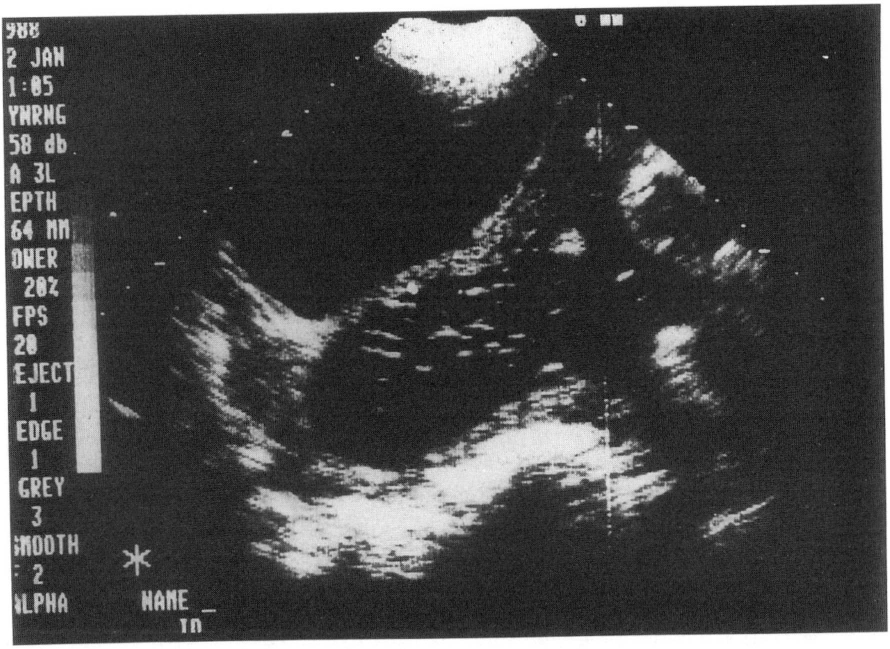

Figure 14. Cord presentation, 32 weeks' gestation. The patient was an asymptomatic primigravida referred for biophysical profile scoring because of suspected IUGR. BPS was 10/10, biometry showed the fetus on the 50th percentile, and birthweight was 2.1 kg. The "accidental finding" of this complete prolapse of the cord through hourglass membranes into the vagina allowed safe delivery by emergency cesarean section and saved this baby's life.

evolving abruptions, silent dilatation of the cervix with prolapsed membranes, oligohydramnios as the first sign of fetal compromise, detection of treatable abnormalities, untreatable anomalies, and diversion of surgical fetal cases all have significant impact on the perinatal mortality of the tested population. Such fortunate "accidents" assume an increasing proportion of serious impacts, as the risk of mortality of the normally formed fetus declines. This means that in some cases, successful intervention is facilitated by the patient being referred for BPS, but not determined by the actual score. Further, as has been noted above, the expertise acquired while using biophysical profile scoring may lead to many other *observer characteristics* which favor prompt and effective intervention, outside the variables of BPS themselves. That mothers have to attend one of two fetal assessment units in our province and are therefore within the walls of a tertiary-care facility with intensive neonatal care, means that intrauterine emergencies can be attended without maternal transport. Undoubtedly this is a contributing factor in some interventions. In short, the context of biophysical profile scoring may provide the compromised fetus many opportunities to make his/her wishes known. These explanations provide evidence about the superiority of ultrasound-based multiple-variable methods of fetal surveillance, regardless of the parameters chosen.

SUMMARY

Biophysical Profile Scoring and the Detection of Fetal Asphyxia

1. Human fetuses show progressive reduction in activity in response to worsening hypoxemia, intensified by acidemia.
2. Because it uses multiple parameters, with different time scales, in a binary format, with simple methodology, biophysical profile scoring is able to depict fetal status accurately. This is particularly true in the detection of fetal asphyxia with a low BPS and in the assurance of fetal well-being with a normal score.
3. Accurate detection of acute, acute-on-chronic, and chronic asphyxia by biophysical profile scoring enables intervention which can lower perinatal mortality and morbidity, including reducing the rate of serious neurologic handicap.
4. The accuracy and impacts of BPS may be difficult to separate from other benefits of comprehensive fetal assessment.
5. BPS provides a basic format for ongoing research in human fetal behavior and applied fetal medicine.

REFERENCES

1. Manning FA, Platt LD, Sipos L. Antepartum fetal evaluation: development of a fetal biophysical profile score. *Am J Obstet Gynecol* 1980;136:787–795.
2. Prechtl HFR. The behavioral states of the newborn infant (a review). *Brain Res* 1974; 76:185–212.
3. Nijhuis JG, Prechtl HFR, Martin CB Jr, et al. Are there behavioural states in the human fetus? *Early Hum Dev* 1982;6:177–195.
4. Pillai M, James D. Human fetal mouthing movements: a potential biophysical variable for distinguishing state 1F from abnormal fetal behaviour; report of 4 cases. *Eur J Obstet Gynecol Reprod Biol* 1991;38(2):151–156.
5. Natale R, Patrick JE, Richardson BS. Effects of maternal venous plasma glucose concentrations on fetal breathing movements. *Am J Obstet Gynecol* 1978;132:36–42.
6. Chamberlain PF, Manning FA, Morrison I, et al. Circadian rhythm in bladder volumes in the term human fetus. *Obstet Gynecol* 1984;64:657–660.
7. Arduini D, Rizzo G, Parlati E, et al. Modifications of ultradian and circadian rhythms of fetal heart rate after fetal–maternal adrenal gland suppression: a double blind study. *Prenat Diagn* 1986;6:409–417.
8. de Vries JIP, Visser GHA, Mulder EJH, et al. Diurnal and other variations in fetal movement and heart rate patterns at 20 to 22 weeks. *Early Hum Dev* 1987;15:333–348.
9. Pillai M, James D. Development of human fetal behaviour: a review. *Fetal Diagn Ther* 1990;5:15–32.
10. Pillai M, James D. The development of fetal heart rate patterns during normal pregnancy. *Obstet Gynecol* 1990;76:812–816.
11. Manning FA, Morrison I, Harman CR, Menticoglou SM. The abnormal fetal biophysical profile score. V. Predictive accuracy according to score composition. *Am J Obstet Gynecol* 1990;162(4):918–927.

12. Manning FA. *Fetal biophysical profile scoring: theoretical considerations and clinical application. Fetal medicine,* vol 6. Norwalk: Appleton & Lange, 1995:221–305.
13. Nageotte MP, Towers CV, Asrat T, Freeman RK, Dorchester W. The value of a negative antepartum test: contraction stress test and modified biophysical profile. *Obstet Gynecol* 1994;84:231–234.
14. Miller DA, Rabello YA, Paul RH. The modified biophysical profile: antepartum testing in the 1990s. *Am J Obstet Gynecol* 1996;174:812–817.
15. Walkinshaw S, Cameron H, MacPhail S, Robson S. The prediction of fetal compromise and acidosis by biophysical profile scoring in the small for gestational age fetus. *J Perinat Med* 1992;20:227–232.
16. Richardson BS. Fetal adaptive responses to asphyxia. *Clin Perinatol* 1989;16(3):595–611.
17. Rurak DW, Selke P, Fisher M, et al. Fetal oxygen extraction: comparison of the human and sheep. *Am J Obstet Gynecol* 1987;156:360–366.
18. Sheldon RE, Peeters LLH, Jones MD, et al. Redistribution of cardiac output and oxygen delivery in the hypoxemic fetal lamb. *Am J Obstet Gynecol* 1979;135:1071–1078.
19. Rudolph AM. The fetal circulation and its response to stress. *J Dev Physiol* 1984;6:11–19.
20. Bocking AD, Gagnon R, White SE, et al. Circulatory responses to prolonged hypoxemia in fetal sheep. *Am J Obstet Gynecol* 1988;159:1418–1424.
21. Jones MD, Traystman RJ, Simmons MA, Molteni A. Effects of changes in arterial O_2 content on cerebral blood flow in the lamb. *Am J Physiol* 1981;240:209–215.
22. Nicolaides KH, Peters MT, Vyas S, et al. Relation of rate of urine production to oxygen tension in small-for-gestational-age fetuses. *Am J Obstet Gynecol* 1990;162:387–391.
23. Natale R, Clewlow F, Dawes GS. Measurement of fetal forelimb movements in the lamb in utero. *Am J Obstet Gynecol* 1981;140:545–551.
24. Rurak DW, Gruber NC. Effect of neuromuscular blockade on oxygen consumption and blood gases. *Am J Obstet Gynecol* 1983;145:258–262.
25. Van Vliet MAT, Martin CB Jr, Nijhuis JG, et al. Behavioural states in growth retarded human fetuses. *Early Hum Dev* 1985;12:183–197.
26. Arduini D, Rizzo G. Fetal behavioural states. In Dawes GS, Burruto F, Zacutti A, Zacutti A Jr (eds). *Fetal autonomy and adaptation.* Chichester, England: Wiley, 1990:117–124.
27. Vintzileos AM, Flemming AD, Scorza WE, Wolf EJ, Balducci J, Campbell WA, Rodis JF. Relationship between fetal biophysical activities and umbilical cord blood gas values. *Am J Obstet Gynecol* 1991;165(3):707–713.
28. Anderson DF, Parks CM, Faber JJ. Fetal O_2 consumption in sheep during controlled long-term reductions in umbilical blood flow. *Am J Physiol* 1986;250:H1037–H1042.
29. Rurak DW, Richardson BS, Patrick JE, et al. Oxygen consumption in the fetal lamb during sustained hypoxemia with progressive acidemia. *Am J Physiol* 1990;258:1108–1115.
30. Harman C, Menticoglou S, Manning F, Albar H, Morrison I. Prenatal fetal monitoring: abnormalities of fetal behaviour. In James DR, Steer PJ, Weiner CP, Gonik B (eds). *High risk pregnancy management options.* London: WB Saunders, 1994;39:693–734.
31. Chamberlain PF, Manning FA, Morrison I, et al. Ultrasound evaluation of amniotic fluid volume. I. The relationship of marginal and decreased amniotic fluid volumes to perinatal outcome. *Am J Obstet Gynecol* 1984;150(3):245–249.
32. Chamberlain PF, Manning FA, Morrison I, et al. Ultrasound evaluation of amniotic fluid volume. II. The relationship of increased amniotic fluid volume to perinatal outcome. *Am J Obstet Gynecol* 1984;150(3):250–254.

33. Bastide A, Manning F, Harman CR, et al. Ultrasound evaluation of amniotic fluid: outcome of pregnancies with severe oligohydramnios. *Am J Obstet Gynecol* 1986;154:895–900.
34. Lavado M, Harman CR, Menticoglou S, Khan R. Obstetrical impacts of oligohydramnios. *Am J Obstet Gynecol* 1998;in press.
35. Dawes GS, Moulden M, Redman CWG. System 8000: computerized antenatal FHR analysis. *J Perinat Med* 1991;19:47–51.
36. Yoon BH, Syn HC, Kim SW. The efficacy of Doppler umbilical artery velocimetry in identifying fetal acidosis. A comparison with fetal biophysical profile. *J Ultrasound Med* 1992;11:1–6.
37. Johnson J, Harman CR. Biophysical profile scoring. In Rumack CM, Wilson SR, Charboneau JW (eds). *Diagnostic Ultrasound.* Philadelphia: Mosby, 1998:1033–1042.
38. Manning FA, Harman CR, Menticoglou S, Morrison I. Assessment of fetal well-being with ultrasound. *Obstet Gynecol Clin North Am* 1991;18(4):891–905.
39. Vintzileos AM, Campbell WA, Ingardia CJ, Nochimson DJ. The fetal biophysical profile and its predictive value. *Obstet Gynecol* 1983;62(3):271–278.
40. Manning FA, Baskett TF, Morrison I, Lange I. Fetal biophysical profile scoring: a prospective study in 1,184 high-risk patients. *Am J Obstet Gynecol* 1981;140(3):289–294.
41. Manning FA, Harman CR, Morrison I, Menticoglou S. Fetal assessment based on fetal biophysical profile scoring. III. Positive predictive accuracy of the very abnormal test (biophysical profile score = 0). *Am J Obstet Gynecol* 1990;162(2):398–402.
42. Manning FA. Fetal biophysical profile score. In Fleischer AC, Manning FA, Jeanty P, Romero R (eds). *Sonography in obstetrics and gynecology. Principles and practice,* 5th ed. Stanford, CT: Appleton & Lange 1996:611–619.
43. Stearns E. *Perinatal and Maternal Welfare Committee 1995 Report.* College of Physicians and Surgeons of Manitoba, 1996.
44. Manning FA, Morrison I, Harman CR, Lange IR, Menticoglou S. Fetal assessment based on fetal biophysical profile scoring: experience in 19,221 referred high-risk pregnancies. II. An analysis of false-negative fetal deaths. *Am J Obstet Gynecol* 1987;157:880–884.
45. Manning FA, Morrison I, Lange IR, et al. Fetal biophysical profile scoring: selective use of the nonstress test. *Am J Obstet Gynecol* 1987;156(3):709–712.
46. Manning FA, Lange IR, Morrison I, Harman CR. Fetal biophysical profile score and the nonstress test: a comparative trial. *Obstet Gynecol* 1984;64(3):326–331.
47. Harman CR, Menticoglou SM. Fetal surveillance in diabetic pregnancy. *Curr Opin Obstet Gynecol* 1997;9:83–97.
48. Johnson JM, Harman CR, Lange IR, Manning FA. Biophysical profile scoring in the management of the postterm pregnancy: an analysis of 307 patients. *Am J Obstet Gynecol* 1986;154(2):269–273.
49. Harman CR. Ultrasound in the management of the alloimmunized pregnancy. In Fleischer AC, Manning FA, Jeanty P, Romero R (eds). *Sonography in obstetrics and gynecology. Principles and practice,* 5th ed, Stamford: Appleton & Lange, 1996:583–609.
50. Vintzileos AM, Campbell WA, Rodis JF. Fetal biophysical profile scoring: current status. *Clin Perinatol* 1989;16:661–689.
51. Manning FA, Lange IR, Morrison I, Harman CR. Fetal biophysical profile score and the nonstress test: a comparative trial. *Obstet Gynecol* 1984;64:326–331.
52. Manning FA, Platt LD. Fetal breathing movements and the abnormal contraction stress test. *Am J Obstet Gynecol* 1979;133:590–593.

53. Morrison I, Menticoglou S, Manning FA, Harman CR, Cheang M. Comparison of antepartum test results to perinatal outcome. *J Matern Fet Med* 1994;3:75–83.

54. Arabin B, Snyjders R, Mohnhaupt A, Ragosch V, Nicolaides K. Evaluation of the fetal assessment score in pregnancies at risk for intrauterine hypoxia. *Am J Obstet Gynecol* 1993;169:549–554.

55. Sener T, Ozalp S, Hassa H, Yildirim A. Doppler and B-mode ultrasonography in biophysical profile scoring. *Int J Gynaecol Obstet* 1996;54:231–236.

56. Schifrin BS, Guntes V, Gergley RC, et al. The role of real-time scanning in antenatal surveillance. *Am J Obstet Gynecol* 1981;140:525–530.

57. Bates JA, Evans JA, Mason G. Differentiation of growth retarded from normally grown fetuses and prediction of intrauterine growth retardation using Doppler ultrasound. *Br J Obstet Gynecol* 1996;103:670–675.

58. Soothill PW, Nicolaides KH, Campbell S. Prenatal asphyxia, hyperlacticacidemia, hypoglycemia and erythroblastosis in growth retarded fetuses. *Br Med J* 1987;297:1051–1053.

59. Soothill PW, Ajayi RA, Campbell S, Nicolaides LH. Prediction of morbidity in small and normally grown fetuses by fetal heart rate variability, biophysical profile score and umbilical artery Doppler studies. *Br J Obstet Gynecol* 1993;100:742–745.

60. Vintzileos AM, Gaffney SE, Salinger LM, et al. The relationship between fetal biophysical profile and cord pH in patients undergoing caesarian section before the onset of labour. *Obstet Gynecol* 1987;70:196.

61. Vintzileos AM, Gaffney SE, Salinger LM, Kontopoulos VG, Campbell WA, Nochimson OJ. The relationship among the fetal biophysical profile, umbilical cord pH, and Apgar scores. *Am J Obstet Gynecol* 1987;157(3):627–631.

62. Vintzileos AM, Campbell WA, Rodis JF, McLean DA, Fleming AD, Scorza WE. The relationship between fetal biophysical assessment, umbilical artery velocimetry, and fetal acidosis. *Obstet Gynecol* 1991;77:622–626.

63. Ribbert LSM, Nicolaides KH, Visser GHA. Prediction of fetal acidaemia in intrauterine growth retardation: comparison of quantified fetal activity with biophysical profile score. *Br J Obstet Gynecol* 1993;100:653–656.

64. Manning FA, Harman CR, Morrison I, Menticoglou SM, Lange IR, Johnson JM. Fetal assessment based on fetal biophysical profile scoring. IV. An analysis of perinatal morbidity and mortality. *Am J Obstet Gynecol* 1990;162(3):703–709.

65. Manning FA, Snijders R, Harman CR, et al. Fetal biophysical profile scoring. VI. Correlations with antepartum umbilical venous pH. *Am J Obstet Gynecol* 1993;169:755–763.

66. Ribbert LSM, Snijders RJM, Nicolaides KH, Visser GHA. Relationship of fetal biophysical profile and blood gas values at cordocentesis in severely growth-retarded fetuses. *Am J Obstet Gynecol* 1990;163(2):569–571.

67. Okamura K, Watanabe T, Endo H, Tanigawara S, Iwamoto M, Murotsuki J, Uehara S, Yajima A. Biophysical profile and its relation to fetal blood gas level obtained by cordocentesis. *Acta Obstet Gynaecol Jpn* 1991;43(11):1573–1577.

68. Montenegro CA, Meirelles-Filho J, Fonseca AL, Netto HC, Amim J Jr, Rezende-Filho J, Jacyntho C. Cordocentesis and evaluation of fetal wellbeing in a very high-risk population (a very reliable index). *Rev Fr Gynecol Obstet* 1992;87:467–477.

69. Shalev E, Zalel Y, Weiner E. A comparison of the nonstress test, oxytocin challenge test, Doppler velocimetry and biophysical profile in predicting umbilical vein pH in growth-retarded fetuses. *Int J Gynaecol Obstet* 1993;43:15–19.

70. Yoon BH, Romero R, Roh CR, Kim SH, Ager JW, Syn HC, Cotton D, Kim SW. Relationship between the fetal biophysical profile score, umbilical artery Doppler velocimetry, and fetal blood acid–base status determined by cordocentesis. *Am J Obstet Gynecol* 1993;169:1586–1594.
71. Salvesen DR, Freeman J, Brudenell JM, Nicolaides KH. Prediction of fetal acidaemia in pregnancies complicated by maternal diabetes mellitus by biophysical profile scoring and fetal heart rate monitoring. *Br J Obstet Gynecol* 1993;100:227–233.
72. Harman CR, Manning F, Menticoglou S. Class 4 hydrops: restoration of biophysical activities with IVT. *Am J Obstet Gynecol* 1997;176:S85.
73. Manning FA, Morrison I, Lange IR, et al. Fetal assessment based on fetal biophysical profile scoring: experience in 12,620 referred high-risk pregnancies. I. Perinatal mortality by frequency and etiology. *Am J Obstet Gynecol* 1985;151(3):343–350.
74. Chamberlain PF. Later fetal death—has ultrasound a role to play in its prevention? *Irish J Med Sci* 1991;160:251–254.
75. Baskett TG, Allen AC, Gray JH, Prewett SJ, et al. Fetal biophysical profile and perinatal death. *Obstet Gynecol* 1987;70:357–360.
76. Ou XD, Liu XX, Liang RX. The application of modified fetal biophysical profile scoring for prenatal monitoring. *Chung Hua Fu Chan Ko Tsa Chih* 1994;29:213–6,252.
77. Johnson JM, Harman CR, Lange IR, Manning FA. Biophysical profile scoring in the management of the postterm pregnancy: an analysis of 307 patients. *Am J Obstet Gynecol* 1986;154(2):269–273.
78. Bresadola M, Lo-Mastro F, Arena V, Bellaveglia L, Di-Gennaro D. Prognostic value of biophysical profile score in post-date pregnancy. *Clin Exp Obstet Gynecol* 1995;22:330–338.
79. Johnson JM, Lange IR, Harman CR, Torchia MG, Manning FA. Biophysical profile scoring in the management of the diabetic pregnancy. *Obstet Gynecol* 1988;72(6):841–846.
80. Lodeiro JG, Vintzileos AM, Feinstein SJ, et al. Fetal biophysical profile in twin gestations. *Obstet Gynecol* 1986;67(6):824–827.
81. Elliott JP, Finberg HJ. Biophysical profile testing as an indicator of fetal well-being in high-order multiple gestations. *Am J Obstet Gynecol* 1995;172:508–512.
82. Merrill PA, Porto M, Lovett SM, Dorchester W, Nageotte MP, Garite TJ, Freeman RK. Evaluation of the nonreactive positive contraction stress test prior to 32 weeks: the role of the biophysical profile. *Am J Perinatol* 1995;12:229–231.
83. Vintzileos AM, Bors-Koefoed R, Pelegano JF, et al. The use of fetal biophysical profile improves pregnancy outcome in premature rupture of the membranes. *Am J Obstet Gynecol* 1987;157:236–240.
84. Carroll SG, Papaioannou S, Nicolaides KH. Assessment of fetal activity and amniotic fluid volume in the prediction of intrauterine infection in preterm prelabour amniorrhexis. *Am J Obstet Gynecol* 1995;172:1427–1435.
85. Devoe LD, Youssef AA, Gardner P, Dear C, Murray C. Refining the biophysical profile with a risk-related evaluation of test performance. *Am J Obstet Gynecol* 1992;167(2):346–352.
86. Donner C, Vermeylen D, Kirkpatrick C, de Maertelaer V, Rodesch F. Management of the growth-restricted fetus: the role of non invasive tests and fetal blood sampling. *Obstet Gynecol* 1995;85:965–970.
87. James DK, Parker MJ, Smoleniec JS. Comprehensive fetal assessment with three ultrasonographic characteristics. *Am J Obstet Gynecol* 1992;166:1486–1495.

88. Pharoah POD. Cerebral palsy and perinatal care. *Br J Obstet Gynecol* 1995;102: 356–358.

89. Murphy DJ, Sellers S, MacKenzie IZ, Yudkin PL, Johnson AM. Case-control study of antenatal and intrapartum risk factors for cerebral palsy in very preterm singleton babies. *Lancet* 1995;346:1449–1454.

90. Manning, FA, Bondagji N, Harman CR, Casiro O, Menticoglou S, Morrison I. Fetal assessment based on the fetal biophysical profile score. VII. Relationship of last BPS result to subsequent cerebral palsy. *J Gynecol Obstet Biol Reprod* 1997;26:720–729.

91. Manning FA, Bondagji N, Harman CR, Menticoglou SM, Casiro O, Morrison I, Burck DJ. Fetal assessment based on biophysical profile scoring. VIII. The incidence of cerebral palsy in tested and non-tested perinates. *Am J Obstet Gynecol* 1998;in press.

92. Nelson KB, Ellenberg JH. Antecedents of cerebral palsy: multivariate analysis of risk factors. *New Engl J Med* 1986;315:81–86.

93. Pattinson RC, Norman K, Kirsten G, Odendaal HJ. Relationship between the fetal heart rate pattern and perinatal mortality in fetuses with absent end-diastolic velocities of the umbilical artery: a case-controlled study. *Am J Perinatol* 1995;12:286–289.

94. Weiner Z, Farmakides G, Schulman H, Lopresti S, Schneider E. Surveillance of growth-retarded fetuses with computerized fetal heart rate monitoring combined with doppler velocimetry of the umbilical and uterine arteries. *J Reprod Med* 1996;41:112–118.

95. Guzman ER, Vintzileos AM, Martins M, Benito C, Houlihan C, Hanley M. The efficacy of individual computer heart rate indices in detecting acidemia at birth in growth-restricted fetuses. *Obstet Gynecol* 1996;87:969–974.

96. Divon MY, Girz BA, Lieblich R, Langer O. Clinical management of the fetus with markedly diminished umbilical artery end-diastolic flow. *Am J Obstet Gynecol* 1989; 161:1523–1527.

97. Rocca MM, Said MS, Khamis MY, Ghanem IA, Karkour TA. The value of doppler study of the umbilical artery in predicting perinatal outcome in pre-eclamptic patients. *J Obstet Gynecol* 1995;21:427–431.

98. Zelop CM, Richardson DK, Heffner LJ. Outcomes of severely abnormal umbilical artery doppler velocimetry in structurally normal singleton fetuses. *Obstet Gynecol* 1996;87: 434–438.

99. Tsang H, Manning FA, Menticoglou SM, Harman CR. Management of pregnancies with absent umbilical artery diastolic velocity and normal biophysical profile. *Proc Soc Obstet Gynecol Canada June,* 1989.

100. Bracero LA, Figueroa R, Byrne DW, Han HJ. Comparison of umbilical Doppler velocimetry, nonstress testing, and biophysical profile in pregnancies complicated by diabetes. *J Ultrasound Med* 1996;15:297–300.

101. Johnstone FD, Steel JM, Haddad NG, Hoskins PR, Greer IA, Chambers S. Doppler umbilical artery flow velocity waveforms in diabetic pregnancy. *Br J Obstet Gynecol* 1992;99:135–140.

102. Hecher K, Campbell S, Doyle P, Harrington K, Nicolaides K. Assessment of fetal compromise by doppler ultrasound investigation of the fetal circulation. *Circulation* 1995;91: 129–138.

103. Chan FY, Pun TC, Lam P, Lam C, Lee CP, Lam YH. Fetal cerebral doppler studies as a predictor of perinatal outcome and subsequent neurologic handicap. *Obstet Gynecol* 1996;87:981–988.

104. Rizzo G, Capponi A, Soregaroli M, Arduini D, Romanini C. Umbilical vein pulsations and acid-base status at cordocentesis in growth-retarded fetuses with absent end-diastolic velocity in umbilical artery. *Biol Neonate* 1995;68:163–168.

105. Shalev E, Blondheim O, Peleg D. Use of cordocentesis in the management of preterm or growth-restricted fetuses with abnormal monitoring. *Obstet Gynecol Survey* 1995;50: 839–844.

106. Harman CR, Menticoglou SM, Manning FA, Pillai M. Fetal oxygen uptake: a test of placental reserve [Abstract]. *Proc Soc Obstet Gynecol Ottawa* June 1993.

17

COMPARATIVE EVALUATION OF DOPPLER WAVEFORM IN ARTERIES AND VEINS EVALUATED WITH NONSTRESS TEST, CONTRACTION STRESS TEST, AND CORD BLOOD SAMPLING IN GROWTH-RETARDED OR HYDROPIC FETUSES

Yoshihide Chiba, M.D., Ph.D.

Department of Clinical Physiology, Clinical Chemistry, and Perinatology, National Cardiovascular Center, Suita, Osaka, Japan

Although it is well known that the resistance index (RI) (1), A/B ratio (2), and pulsatility index (PI) (3) of the umbilical artery are generally elevated, these indices for the middle cerebral artery may be depressed in fetal growth retardation or fetal distress

Asphyxia and Fetal Brain Damage, Edited by Dev Maulik, M.D., Ph.D.
ISBN 0-471-18427-6

(4–6). We reported the utility of Doppler examinations, Contraction Stress Test (CST), and Nonstress Test (NST) compared to that of cord blood sampling in a prospective study of growth retarded fetuses (7). On the other hand, Doppler examinations in the fetal vein have indicated that various blood flow dynamics are present during fetal breathing movements (8), during labor (9), in early pregnancy (10), and in cases of hydropic fetuses (11).

In this chapter the relationship between the hyper-preload condition and the high-resistance condition is discussed.

HYPER-PRELOAD IN PATHOLOGICAL AND PHYSIOLOGICAL STATES

From our published study we can conclude that hyper-preload conditions of fetuses are observed in cardiogenic hydrops, noncardiogenic hyper-preload hydrops, in early pregnancy around 12 weeks, and during labor, particularly at the recovery period from cord compression and the bottom of late deceleration (Table 1).

Preload Index (PLI)

Doppler waveform in the fetal inferior vena cava under normal sinus rhythm shows a pulsating pattern synchronized with the cardiac motions. There are three components in a cardiac cycle. They are monophasic blood flow retrograding from the right atrium to the inferior vena cava, the initial forward flow, and the second forward flow. The reverse flow (A) occurs during atrial contraction. The initial forward flow (S_f) coincides with atrial diastole and ventricular systole, and the second forward flow (D_f), with ventricular diastole (Figure 1) (11,12).

A new index, the preload index (PLI) (11), is defined as follows:

$$\text{PLI} = A/S_f$$

where A is reverse blood flow from the right atrium, and S_f is forward blood flow into the right atrium coinciding with ventricular systole. PLI is independent of the angle between the Doppler beam incidence and the blood flow (Figure 2).

Table 1. Hyper-preload condition of fetuses in pathological and physiological states (9–11)

Pathological	Cardiogenic hydrops Noncardiogenic hyper-preload hydrops	PLI[a] > 0.4 PLI > 0.4
Physiological	Around 12 weeks	PLI = 0.85(SD = 0.16)
During labor	Recovering from cord compression During late deceleration	Pulsation in UV PLI increase
Normal	After 24 weeks	PLI; 0 to 0.35

[a]PLI, preload index.

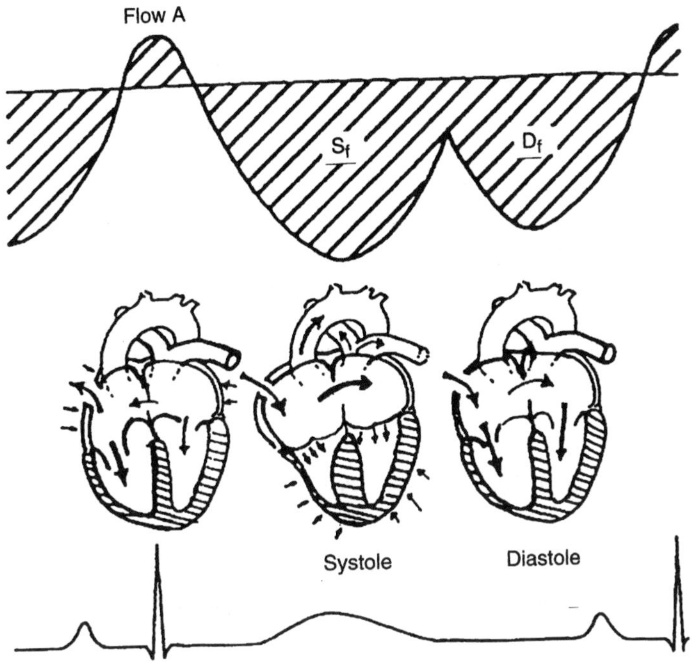

Figure 1. Time relation of venous return in the inferior vena cava with a cardiac cycle. Flow *A* is the reverse flow of atrial contraction. S_f is the initial forward flow by ventricular systole. D_f is the second forward flow by ventricular diastole.

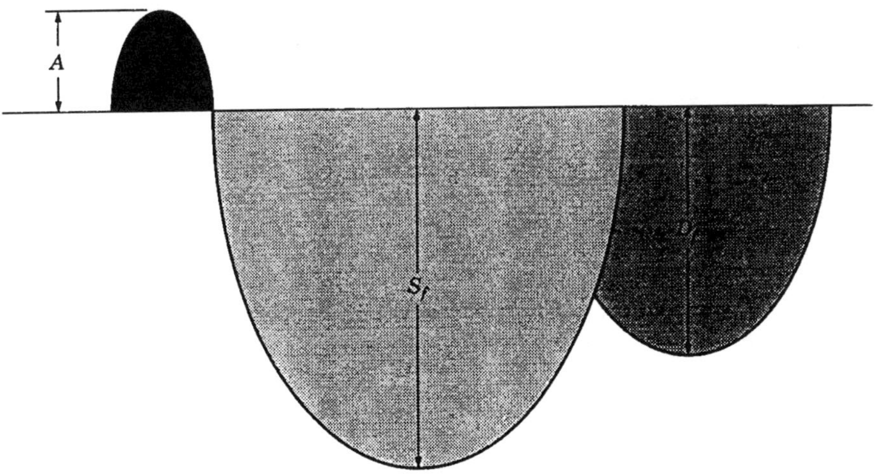

Figure 2. The definition of the preload index (PLI). Flow *A* is the blood flow from the right atrium occurring at atrial contraction. Flow S_f is the blood flow into the right atrium coinciding with the ventricular systole. Flow D_f is the blood flow into the right atrium coinciding with the ventricular diastole. (From reference 11, reproduced with permission.)

Preload Index of Hydropic Fetuses

We compared PLI values in the three groups of fetal disease (Figure 3) (11). The PLI values of hydrops associated with heart disease were significantly higher than those of normal fetuses and were also higher than the group with heart disease without hydrops. All values of PLI of cardiogenic hydrops showed more than 0.5. PLI values of the hydrops without heart disease showed a very wide range from 0 to 1.08. According to the results of our study, cardiogenic hydrops showed significantly higher PLI in the inferior vena cava. Another study has shown that umbilical venous pressure is higher in hydrops fetalis (13). Thus, it is logical to assume that excessive preload was present in cases of cardiogenic hydrops. Half of the cases of hydrops without heart disease had higher PLI. They might have had secondary hyper-preload condition, although they were not primarily cardiogenic hydrops. We can label them as a new group that is non-cardiogenic hyper-preload hydrops.

Hyper-Preload Condition in Early Pregnancy

From the results of our Doppler study in early pregnancy, it appeared that the placental vascular resistance decreased after 12 weeks of pregnancy. The resistance index began to decrease from 1.0 at 12 weeks. At the same gestational age of 12

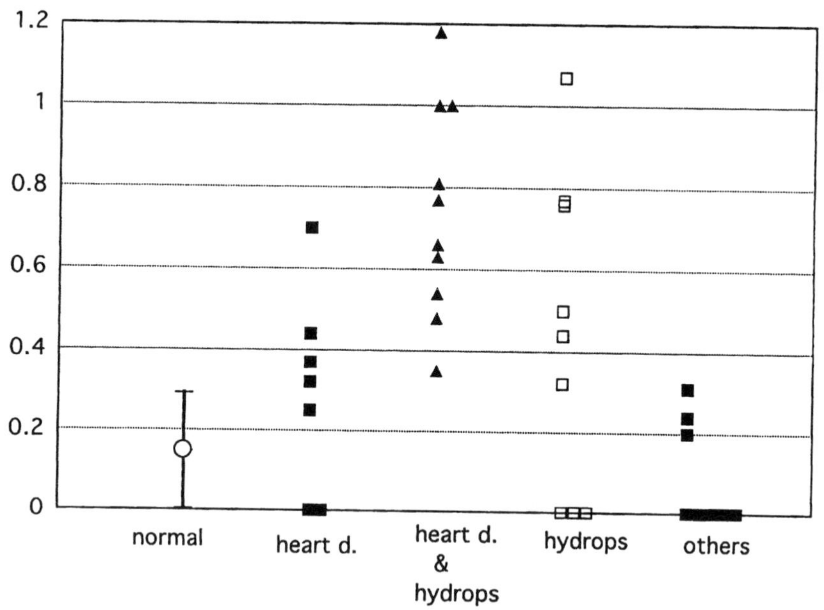

Figure 3. Values of preload index (PLI) among controls, group 1, group 2, group 3, and group 4. Group 1: Structural heart disease without hydrops. Group 2: Hydrops associated with heart disease. Group 3: Hydrops without heart disease. Group 4: Other malformations. (From reference 11, reproduced with permission.)

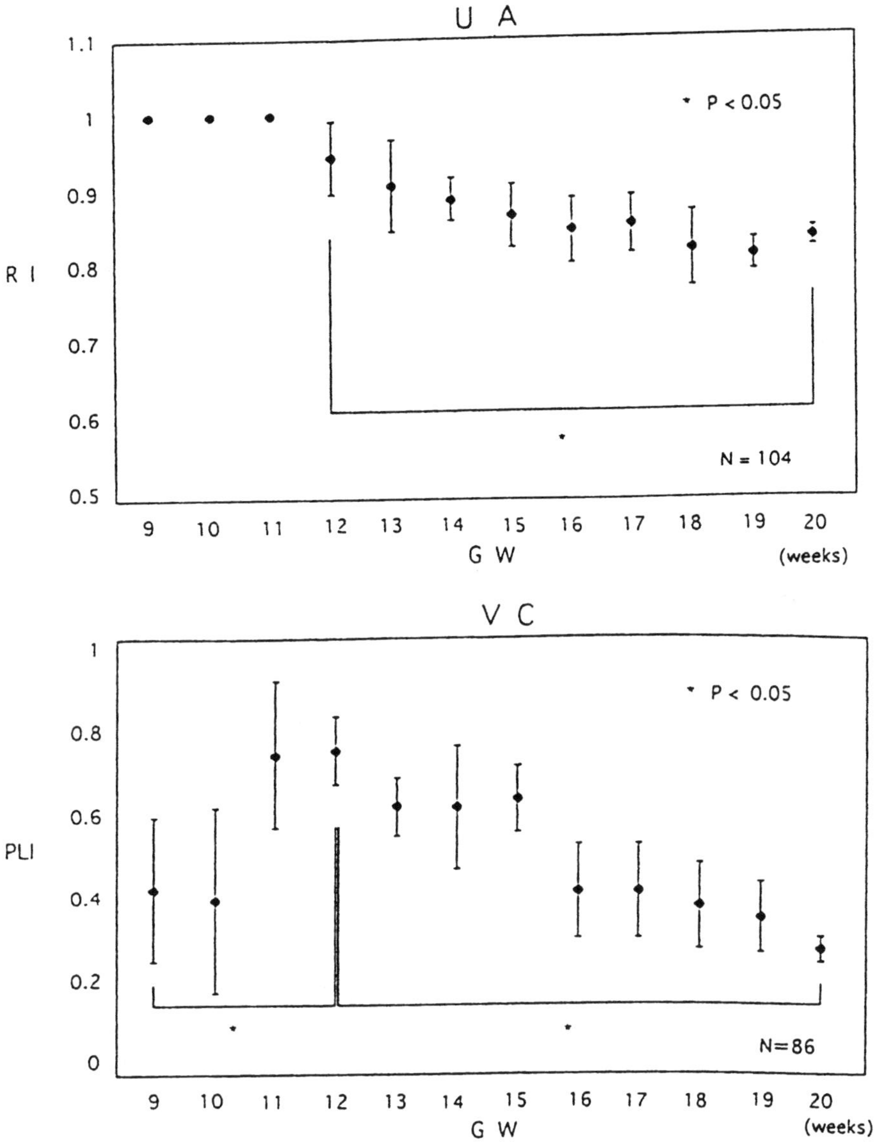

Figure 4. The dynamics of the umbilical arterial RI (*upper*) and PLI of the inferior vena cava from 9 to 20 weeks of pregnancy. (From reference 10, reproduced with permission.)

weeks, the PLI of the inferior vena cava showed its peak value (Figure 4). It is estimated that at 12 weeks the venous return from placenta to fetus may increase by the decreasing of placental vascular resistance, and the preload for the fetal heart may increase.

Dynamics of Venous Doppler during Labor

In the developmental stage of fetal Doppler, we recognized pulsations of the Doppler waveform in the umbilical vein. The physiological cause of these pulses are generally fetal breathing movements (8). During labor, we observed another cycle of pulsation showing the blood flow pattern synchronized with heart movements (9).

They appeared at the recovery period from variable deceleration of the heart rate pattern and during late deceleration. Figure 5 shows an example of the change in Doppler waveform detected in the umbilical vein at variable deceleration. This figure reveals the gradual decrease of maximum blood flow and shows gradual recovery. Before the cord compression the blood flow shows pulsation synchronized with fetal breathing movements, and after the compression it shows another cycle synchronized with heart movements. During the late deceleration, the Doppler waveform in the umbilical vein also shows pulsation synchronized with heart rate (Figure 6). In addition, the PLI of the inferior vena cava shows its higher level during late decelerations (Figure 7).

DOPPLER EXAMINATIONS FOR GROWTH-RETARDED FETUSES

Doppler Waveform in Arteries Evaluated with Nonstress Test, Contraction Stress Test, and Cord Blood Sampling in Growth-Retarded Fetuses

For the purpose of assessing the utility of Doppler examinations of the umbilical and fetal middle cerebral arteries, we performed a prospective study. The utility of Doppler examinations was compared to that of CST, NST, and cord blood sampling

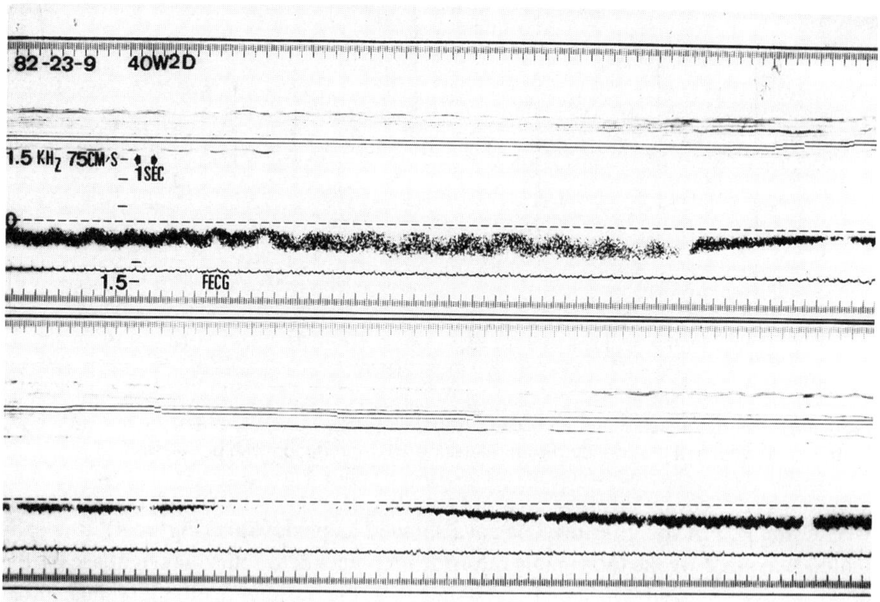

Figure 5. An example of the change in Doppler waveform in the umbilical vein at variable deceleration.

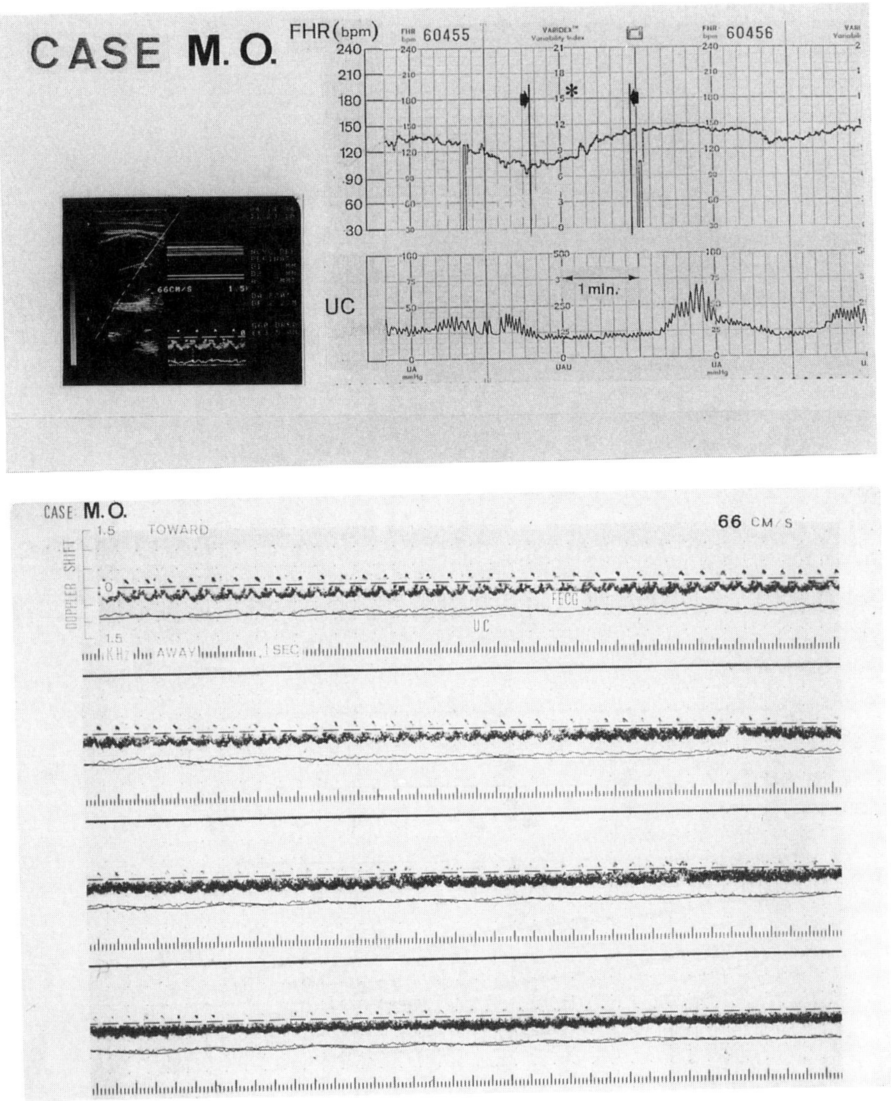

Figure 6. Pulsation of Doppler waveform in the umbilical vein synchronized with heart rate during the late deceleration.

for growth-retarded fetuses (7). We concluded that cordocentesis is the most direct method of identification of fetal acidemia. However, there is a risk of continuous bradycardia in approximately 5% of growth-retarded fetuses. In this study, CST provided an estimation of fetal acidemia with the highest accuracy. Doppler examination of the umbilical artery can also be used as an alternative to CST. In this study a total of 101 examinations were carried out on 65 patients. We designed the study to keep to conventional decision-making, which is performed depending on the last result of

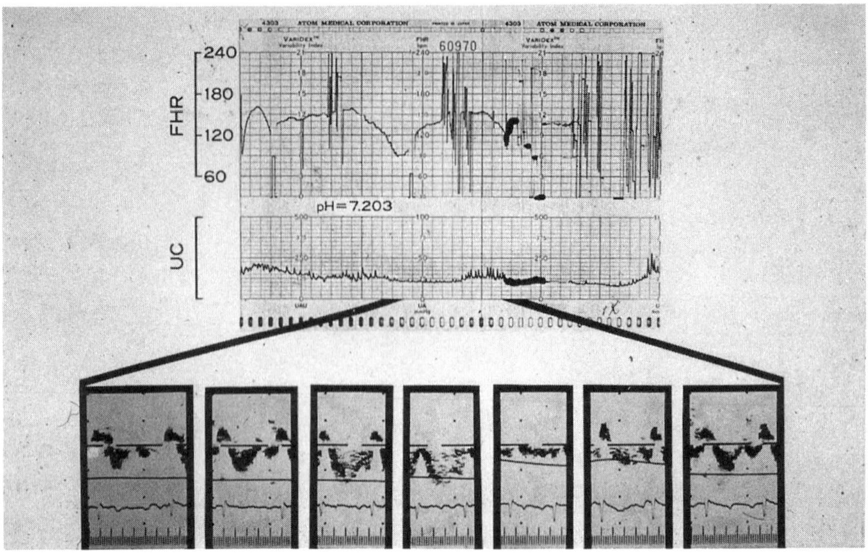

Figure 7. The reverse flow in the inferior vena cava shows its higher level during late decelerations.

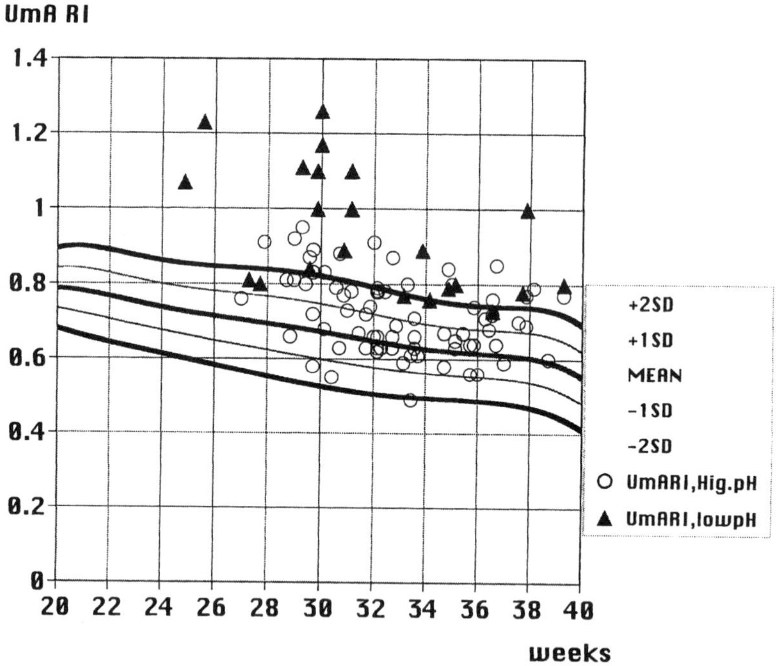

Figure 8. Resistance index of the umbilical artery in each subject of growth-retarded fetus with acidemia and nonacidemia, indicated with the normal level. UmARI is the umbilical artery resistance index. High pH value is >7.318, low pH value is <7.318. (From reference 7, reproduced with permission.)

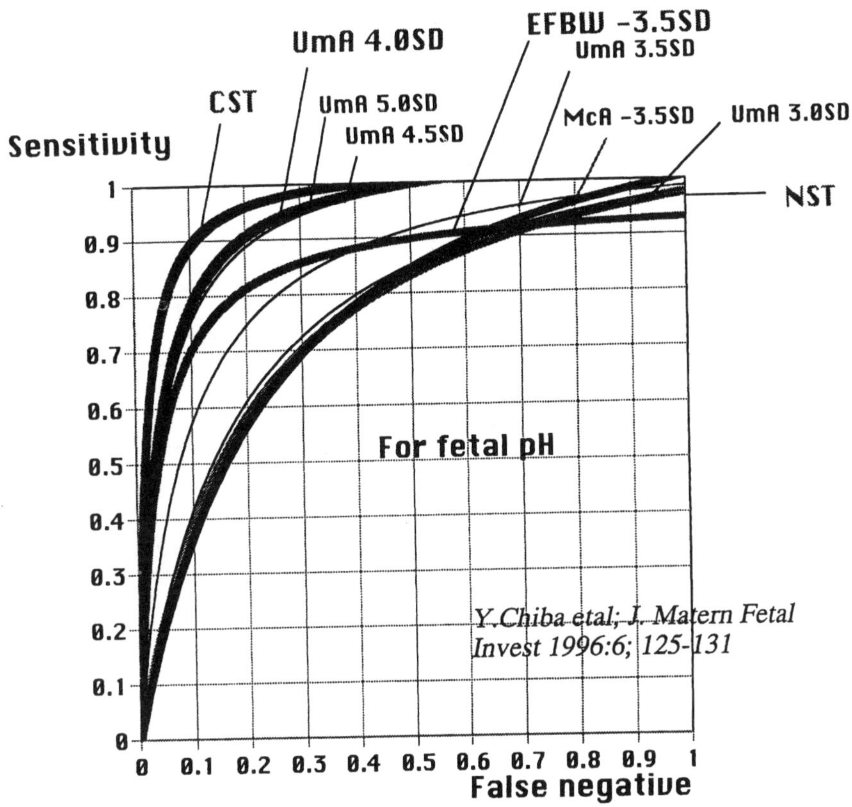

Figure 9. Sensitivity to false negativity (1 – specificity) ratio of each test in prediction of fetal pH. The CST showed the highest sensitivity with the lowest false negativity in the prediction of fetal pH. Doppler examinations of the umbilical artery at the cutoff SD of 4.0, 4.5, and 5.0 also showed high diagnostic accuracy. (From reference 7, reproduced with permission.)

CST. At each examination, NST was followed by Doppler examinations, fetal blood sampling, and CST, respectively. All tests were carried out on the same day during one examination, after informed consent was obtained.

The resistance index (RI) of the umbilical artery (UmARI) in each subject according to venous pH (<7.318 or >7.318) is shown with the nomogram in Figure 8. The sensitivity to false negative (1– specificity) ratio of each test was evaluated using a sensitivity to false negative curve, a hyperbolic curve calculated by the minimum square method (Figure 9). The CST showed the highest sensitivity with the lowest false-negativity, and thus the highest specificity, in the prediction of fetal pH. Doppler examinations of the umbilical artery at the cutoff SD of 4.0, 4.5, and 5.0 also showed high diagnostic accuracy. The diagnostic accuracy in the prediction of fetal pH was relatively lower for the NST and for Doppler examinations of the middle cerebral artery and the umbilical artery at the cutoff SD of 3.0, 2.5, and 2.0. The accuracy of NST in the prediction of fetal pH was lower than that of the estimated fetal body weight (EFBW) of –3.5 SD.

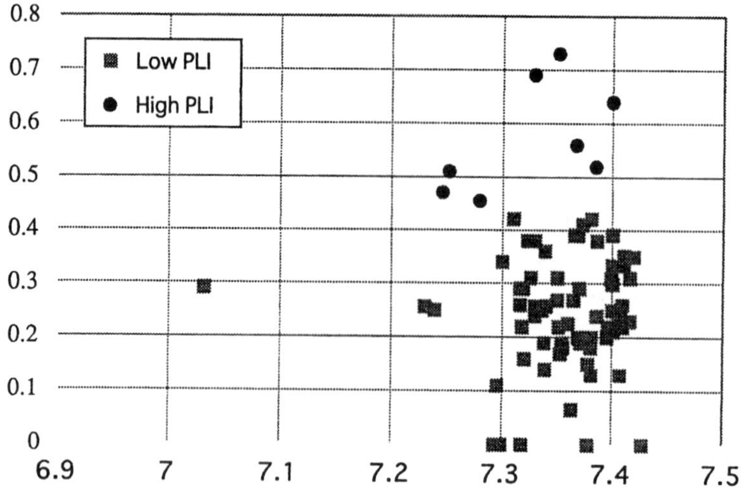

Figure 10. There is no significant correlation efficient between PLI and venous pH in growth-retarded fetuses.

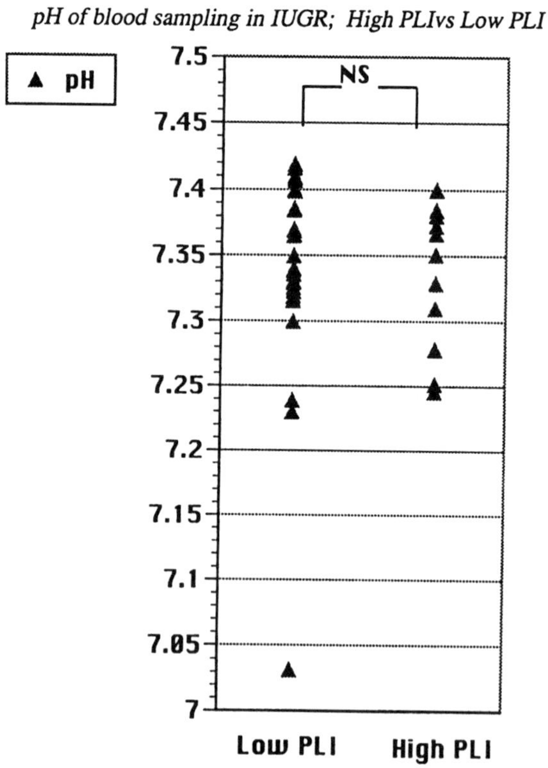

Figure 11. There are no significant differences between pH values of high PLI group and those of lower PLI group in growth-retarded fetuses.

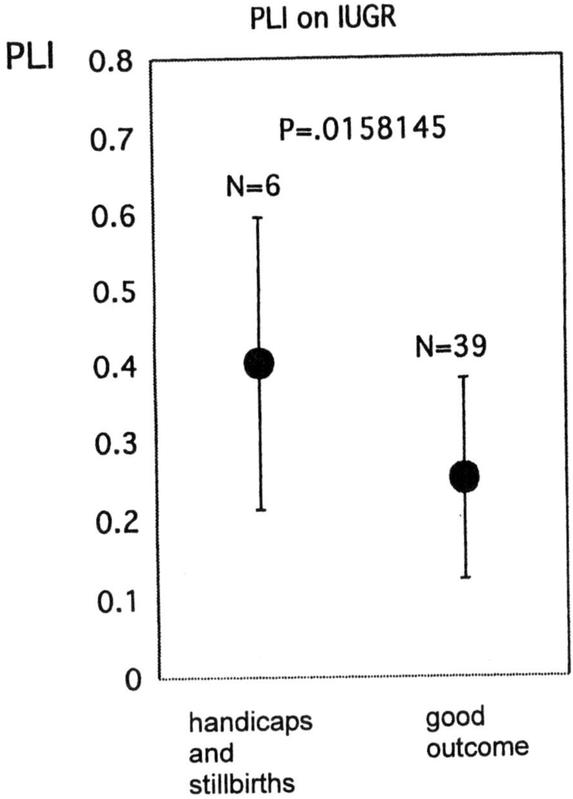

Figure 12. In the study of growth-retarded fetuses, there are significant differences in PLI values in cases of stillbirth or handicap and those with good outcome cases.

Preload Index of Growth-Retarded Fetuses

The utility of the preload index (PLI) for estimation of fetal pH was also evaluated in cases of growth-retarded fetuses. The relationship between the PLI and the pH of the cord vein was evaluated. Several cases in IUGRs showed a higher PLI. However, there was no significant correlation between the PLI and the pH (Figures 10 and 11). When we divided growth-retarded fetuses into two groups according to their prognoses, values of PLI in cases resulting in fetal death or handicap were significantly higher than those with good prognosis (Figure 12). There is some possibility to estimate the prognosis by Doppler examinations in the fetal vein.

CONCLUSIONS

We should not discuss whether venous Doppler or arterial Doppler is better for detecting fetal well-being. The venous Doppler shows good accuracy when the fetus has a hyper-preload condition. We can understand that the most typical pathologic state of the hyper-preload is a hydropic fetus. When we discuss the placental vascular resistance of growth-retarded fetuses, the resistance index of the umbilical vein shows a high accuracy for the detection of fetal blood pH. It is logical to believe that venous Doppler waveforms and arterial Doppler patterns are, in general, independent of each other. However, in early pregnancy we recognized both dynamics of arterial and venous blood flow at the same gestational age of 12 weeks. We can also pay attention to the result of the study that showed that PLI in cases of fetal death or handicap are significantly higher than those of good prognoses in growth-retarded fetuses. This result suggests that the fetus showing a bad prognosis and higher preload index may have a different circulatory dysfunction compared with other growth-retarded fetuses.

REFERENCES

1. Pourcelot L. Applications clinique de l'examen Doppler transcutane. *Velocimetric Ultrasonore Doppler INSERM* 1974;34:213–240.
2. Trudinger BJ, Gill WB, Cook CM. Flow velocity waveforms in the maternal uteroplacental and fetal umbilical placental circulations. *Am J Obstet Gynecol* 1985;152:155–163.
3. Gosling RJ, King DH. Arteries and veins. In Marcus AW, Adamson L (eds). *Ultrasound angiology.* Edinburgh: Churchill Livingstone, 1975:61–98.
4. Trudinger BJ, Giles WB, Cook CM. Fetal umbilical artery flow waveforms and placental resistance: clinical significance. *Br J Obstet Gynaecol* 1985;92:23–30.
5. Wladimiroff JW, Wijndaard SD, von Eyck NJ, Tonge HM. Cerebral and umbilical arterial blood flow velocity waveforms in normal and growth-retarded pregnancies; a comparative study. *Obstet Gynecol* 1986;69:705–709.
6. Satoh S, Koyanagi T, Hara K, Shimokawa H, Nakano H. Developmental characteristics of blood flow in the middle cerebral artery in the human fetus in utero, assessed using the linear-array pulsed Doppler method. *Early Hum Dev* 1988;17:195–203.
7. Chiba Y, Murakami M, Murakami N, Kobayashi H, Ohmichi M. Comparative evaluation of non-stress test, Doppler examinations, and contraction stress test; evaluated with cord blood sampling in growth-retarded fetuses. *J Matern Fetal Invest* 1996;6:125–131.
8. Chiba Y, Utsu M, Kanzaki T, Hasegawa T. Changes in venous flow and intra-tracheal flow in fetal breathing movements. *Ultrasound Med Biol* 1983;11:43–49.
9. Murakami M, Kanzaki T, Utsu M, Chiba Y. Changes in the umbilical venous flow of human fetuses in labor. *Acta Obstet Gynecol Jpn* 1985;37:776–782.
10. Itoh S, Chiba Y, Kanzaki T, Kobayashi H, Murakami N. The dynamics of blood flow in fetal inferior vena cava in early pregnancy, evaluated with those in the umbilical artery, the middle cerebral artery and the descending aorta. *J Matern Fetal Invest* 1995;5:20–24.
11. Kanzaki T, Chiba Y. Evaluation of the preload condition of the fetus by inferior vena caval blood flow pattern. *Fetal Diagn Ther* 1990;5:168–174.
12. Chiba Y, Kanzaki T, Weiner Z. Doppler investigation of the fetal inferior vena cava. In Maulik D (ed). *Doppler ultrasound in obstetrics and gynecology.* New York: Springer, 1996:392–402.
13. Weiner CP, Heilskov J, Pelzer G, Grant S, Wenstrom K, Williamson R. Normal values for human umbilical venous and amniotic fluid pressure and their alteration by fetal disease. *Am J Obstet Gynecol* 1989;161:714–717.

18

MONITORING THE GROWTH-RETARDED FETUS

Gerard H. A. Visser, Ph.D. and Robert H. Stigter, M.D.
Department of Obstetrics and Gynecology, University Hospital, Utrecht, The Netherlands

INTRODUCTION

There are a number of "antenatal assessment techniques" that are suitable to identify the abnormal pregnancy: assessment of the fundal height, kick-chart, ultrasound biometry, Doppler examination of the uterine artery, measurement of the maternal blood pressure, and so forth. Having thus identified the fetus with inadequate growth as a result of impaired uteroplacental function, a number of tools are available to monitor fetal well-being. All these techniques can contribute to our understanding of the fetal condition, and one is not superior to another. Combining information obtained from a number of tests is superior to the use of a single technique, since it reduces the risk of false positives leading to inappropriate intervention.

With progressive deterioration of the fetal condition a certain rank order can be determined in which test results become abnormal. Changes in flow velocity waveforms (FVWs) of the umbilical artery, for example, usually precede fetal heart rate (FHR) abnormalities. It is useful to be informed about the rank order of these changes in various test results. It helps the clinician in determining the degree of deterioration.

Asphyxia and Fetal Brain Damage, Edited by Dev Maulik, M.D., Ph.D.
ISBN 0-471-18427-6

Decisions on intervention can be made after carefully weighing the risks of prolonged exposure to a less favorable intrauterine environment against the risks the infant is exposed to when delivered. It helps us to understand the gradual process of compensation and adaptation through decompensation. Awareness of the rank order may also be helpful when assessing the effect of treatment modalities.

In this chapter the rank order of changes occurring with progressive deterioration of the condition of the intrauterine growth-retarded (IUGR) fetus is discussed and related to the timing of delivery of these fetuses.

RANK ORDER OF CHANGES OCCURRING WITH PROGRESSIVE DETERIORATION OF THE FETAL CONDITION

Figure 1 shows the rank order in which changes occur in the various assessment tests, with progressive deterioration of the condition of the IUGR fetus. This rank order is based on longitudinal and cross-sectional studies in which the result of tests for fetal well-being were related to blood gases obtained by cordocentesis or from cord blood immediately after cesarean section. The sequence of events shown in Figure 1 applies to the entire population of IUGR fetuses studied, and it is wise to consider that individual fetuses may show different patterns. The various studies that have formed the basis of the rank order proposed have been reviewed in detail before (1,2) and will not be discussed here.

Abnormalities of Doppler waveform patterns of the fetal umbilical artery are usually the first sign of impending deterioration of the fetal condition (3). Abnormal

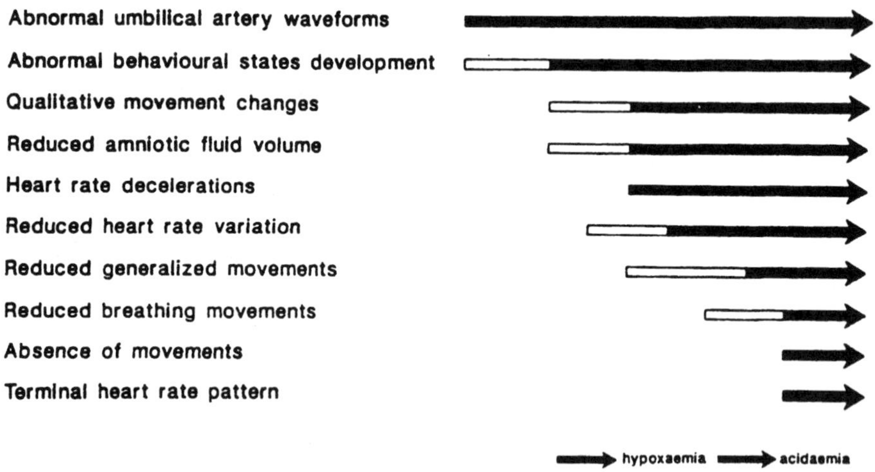

Figure 1. Suggested rank ordering in which blood velocity waveforms, amniotic fluid volume, movements, and heart rate changes occur in growth-retarded human fetuses with progressive deterioration of the fetal condition. Interfetal variation in first occurrence of an abnormal test result is indicated by the open part of the arrow. (From reference 2, reproduced with permission.)

waveform patterns probably reflect inadequate development of the placenta and are most likely an indication of increased impedance to blood flow due to abnormalities in the small capillaries of the terminal villi (4). At approximately the same time, changes can be observed in the FVW forms of fetal cerebral vessels (5) with reduced impedance to flow, suggesting a compensatory mechanism known as "redistribution of the fetal circulation." Changes in umbilical and cerebral artery waveform patterns precede the onset of fetal hypoxemia (6), and in the presence of a normal FHR pattern the pO_2 in fetal cord samples will usually be in the lower part of the normal range (7).

Since abnormal Doppler waveforms occur rather early in the process of deterioration, this technique has been shown to be useful in a high-risk population to identity fetuses at risk of becoming hypoxemic and to distinguish "low-risk" small-for-gestational-age fetuses from "high-risk" IUGR fetuses (8,9). A meta-analysis of randomized trials has shown that Doppler investigation of the umbilical artery reduces perinatal mortality in high-risk populations (10). In low-risk populations, no benefits have been shown thus far (11).

Doppler waveform patterns of the umbilical artery may deteriorate from decreased, to absent, and finally to reversed end-diastolic velocities. This sequence is not indicated in Figure 1, since its occurrence in relation to changes in other tests varies substantially. Prior to 30 weeks' gestation, most fetuses with FHR abnormalities will have had absent end-diastolic velocities of the umbilical artery for a considerable period; after 36 weeks, absent end-diastolic velocities are a rare phenomenon and are associated with signs of severe fetal compromise. Reversed end-diastolic flow in the umbilical artery probably reflects fetal cardiac failure, since cardiac contractility decreases concomitantly (12). It is associated with the occurrence of a terminal FHR pattern (which is indicative of myocardial hypoxemia) (13), and outcome is poor. With progressive deterioration of the fetal condition the changes in waveform patterns of cerebral vessels (e.g., middle cerebral artery) follow a biphasic pattern. Initially there is a progressive increase in end-diastolic velocities (and a decrease in pulsatility index)—that is, a progressive redistribution of blood flow favoring the brain. Later a plateau occurs and finally end-diastolic velocities decrease again (5). The latter may be due to a decrease in cardiac contractility, the occurrence of cerebral edema, or both. It has been reported that this decrease in end-diastolic velocities precedes the occurrence of FHR abnormalities (5), but in our opinion it may be a late sign of impairment coinciding with fetal acidemia.

There is insufficient information available as to the place of changes of Doppler FVW forms in the fetal venous circulation (14,15). Most tests aim at determining early signs of fetal cardiac failure, which is likely to coincide with the appearance of reversed flow in the umbilical artery. A longitudinal study on the place of venous Doppler abnormalities within the proposed model is currently in progress, and an early report has recently been published (16).

Abnormalities of the FHR coincide with the occurrence of fetal hypoxemia. This applies to a reduction of FHR variation below the normal range and to the occurrence of late FHR decelerations (7,17,18). FHR variation usually decreases gradually during the weeks preceding the appearance of late decelerations (and fetal hypoxemia)

(19). Longitudinal FHR recordings may, therefore, indicate a gradual deterioration of the fetal condition, even before the onset of hypoxemia. However, a single recording will not identify the small fetus at risk of becoming hypoxemic, since FHR variation is still within the normal range. This indicates that antenatal FHR monitoring is not a useful screening test. It should be applied longitudinally in a high-risk population. The best indication for serial FHR monitoring is the IUGR fetus with abnormal Doppler waveform patterns, in whom hypoxemia is likely to occur in due course.

In IUGR fetuses the interval between the first abnormal Doppler finding and the onset of FHR abnormalities/hypoxemia varies considerably. The interval is shorter in late than in early gestation and also shorter in IUGR complicated by preeclampsia (2,3,20). Apparently, a tiny fetus in early gestation can cope with a reduced placental supply for much longer than a bigger IUGR fetus later in pregnancy. This seems logical, taking into account the higher oxygen requirements in the latter. From these findings, one may also conclude that in preeclampsia the deterioration of the placental function occurs more rapidly than in IUGR fetuses without preeclampsia. The clinical implication of these observations is that once Doppler waveforms become abnormal, FHR monitoring should be carried out more frequently beyond 30 weeks and in all cases complicated by preeclampsia.

Disturbances in the development of fetal behavioral (sleep) states usually precede the occurrence of FHR abnormalities by some weeks (21,22). With advancing gestation, fetal behavioral states normally become more organized, demonstrated by a decrease in percentage of no-coincidence—that is, a decrease in the percentage of time that FHR patterns and eye and body movement patterns do not fit within a particular state. In IUGR fetuses that eventually become hypoxemic, this decrease in no-coincidence does not take place (22). Monitoring of fetal behavioral states is clinically not feasible, since it is time-consuming and requires considerable experience. However, these data indicate that in IUGR fetuses, disturbances in brain function antedate the occurrence of fetal hypoxemia. Apart from these disturbances in development of sleep states, there is also a redistribution in the incidence of occurrence of the different states, with an increase of state 1F (quiet sleep) and a decrease of state 2F (active sleep) (23). The latter phenomenon may be considered as a sign of fetal adaptation. Abnormalities in the quality of fetal movements (monotonous, reduced speed and amplitude) also precede the occurrence of FHR decelerations (24). These disturbances of the functioning of the fetal nervous system in IUGR fetuses could well be the result of prolonged malnutrition rather than merely an effect of fetal hypoxemia. This is in line with observations from cord blood analysis in IUGR fetuses where hypoglycemia and abnormally low levels of essential amino acids were shown even before the occurrence of hypoxemia (7,25).

In IUGR fetuses, oligohydramnios is most likely due to a reduced renal blood flow (caused by blood flow redistribution) and decreased urine output (26). In most third-trimester IUGR fetuses, oligohydramnios occurs before the onset of FHR abnormalities (and hypoxemia) (13). Therefore, its occurrence is an important finding which warrants intensive fetal monitoring. Before 32 weeks of gestation, oligohydramnios usually occurs after the onset of FHR abnormalities (13,27). Data from immature sheep fetuses indicate that induced hypoxemia does not result in a decrease of blood flow to the kidneys (28); this is in contrast to findings in term fetuses. Relative immaturity in chemoreceptor functioning might explain this absence of adaptation.

The incidence of fetal movements usually only falls below the normal range after the occurrence of FHR abnormalities, and this reduction is associated with impending acidemia (27,29). Longitudinal observations of fetal movements in IUGR fetuses have also shown that the incidence of body movements declines when FHR variation has reached the lower limit of the normal range—that is, at the time the fetus is likely to have become hypoxemic (13). Thereafter, FHR variation usually remains constant over a certain period of time during which the incidence of body movements continues to fall. Eventually, FHR variation is reduced further, and body and breathing movements disappear: The fetus becomes progressively hypoxemic and acidemic. These data suggest that a constant level of fetal pO_2 is maintained for some time by the reduction in body movements. Reduction of fetal movements when oxygen supply is limited aids in maximizing delivery of oxygen to vital organs and may be considered a sign of fetal adaptation. In the fetal sheep it has been shown that oxygen consumption fell by 17% after neuromuscular blockade (30) while pO_2 values rose by a similar percentage (30,31).

It is also known from subjective fetal movement records kept by pregnant women that, before the sudden decline in movements which may indicate impending fetal death, the movement incidence is still within the normal range (32,33). Recording of movements by pregnant women ("kick chart") does not have a high sensitivity or specificity with regard to fetal compromise; however, it is cheap and may identify the small and compromised fetus that was not identified by routine prenatal care.

TIMING OF DELIVERY

When should the small fetus, in which growth restriction is likely to be due to a reduced supply line, be delivered? At present, it is impossible to answer this question since randomized trials, in which early versus late delivery are compared, have not yet been completed (34). There is evidence that IUGR fetuses delivered when severe waveform abnormalities of fetal vessels are present have a greater morbidity and mortality than those with end-diastolic frequencies still present (3,35,36). Growth-retarded fetuses that had antepartum FHR decelerations are more likely to develop a severe degree of intraventricular hemorrhage or show abnormal neurological signs during the newborn period than those that had been delivered before decelerations had occurred (37–39). Fetuses delivered before 34 weeks of gestation have poorer cognitive development at age 2 years when antenatal FHR abnormalities had been present than when only abnormal Doppler results had been obtained (40). Moreover, IUGR fetuses who were acidemic at cordocentesis (41) or at elective cesarean section (39) have a poorer neonatal and subsequent neurological development than nonacidemic fetuses. These data may lead to the conclusion that IUGR fetuses should be delivered before antenatal test results become severely abnormal (35). However, in none

Table 1. Studies indicating that small-for-gestational-age fetuses delivered when (severely) abnormal Doppler waveforms or fetal heart rate (FHR) abnormalities had been present antenatally or when pH at cordocentesis was abnormal have a greater mortality and morbidity than less severely compromised fetuses. Note that mean gestational age and/or birthweight are lower in the population with abnormal antenatal test results.

		Age (weeks)		Weight (g)	
Authors	Test (Result)	Normal	Abnormal	Normal	Abnormal
Hackett et al. (35)	Doppler	33.1	31.8	1465	1045
Bekedam et al. (3)	Doppler	33.2	31.1	1365	991
Karsdorp et al. (36)	Doppler	36.3	31.5(29)[a]	2204	1209(769)[a]
Westgren et al. (37)	FHR	29.9	29.8	1400	1023
Dijxhoorn et al. (38)	FHR	38.6	37.5	2601	2271
Visser (39)	FHR	36	35	1739	1392
Soothill et al. (41)	pH	36	34.5	1824	1559

[a]Data in parentheses are from the study of Karsdorp et al. (36) on reversed end-diastolic velocities.

of these studies were patients randomized, and gestational age was lower and growth retardation more severe in the populations with the poorest outcome (Table 1). When we matched IUGR fetuses with and without end-diastolic velocities in the umbilical artery for gestational age and birthweight, no differences in outcome were found (3). This seems to indicate that absence of end-diastolic velocities is a marker of early and severe IUGR—which by itself has an effect on outcome—rather than a marker purely related to outcome.

So, when should the growth-restricted fetus be delivered, taking into account the fact that delivery at an earlier age may increase the risk of prematurity-related neonatal complications? A small fetus with an estimated weight of 900 g at 31 weeks is bound to be at risk for neurological handicap. The obstetrician may decide to deliver this fetus before signs of hypoxemia occur, let us say at about 29 or 30 weeks, but handicap may then result from pulmonary problems during the neonatal period. He may also decide to leave the fetus in utero longer, in the hope of improving maturation, but then the impact of prolonged malnutrition, particularly on the brain, may offset these benefits.

The timing of delivery of IUGR fetuses depends on many aspects: gestational age, degree of growth retardation, growth rate at repeated serial ultrasonography, amount of amniotic fluid, FHR pattern, Doppler waveforms, and, last but not least, the severity of a possible coexisting maternal disease (e.g., preeclampsia). The presence of so many variables requires individualization of management and of the timing of delivery. A proposal for the timing of delivery of the IUGR fetus, based on only three of these variables (gestational age, FHR, and Doppler), is shown in Figure 2. This scheme is a modification of a proposal published previously (42); and although rigid, it may contribute to decision-making in clinical situations of an extremely complex nature.

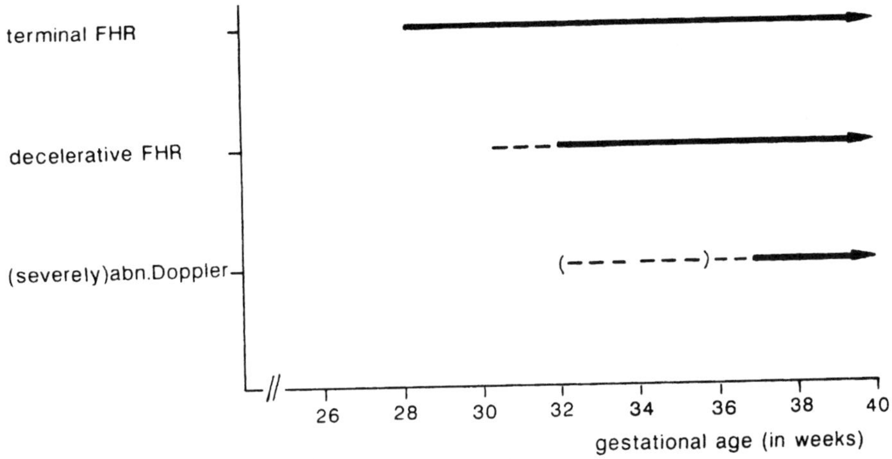

Figure 2. Timing of delivery of intrauterine growth-retarded fetuses, according to gestational age and fetal heart rate and Doppler waveform abnormalities. Solid arrow: delivery indicated. Dashed arrows: delivery may be considered. (Modified from reference 42.)

CONCLUDING REMARKS

The condition of the compromised fetus can be adequately assessed with the tools available, given that clinicians are well aware of the physiological processes underlying the tests performed. Being aware of the usual course of events in the process of deterioration can be of help in clinical decision making. The various tests available have different properties, and a combination of tests is superior to a single test (Figure 3). All tests show considerable variation and false-positive results remain a problem. Consistent signs of deterioration in all tests applied form a safer basis for intervention. It would appear prudent to deliver the IUGR fetus before signs of acidemia or severe hypoxemia emerge unless the fetus is extremely premature. If one decides to defer delivery, serial computer FHR recordings performed frequently can be helpful in determining a trend towards impending hypoxemia, using each fetus as its own control.

Doppler recordings of the umbilical artery and assessment of amniotic fluid volume are useful in at-risk populations to identify fetuses who are likely to become hypoxemic. In the case of consistent abnormal test results and sufficient duration of gestation, delivery may be undertaken.

In IUGR fetuses, changes in heart rate and motility are rather late signs of impairment. In general a growth-retarded fetus will have a normal heart rate pattern and a normal incidence of fetal body movements. It is not growth retardation that is detected with these assessment techniques, but instead hypoxemia and beginning acidemia. The lack of identification of fetuses with a pO_2 in the lower normal range indicates that antepartum FHR monitoring is not a reliable screening method for the

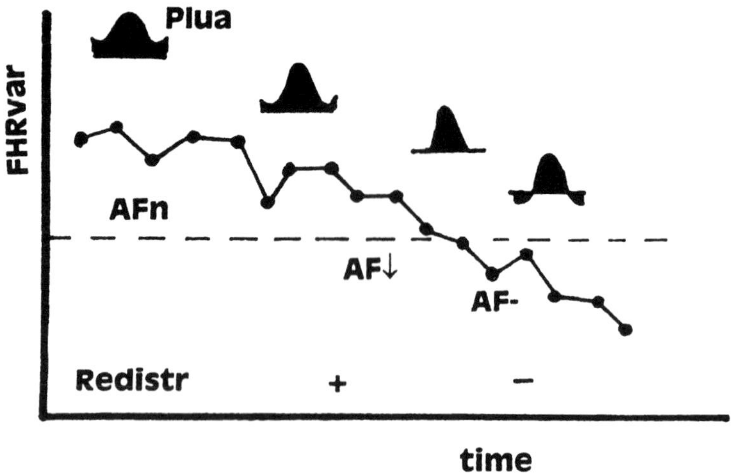

Figure 3. Schematic representation of changes occurring with time in umbilical artery velocity waveform patterns (Plua), fetal heart rate variation (FHR var), amniotic fluid (AF) volume, and presence (+) or absence (-) of redistribution of blood flow to the fetal head in an individual IUGR fetus. The dashed line indicates the lower normal range of FHR var. Monitoring of trends from a number of tests provides the best information on actual fetal condition and rate of deterioration and therefore also on the timing of delivery.

detection of future impairment. With progressive deterioration of the fetal condition the different components of FHR pattern (accelerations, baseline variation, decelerations) change at about the same time as decelerations occur (18,19). However, there is considerable variation between individuals. It has been shown in both normal and IUGR fetuses that FHR variation within the same individual remains within a range (19,43); hence it is advisable to follow IUGR fetuses longitudinally.

The incidence of movements usually falls below the normal range after the occurrence of FHR abnormalities. This implies that monitoring of movements is of limited value. Possible applications include assessment of fetal well-being in cases of suspect (i.e., suboptimal) FHR patterns and in assessing the degree of impairment in fetuses with abnormal FHR patterns in whom further maturation in utero must be considered, particularly at early gestation.

Timing of intervention remains dependent on expected chances of survival in postnatal life, and this depends to a considerable degree on management in the neonatal intensive care unit. The results of a large multicenter study are eagerly awaited and will hopefully provide some answers as to whether an attempt to obtain maximal maturity is still a good objective even in the very premature growth-retarded fetus.

It would be even better if growth restriction would be amenable to prevention since current knowledge implies that the process of prolonged malnutrition may result in neurological impairment well prior to the onset of hypoxemia. Fetal monitoring seems capable of preventing mortality, but its potential impact on the prevention of neurological handicap appears to be limited.

REFERENCES

1. Visser GHA. Fetal health assessment. *Curr Opin Obstet Gynecol* 1991;3:242–247.
2. Visser GHA. Assessment of fetal well being in growth retarded fetuses. In Hanson MA, Spencer JAD, Rodeck CH (eds). *Fetuses and neonate,* vol 3: *Growth.* Cambridge: Cambridge University Press 1995:327–345.
3. Bekedam DJ, Visser GHA, van der Zee AGJ, Snijders RJM, Poelmann-Weesjes G. Abnormal velocity waveforms of the umbilical artery in growth retarded fetuses: relationship to antepartum late heart rate decelerations and outcome. *Early Hum Dev* 1990;24:79–90.
4. Krebs C, Macara LM, Leiser R, Bowman AWF, Greer IA, Kingdom JCP. Intrauterine growth restriction with absent end-diastolic flow velocity in the umbilical artery is associated with maldevelopment of the terminal placental villous tree. *Am J Obstet Gynecol* 1996;175:1534–1542.
5. Arduini D, Rizzo G, Romanini C. Changes of pulsatility index from fetal vessels preceding the onset of late decelerations in growth retarded fetuses. *Obstet Gynecol* 1992;79: 605–610.
6. Bilardo CM, Nicolaides KH, Campbell S. Doppler measurements of fetal and uteroplacental circulation: relationship with umbilical venous blood gases measured at cordocentesis. *Am J Obstet Gynecol* 1990;163:115–120.
7. Pardi G, Cetin I, Marconi AM, Langranchi A, Bozzeti P, Ferrazzi E, Buscaglia M, Battaglia FC. Diagnostic value of blood sampling in fetuses with growth retardation. *New Engl J Med* 1993;328:692–696.
8. Reuwer PHJM, Rietman GW, Sijmons EA, van Tiel MWM, Bruinse HW. Intrauterine growth retardation: prediction of perinatal distress by Doppler ultrasound. *Lancet* 1987;1:415–418.
9. Beattie RB, Dordan JC. Antenatal screening for intrauterine growth retardation with umbilical artery Doppler ultrasonography. *Br Med J* 1989;298:631–635.
10. Divon MY. Randomized controlled trials of umbilical artery Doppler velocimetry: how many are too many. *Ultrasound Obstet Gynecol* 1995;6:377–379.
11. Goffinet F, Paris-Llado J, Nisand I, Bréart G. Umbilical artery Doppler velocimetry in unselected and low risk pregnancies: a review of randomised controlled trials. *Br J Obstet Gynaecol* 1997;104:425–430.
12. De Vore GR. Examination of the fetal heart in the fetus with intrauterine growth retardation. *Semin Perinatol* 1988;12:66–79.
13. Ribbert LSM, Visser GHA, Mulder EJH, Zonneveld MF, Morssink LP. Changes with time in fetal heart rate variation, movement incidences and haemodynamics in intrauterine growth retarded fetuses; a longitudinal approach to the assessment of fetal wellbeing. *Early Hum Dev* 1993;31:195–208.
14. Hecher K, Snijders RJM, Campbell S, Nicolaides KH. Fetal venous, intracardiac and arterial blood flow in intrauterine growth retardation. Relationship with blood gases. *Am J Obstet Gynecol* 1995;173:10–15.
15. Rizzo G, Capponi A, Talone P, Arduini D, Romanini C. Doppler indicates from inferior vena cava and ductus venosus in predicting PH and oxygen tension in umbilical blood at cordocentesis in growth-retarded fetuses. *Ultrasound Obstet Gynecol* 1996;7:401–410.
16. Hecher K, Hackelöer BJ. Cardiotocogram compared to Doppler investigation of the fetal circulation in the premature growth-retarded fetus: longitudinal observations. *Ultrasound Obstet Gynecol* 1997;9:152–161.

17. Bekedam DJ, Visser GHA, Mulder EJH, Poelmann-Weesjes G. Heart rate variation and movements incidence in growth-retarded fetuses: the significance of antenatal late heart rate decelerations. *Am J Obstet Gynecol* 1987;157:126–133.
18. Visser GHA, Sadovsky G, Nicolaides KH. Antepartum heart rate patterns in small-for-gestational-age third trimester fetuses: correlations with blood gas values obtained at cordocentesis. *Am J Obstet Gynecol* 1990;162:698–703.
19. Snijders RJM, Ribbert LSM, Visser GHA, Mulder EJH. Numeric analysis of heart rate variation in intrauterine growth-retarded fetuses: a longitudinal study. *Am J Obstet Gynecol* 1992;166:22–27.
20. Arduini D, Rizzo G, Romanini C. The development of abnormal heart rate patterns after absent end-diastolic velocity in umbilical artery. *Am J Obstet Gynecol* 1988;168:43–48.
21. Van Vliet MAT, Martin CB, Nijhuis JG, Prechtl HFR. Behavioural states in growth-retarded fetuses. *Early Hum Dev* 1985;12:183–198.
22. Arduini D, Rizzo G, Caforio L, Boccolini MR, Romanini C, Mancuso S. Behavioural state transitions in healthy and growth retarded fetuses. *Early Hum Dev* 1989;19:155–165.
23. Gazzolo D, Visser GHA, Santi F, Magliano CP, Scopesi F, Russo A, Pittaluga C, Nigro M, Camoriano R, Bruschettini PL. Behavioural development and Doppler velocimetry in relation to perinatal outcome in small for dates fetuses. *Early Hum Dev* 1995;43:185–195.
24. Sival DA, Visser GHA, Prechtl HFR. The effect of intrauterine growth retardation on the quality of general movements in the human fetus. *Early Hum Dev* 1992;28:119–132.
25. Cetin I, Ronzoni S, Marconi AM, Perugino G, Corbetta C, Battaglia FC, Pardi G. Maternal concentrations and fetal–maternal concentration differences of plasma amino acids in normal and intrauterine growth-retarded pregnancies. *Am J Obstet Gynecol* 1996;174: 1575–1583.
26. Arduini D, Rizzo G. Fetal renal artery velocity waveforms and amniotic fluid volume in growth-retarded and post-term fetuses. *Obstet Gynecol* 1991;72:370–373.
27. Ribbert LSM, Snijders RJM, Nicolaides KH, Visser GHA. Relationship of fetal biophysical profile and blood gas values at cordocentesis in severely growth-retarded fetuses. *Am J Obstet Gynecol* 1990;163:569–571.
28. Iwamoto HS, Kaufman T, Keil LC, Rudolph AM. Responses to acute hypoxemia in fetal sheep at 0.6–0.7 gestation. *Am J Physiol* 1989;256:613–620.
29. Ribbert LSM, Nicolaides KH, Visser GHA. Prediction of fetal acidaemia in intrauterine growth retardation: comparison of quantified fetal activity with biophysical profile score. *Br J Obstet Gynaecol* 1993;100:653–656.
30. Rurak DW, Gruber NC. Effect of neuromuscular blockade on oxygen consumption and blood gases in the fetal lamb. *Am J Obstet Gynecol* 1983;145:258–262.
31. Nathanielsz PW, Yu HK, Calabum TC. Effect of abolition of fetal movements on intravascular PO_2 and incidence of tonic myometrial contractures in the pregnant ewe at 114 to 134 days gestation. *Am J Obstet Gynecol* 1982;144:614–618.
32. Sadovsky E, Yaffe H, Polishuk WZ. Fetal movement monitoring in normal and pathologic pregnancy. *Int J Obstet Gynecol* 1974;12:75–79.
33. Pearson JF, Weaver JB. Fetal activity and fetal well-being; an evaluation. *Br Med J* 1976;1:1305–1307.
34. The GRIT Study Group. When do obstetricians recommend delivery for a high-risk preterm growth-retarded fetus? *Eur J Obstet Gynecol Reprod Biol* 1996;67:121–126.

35. Hackett GA, Campbell S, Gamsu H, et al. Doppler studies in the growth retarded fetus and prediction of neonatal necrotising enterocolitis, haemorrhage and neonatal morbidity. *Br Med J* 1987;294:13–16.

36. Karsdorp VHM, Van Vugt JMG, Van Geijn HP, Kostense PJ, Arduini D, Montenegro N, Todros T. Clinical significance of absent or reversed end diastolic velocity waveforms in umbilical artery. *Lancet* 1994;344:1664–1668.

37. Westgren LMR, Malcus P, Svenningsen NW. Intra-uterine asphyxia and long-term outcome in preterm fetuses. *Obstet Gynecol* 1986;67:512–516.

38. Dijxhoorn MJ, Visser GHA, Touwen BCL, Huisjes HJ. Apgarscore, meconium and acidaemia at birth in small-for-gestational age infants born at term, and their relationship to neonatal neurological morbidity. *Br J Obstet Gynaecol* 1987;94:873–879.

39. Visser GHA. Abnormal antepartum fetal heart rate patterns and subsequent handicap. In Patel N (ed). *Antenatal and perinatal causes of handicap. Baillière's clinical obstetrics and gynaecology,* vol 2(1), London: Baillière Tindall 1988:117–124.

40. Todd AL, Trudinger BJ, Cole MJ, Cooney GH. Antenatal tests of fetal welfare and development at age 2 years. *Am J Obstet Gynecol* 1992;167:1661–1671.

41. Soothill PW, Ajaji RA, Campbell S, Ross EM, Candy DCA, Snijders RJM, Nicolaides KH. Relationship between fetal acidaemia at cordocentesis and subsequent neurodevelopment. *Ultrasound Obstet Gynecol* 1992;2:80–84.

42. Visser GHA, Stigter RH, Bruinse HW. Management of the growth-retarded fetus. *Eur J Obstet Gynecol Reprod Biol* 1991;42:S73–S78.

43. Visser GHA, Dawes GS, Redman CWG. Numerical analysis of the normal human antenatal fetal heart rate. *Br J Obstet Gynaecol* 1981;88:792–802.

19

EMERGING TECHNOLOGIES: FETAL OPTICAL MONITORING

Miljan R. Stankovic, M.D., Ph.D., Dev Maulik, M.D., Ph.D.,
David Boas, Ph.D., and Phillip G. Stubblefield, M.D.

Department of Obstetrics and Gynecology, Boston University School of Medicine, Boston, Massachusetts (MRS, PGS); and Electro-Optics Technology Center, Tufts University School of Engineering and Computer Science, Medford, Massachusetts (DB); and Department of Obstetrics and Gynecology, Winthrop-University Hospital, Mineola, New York (DM).

INTRODUCTION

Shine a flashlight at your finger, and your finger will glow red—a demonstration that red and near-infrared light penetrate deeply into tissue (1). We are devoting this chapter to optical spectroscopy—a noninvasive real-time method that uses red and/or near-infrared light to assess fetal hemodynamics and oxygenation.

Numerous studies in humans and animals have demonstrated the importance of disturbances in cerebral hemodynamics and oxygenation in the pathogenesis of perinatal "hypoxic-hemodynamic" brain injury leading to cerebral palsy, mental retardation, and seizures (2–8). It is assumed that at least some of the injuries could be prevented (or ameliorated) if information on cerebral hemodynamics and oxygenation were available (3). Unfortunately, none of the presently available diagnostic techniques can

Asphyxia and Fetal Brain Damage, Edited by Dev Maulik, M.D., Ph.D.
ISBN 0-471-18427-6

afford this type of information in a continuous and noninvasive manner (9,10). Assessment of cerebral blood flow autoregulation, as well as monitoring of the brain hemodynamics and oxygenation from labor, through delivery and then in the neonatal intensive care unit could be crucial and could help us to ensure normal brain oxygenation throughout, and this might help us prevent oxygenation–perfusion-related brain injury in high-risk babies. Optical spectroscopy might have a potential to fulfill this need (11).

Although the majority of data show that timing of brain injury is primarily postnatal, 12% to 23% of cerebral palsy can be related to intrapartum asphyxia (12). Avoiding significant hypoxia (and/or perturbations in hemodynamics) intrapartum is of paramount importance (6,13). In addition, a wide variety of therapeutic strategies are currently in use, aiming to reduce perinatal neurological morbidity and mortality in the fetus and neonate. Magnesium sulfate, a drug routinely used to prevent preterm labor and delivery, reportedly decreased the incidence of cerebral palsy (14). Antenatal corticosteroids for fetal maturation reduced mortality, respiratory distress syndrome, and intraventricular hemorrhage in preterm infants (15). The ability of some other drugs to decrease the incidence and severity of intracranial hemorrhage (i.e., phenobarbital, vitamin K, indomethacin, and vitamin E injections) is still controversial, including their impacts on fetal and neonatal cerebral hemodynamics (16,17). Monitoring of their efficacy and side effects on cerebral perfusion and oxygenation will be important. These diagnostic and therapeutic modalities emphasize the potential importance of optical spectroscopy.

JUSTIFICATION FOR THE INTRODUCTION OF A NEW FETAL MONITORING MODALITY

Antepartum, electronic fetal heart rate (FHR) monitoring, either alone [nonstress test NST)] or as a part of the biophysical profile (BPP), has been the primary means of assessing fetal health in the United States for decades. NST can forecast severe fetal jeopardy (18) with reported false-positive NST rates of 90% (19). High (≥ 8) and low (zero) BPP scores predict normal pH and acidemic babies, respectively, while the BPP score of 6 is a poor predictor of abnormal outcome (20). Intrapartum, FHR monitoring is a standard of care in the United States. Unfortunately, intrapartum FHR monitoring has turned out to be a very poor predictor of neurological outcome, failing to fulfill the major intrapartum diagnostic goal—that is, the avoidance of neurological sequelae. Instead of reducing developmental disabilities, neonatal illness, and death, FHR monitoring has led to unnecessary interference with the birth process, and even to harm through increased rate of cesarean sections (11). Indeed, abnormal intrapartum fetal heart rate patterns have been associated with an increased risk of cerebral palsy, but the false-positive rate was 98.8% (21). Ellison et al. (22) observed that any method (in this case FHR) that describes more than 40% of the patterns as deviant cannot possibly be accurate in predicting a considerably lower-frequency outcome such as neurological abnormality. To increase the accuracy of FHR monitoring, several other methods have been attempted intrapartum. Fetal scalp pH has been utilized clinically for more that three decades, but its invasive nature, together with the necessity for repeated measurements, have seriously limited its use (23). Some other diagnostic tools—for example, continuous tissue pH (24), fetal transcutaneous pO_2 (25), and pCO_2 monitors (26)—have never reached a stage of development appropriate for clinical application (27). Optical spectroscopy can now provide repeated and continuous monitoring and imaging of fetal cerebral hemodynamics and oxygenation in vivo (10,11).

BACKGROUND OF OPTICAL SPECTROSCOPY

Optical spectroscopy is based on (a) relative optical transparency of biological tissues in the red and near-infrared region and (b) the distinct absorption properties of oxyhemoglobin (HbO) and deoxyhemoglobin (Hb) (1,9). It can be used to measure tissue hemodynamics and oxygenation noninvasively and in real time (Figure 1) (9). In tissue, light is both absorbed and scattered, with the scattering dominating in the red and near-infrared region (1). The scattering coefficient is fairly constant between 750 nm and 907 nm, and thus differences in diffuse light intensities can be attributed to differences in the absorption coefficient (9). Optical and biological properties of tissues, as well as characteristics of different clinical settings (e.g., antepartum or intrapartum fetus, neonate, etc.), will define the optimal type of optical instrument probe to be used. All optical spectrometers contain (1) a light source that emits light of a known wavelength and intensity, (2) a light detector (a photodiode or photomultiplier tube) that measures the intensity of scattered light exiting the tissues, and (3) a computer that integrates the input and output signals into clinically useful information (10).

The volume of the investigated tissue beneath the light source(s) and detector(s) depends on (a) optical properties and geometry of the investigated organ(s) or tissue(s)

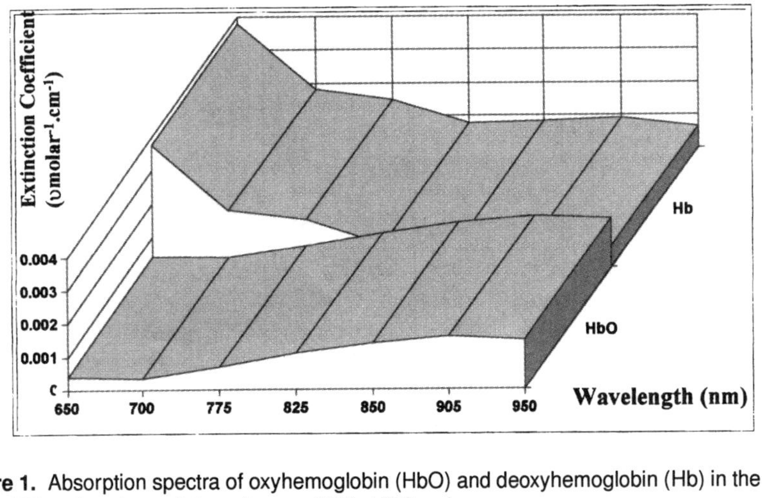

Figure 1. Absorption spectra of oxyhemoglobin (HbO) and deoxyhemoglobin (Hb) in the visible (up to 650 nm) and near-infrared range (650–1000 nm).

(e.g., skin, brain, muscle, etc.), (b) probe–detector separation (i.e., the larger the separation, the deeper the penetration) (Figure 2), and (c) the wavelength (Figure 1) (9,10). While visible light (wavelengths up to 650 nm)—strongly absorbed by hemoglobin and melanin—penetrates up to 1 cm into tissue, near-infrared light (700–1000 nm) can penetrate up to 10 cm through the scalp, skull, and brain (9,10). Light detectors may be placed on the opposite tissue surface (transmission or transillumination mode) or the adjacent surface (reflectance mode) (Figure 2) (10). By increasing the number of light sources and light detectors, optical data can be converted into sophisticated functional and anatomical tissue images (28,29).

There are three basic types of optical instruments (a) continuous-wave (CW), (b) time-domain, and (c) frequency-domain (Figure 3). Each of these can be used for both optical monitoring and imaging. (a) Continuous-wave spectrometers are unable to determine the tissue scattering and optical pathlength (Figure 3C) (30–36). That is, they do not provide absolute concentration measurements but only changes from a baseline with no information about whether the baseline value was normal, high, or low (10,37). Despite this disadvantage, CW spectrometers have been "good enough" to afford pulse oximetry that utilizes ratios (HbO/HbO + Hb) rather than absolute measurements (10,27,38), as well as brain oximetry showing trends and relative changes from baseline (37,39,40). (b) Time-domain instruments [time-of-flight-and-absorbance (TOFA)] provide scattering information from the mean transit time of picosecond light pulses and tissue absorption from the long time decay of the broadened laser pulses (Figure 3B) (28,41–43). (c) Frequency-domain instruments, using radio-frequency-modulated light sources and phase-sensitive detection of the modulated light (which is directly related to the pathlength), enable quantification of tissue absorption and scattering (Figure 3A) (9,29,44,45). Because both time- and

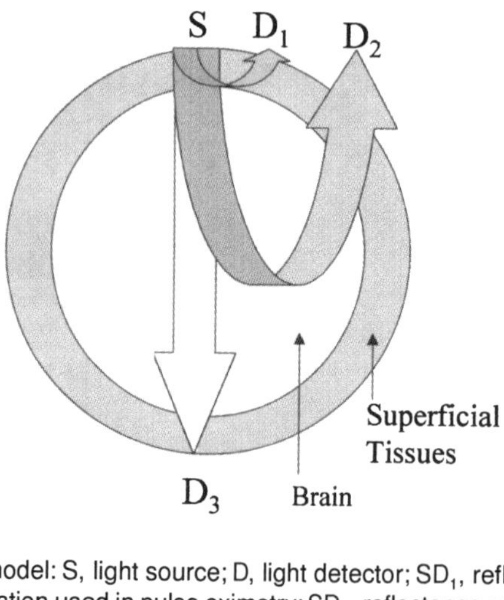

Figure 2. The head model: S, light source; D, light detector; SD_1, reflectance mode with small source–detector separation used in pulse oximetry; SD_2, reflectance mode; and SD_3, transillumination (transmission) mode. Both SD_2 and SD_3 have large source–detector separation, used in cerebral optical spectroscopy.

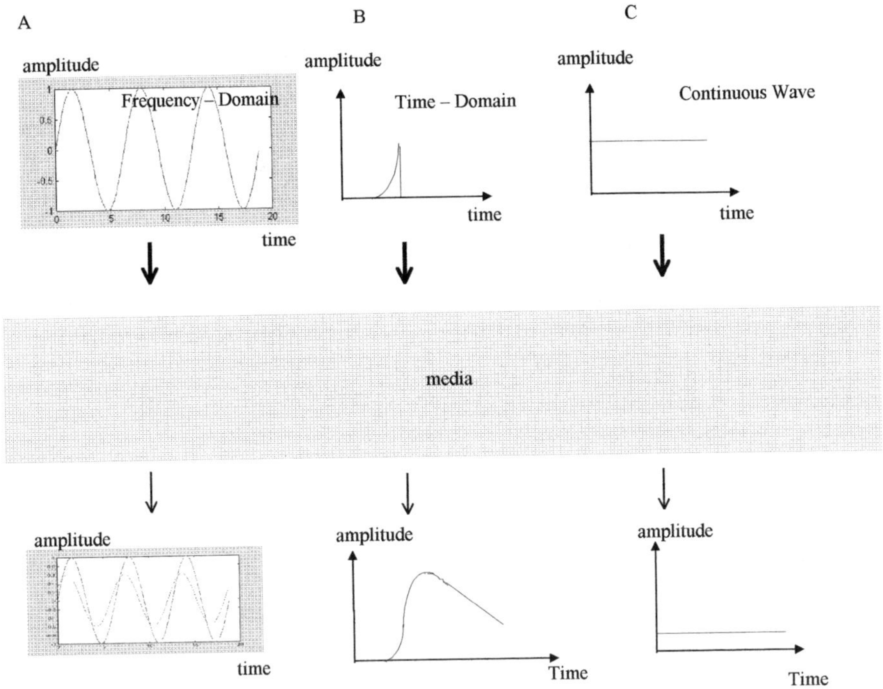

Figure 3. Three basic types of optical instruments: **(A)** frequency-domain, **(B)** time-domain, and **(C)** continuous-wave.

frequency-domain methods enable quantification of tissue absorption and scattering, they thus provide absolute determination of hemoglobin concentration.

Hemoglobin is an intravascular chromophore containing information on tissue hemodynamics (flow/volume) and oxygenation; this information can be appreciated by measuring (a) total hemoglobin concentration (HbT = Hb + HbO), considered to reflect changes in tissue blood flow and volume (46,47), and (b) tissue hemoglobin oxygen saturation (StO_2 = HbO / HbO + Hb), considered to reflect changes in tissue oxygenation (33,34,40,48–54). The absorption curves of adult and fetal hemoglobin slightly differ in the near-infrared range. However, it has been demonstrated that the error arising from the use of absorption coefficients derived from adult Hb is insignificant, irrespective of the level of fetal hemoglobin present (55).

Conventional pulse oximeters are calibrated through controlled hypoxia studies in human volunteers subjected to moderate hypoxia with SaO_2 ranging from 100% to 70%. Pulse oximetry measurements are calibrated to fit those of their arterial blood SaO_2. It is not possible to perform similar calibration studies in the human fetus, nor would it be ethically acceptable to induce SaO_2 changes below 70% in human volunteers to get to the fetal SaO_2 that can be as low as 15%. As opposed to pulse oximetry, the calibration of cerebral optical spectrometers in vivo is currently impossible because there are no "gold standard" techniques for measuring tissue oxygenation (10).

The focus of this chapter will be two clinical applications of fetal optical spectroscopy: cerebral optical spectroscopy [i.e., near-infrared spectroscopy (NIRS)] and intrapartum fetal pulse oximetry.

FETAL CEREBRAL OPTICAL SPECTROSCOPY

Unlike pulse oximetry that uses a pulse-gated signal to measure changes in hemoglobin absorption in the pulsatile vascular bed, cerebral optical spectroscopy samples the entire vascular bed, determining Hb and HbO changes without differentiating in which vascular compartment—venous, arterial, or capillary—the hemoglobin is found (Figure 4) (10). Because more than 70% of cerebral hemoglobin at any time is in the venous blood, it is assumed that cerebral saturation as determined by optical spectroscopy represents predominantly cerebral venous saturation (10).

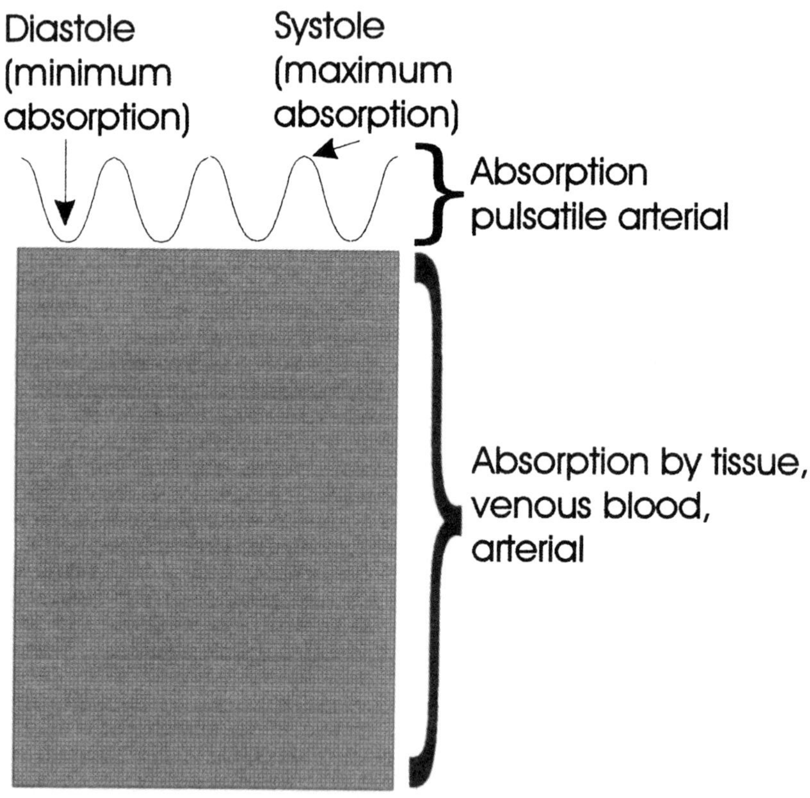

Figure 4. Light absorption by various tissue components during cardiac cycle. Pulse oximetry uses a pulse-gated signal to measure changes in hemoglobin absorption in the pulsatile vascular bed. Cerebral optical spectroscopy samples the entire vascular bed, determining Hb and HbO changes without differentiating in which vascular compartment—venous, arterial, or capillary—the hemoglobin is found.

It has been almost a decade since transvaginal cerebral optical spectroscopy was first demonstrated in the human fetus intrapartum (56). Most of the subsequent intrapartum studies were based on a small number of cases. The researchers at the University College London, using CW optical spectroscopy (Hamamatsu NIRO-500 Monitor), have presented several observations regarding this intrapartum optical application. The authors described the "contraction or parallel pattern,"—that is, decrease in Hb, HbO, and HbT (cerebral blood volume) associated with normal uterine contractions (Figure 5a). Different patterns of cerebral hemoglobin changes—that is, "desaturation or divergent patterns"—were associated with variable, late, and prolonged decelerations, as well as with short contraction intervals (33,34,53,54) (Figure 5b). Similar desaturation patterns have been described in a study conducted in Germany on a small number of patients, reporting a good correlation between CW spectroscopy (56) and pulse oximetry readings (Nellcor-400) recorded simultaneously in

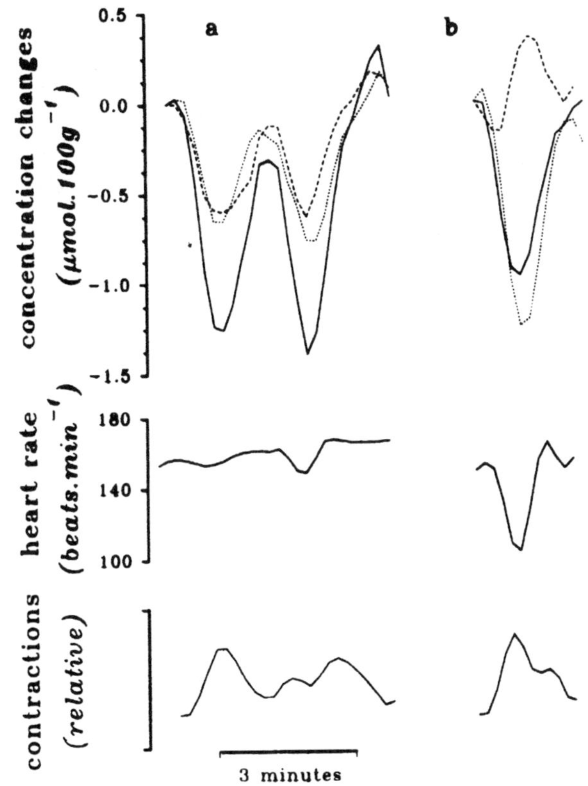

Figure 5. Changes from an arbitrary baseline in the cerebral concentrations of oxyhemoglobin (...), deoxyhemoglobin (– – –), and total hemoglobin (———) in the same fetus during two normal contractions (**a:** contraction or parallel pattern) and a contraction with an early FHR deceleration (**b:** desaturation or divergent pattern). The *x* axis is time. (From reference 33, reproduced with permission.)

the human fetus during labor (57). A significant correlation between cerebral oxygen saturation measured by optical spectroscopy shortly before delivery and fetal umbilical blood gas and acid–base status at birth has been reported (50); a significant rise in fetal cerebral oxygenation after maternal oxygen administration during normal labor has also been reported (51). Changes in maternal posture during labor, in women with effective epidural analgesia, were reportedly associated with a significant decrease in fetal cerebral oxygenation (53). The whole idea of transvaginal optical monitoring was challenged after Hamilton et al. demonstrated the "apparent

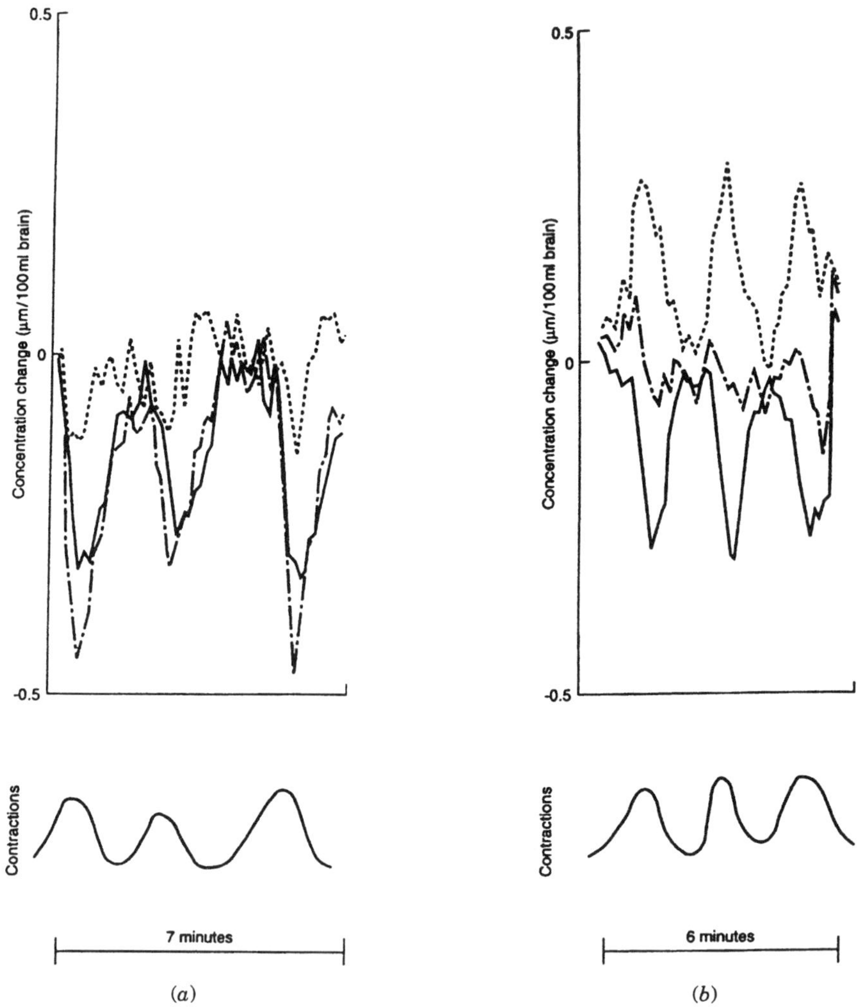

Figure 6. Changes from an arbitrary baseline in the cerebral concentrations of oxyhemoglobin (———), deoxyhemoglobin (– – –), and total hemoglobin (–·–) in a dead fetus during uterine contractions: **(a)** contraction or parallel pattern; **(b)** desaturation or divergent pattern). (From Hamilton et al. (58), reproduced with permission.)

Table 1. Potential advantages/disadvantages of transabdominal and transvaginal fetal optical monitoring

	Type of Optical Spectroscopy	
Facts	Transvaginal	Transabdominal
Obstetrical		
Antepartum	No	Yes
Intrapartum	Yes	Yes
Need for ruptured membranes	Yes	No
Need for cervical dilatation	Yes (2–3 cm or more)	No
Increased risk of maternal–fetal infection, and other complications (placental abruption, maternal or fetal injury, etc.)	Yes	No
Comfortable for patients	No	Yes
Technical		
Probe in direct contact with the fetal head	Yes	No
Overlying maternal and fetal tissues that light has to pass in order to reach fetal brain	Fetal cerebrospinal fluid, skull, and scalp	Fetal cerebrospinal fluid, skull, and scalp; amniotic fluid; placenta (sometimes); uterus; maternal abdominal wall
Type of probe	Monitoring type of probe (one light source and one light detector)	Imaging type of probe (several light sources and detectors)
Type of output clinical information	Cerebral blood volume and oxygenation: continuous or intermittent tracing	Cerebral blood volume and oxygenation: continuous or intermittent tracing + volume and oxygenation images
Incidence of artifacts related to the coupling of the probe and the fetal head	High[a]	N/A
Incidence of motional artifacts	High[a]	To be investigated

[a]Wyatt et al., London, UK, Personal communication.

change in oxygenation in a dead fetus" (i.e., both contraction and desaturation patterns) (Figure 6) (58). This could serve as an illustration of a motion artifact induced by movements of the fiber-optodes during uterine contractions that might have induced the false-positive changes in hemoglobin concentrations.

The sources of errors and potential misinterpretations associated with intrapartum fetal pulse oximetry may apply to fetal cerebral optical spectroscopy as well, particularly those related to the sensor-to-skin contact and motion artifacts. Increased source detector separation (e.g., 4 cm) and a flexible soft rubber probe placed through the cervix of the laboring woman and up against the fetal head to carry small fiber-optic cables transmitting and receiving near-infrared light appears to be very sensitive to contractions or any other source-of-motion artifacts. The possibility to resolve these problems might lead to improved designs of the existing optical instrumentation, as has been recently presented at the NIH Workshop on Near Infrared Spectroscopy in Bethesda, MD, in September 1997. Chance et al. (59) have proposed a totally different approach using a transabdominal optical probe with source detector separation of 10 cm and showed that transabdominal optical spectroscopy is feasible both antepartum and intrapartum. Table 1 summarizes potential advantages/disadvantages of both transvaginal and transabdominal optical spectroscopy. Future clinical trials that will be using improved transvaginal or transabdominal equipment are needed. Such studies will inevitably fuel further development and sophistication of optical spectroscopy, ultimately leading to better understanding of fetal cerebrovascular physiology (59).

FETAL PULSE OXIMETRY

Pulse oximetry uses a pulse-gated signal to measure changes in hemoglobin absorption in the pulsatile vascular bed. Tested for the first time in humans in 1975, pulse oximetry has been embraced by the medical community worldwide, becoming a standard of care during the 1980s in several medical disciplines such as anesthesiology, critical care medicine, and neonatal intensive care (27,60–62). The fetal intrapartum application has been a natural extension of conventional pulse oximetry, aiming to (a) become a useful adjunct to conventional FHR monitoring, (b) provide important and direct information on fetal oxygenation and peripheral perfusion (27,63), (c) improve the specificity of detecting fetal compromise (27), and (d) reassure obstetrical staff in cases of abnormal FHR by demonstrating an adequate fetal oxygenation (38,64). Over the past 10 years, the use of fetal pulse oximetry has been limited to experimental feasibility (62,65), validation (66), and correlation studies (fetal/neonatal acid–base status, FHR, or neonatal outcome) (38,67–70). Most recently, using Nellcor N-400 (wavelengths: red 660 nm and infrared 890–940 nm), a prospective multicenter observational study in 174 patients with abnormal intrapartum FHR tracings has been conducted to (a) correlate antepartum fetal pulse oximetry measurements from the last 30 min of monitoring with fetal oxygen saturation determined from scalp blood analysis and (b) correlate postpartum measurements with cord blood gases and outcome (64). The pulse oximetry reading was considered adequate in 134 cases. The diagnostic value and the ability of both fetal pulse oximetry and scalp blood analysis to correctly predict umbilical cord arterial pH ≤ 7.15 and "abnormal outcome" (i.e., any of the following: 5-min Apgar score ≤ 7, secondary respiratory distress, transfer to a neonatal care unit, arterial blood pH ≤ 7.15, or neonatal death) are presented in Tables 2–4. The conclusion was that the predictive value of pulse oximetry can be favorably compared with that of scalp blood analysis, with a remark that in the general population a low umbilical cord pH is a rare event; and when the event is rare, even a poorly effective diagnostic method can have a good negative predictive value (64). Alshimmiri et al. (71), using a Nellcor N-400 fetal monitor and FS-14 fetal oxygen sensor, conducted a study in 60 patients (54 met the criteria for data analysis) with either nonreassuring fetal heart rate pattern, intrauterine growth

Table 2. Value of fetal pulse oximetry and fetal blood analysis in predicting low umbilical artery blood pH at birth or abnormal neonatal outcome[a,b]

	Fetal Blood Analysis (cutoff pH ≤7.20) (n = 78)		Fetal Oxygen Saturation (cutoff 30%) (n = 134)	
Outcome Variable	Umbilical Arterial pH ≤7.15	Abnormal Neonatal Outcome	Umbilical Arterial pH ≤7.15	Abnormal Neonatal Outcome
PPV (%)	40 (10–70)	50 (22–78)	60 (30–90)	69 (44–94)
NPV (%)	89 (81–97)	83 (74–92)	88 (81–95)	83 (76–90)
Sensitivity (%)	40 (10–70)	35 (12–58)	40 (15–65)	32 (15–49)
Specificity (%)	89 (81–97)	90 (82–98)	94 (89–99)	96 (92–100)

[a]The thresholds used were 7.20 for scalp pH and 30% for fetal oxygen saturation. 95% Confidence intervals are indicated in parentheses. PPV, positive predictive value; NPV, negative predictive value.
[b]From reference 64, with permission.

Table 3. Compared values of fetal pulse oximetry and fetal blood analysis in paired measurements obtained simultaneously before birth for prediction of umbilical artery blood pH ≤7.15 at birth[a,b]

	Pairs of Values (n = 71)		
		Fetal Pulse Oximetry	
Outcome Variable	Fetal Blood Analysis (pH 7.20)	30%	40%
PPV (%)	44 (12–76)	43 (6–80)	27 (11–43)
NPV (%)	88 (79–97)	87 (78–96)	93 (84–100)
Sensitivity (%)	40 (10–70)	30 (2–58)	80 (55–100)
Specificity (%)	90 (82–98)	92 (84–100)	55 (41–69)

[a]Results are given at various cutoff values (30% and 40% for pulse oximetry). PPV, positive predictive value; NPV, negative predictive value.
[b]From reference 64, with permission.

Table 4. Compared values of pulse oximetry and fetal blood analysis in paired measurements obtained simultaneously before birth for prediction of abnormal neonatal outcome[a,b]

	Pairs of Values (n = 71)				
	Fetal Blood Analysis		Fetal Pulse Oximetry		
Outcome Variable	pH 7.20	pH 7.25	30%	35%	40%
PPV (%)	55 (26–84)	31 (16–46)	56 (24–88)	41 (32–51)	36 (20–52)
NPV (%)	82 (72–92)	80 (73–87)	81 (71–91)	82 (75–88)	89 (79–99)
Sensitivity (%)	35 (12–58)	47 (39–56)	29 (7–51)	41 (32–51)	76 (56–96)
Specificity (%)	91 (83–99)	67 (57–77)	93 (86–100)	82 (75–88)	57 (44–70)

[a]Results are given at various cutoff values (pH 7.20 to 7.25 for fetal blood analysis and 30% to 40% for pulse oximetry). PPV, positive predictive value; NPV, negative predictive value.
[b]From reference 64, with permission.

restriction, or thick meconium. Antepartum fetal pulse oximetry measurements from the last 30 min of monitoring were correlated with umbilical artery base excess and pH at birth at different saturation thresholds with use of receiver–operator characteristic curve calculations (Figures 7 and 8). The authors concluded that intrapartum fetal saturation (as monitored in their study) was of limited use as a diagnostic test for predicting acidosis at birth, regardless of the saturation cutoff value used (71).

There are several potential sources of technical and clinical error and possible misinterpretation in fetal pulse oximetry that we would like to emphasize: the accuracy of measurements, calibration, signal-to-noise ratio, optical shunting, motion artifacts, sensor-to-skin contact, and clinical relevance to cerebral physiology.

Conventional pulse oximeters, in general, have limited accuracy at low saturation (below 70%). This limitation does not affect the clinical utility of the system, because such conditions occur relatively rarely in adults and neonates (saturation is usually greater than 90% and rarely below 70%) and are always followed by some form of intervention (72). In the human fetus, normal umbilical venous oxygen saturation declines from 90% at midgestation to 70% or less, concomitantly with an increase in O_2 capacity as gestation progresses towards term (73–75), which raises the question regarding the accuracy of pulse oximetry in the low saturation range (70% to 30% and less). At high saturation the accuracy of pulse oximetry can be achieved with 660 nm (red) and 900 nm (infrared) light emitters (LED), while at low saturation 735 nm and 890 nm should provide better performance (72). The calibration of fetal pulse oximeters is also a problem, because animal models (including the fetal animal models) used to calibrate fetal pulse oximeters may present sources of their inaccuracy.

The signal-to-noise ratio in fetal pulse oximetry is much worse than in conventional pulse oximetry primarily because the amplitude of the fetal pulse signal is much smaller at the available probe application sites (scalp or face) (62).

Conventional pulse oximeters use the transillumination (transmission) probe where light source and detector are on the opposite side of the vascular bed (Figure 2). In the fetus there is a significant restriction in space and number of probe place-

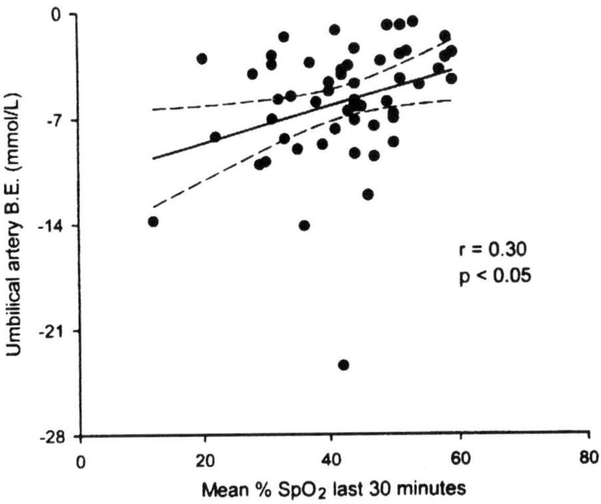

Figure 7. Relationship between umbilical artery base excess (B.E.) at birth and mean percent fetal saturation (SpO_2) for the last 30 min of monitoring. (From reference 71, reproduced with permission.)

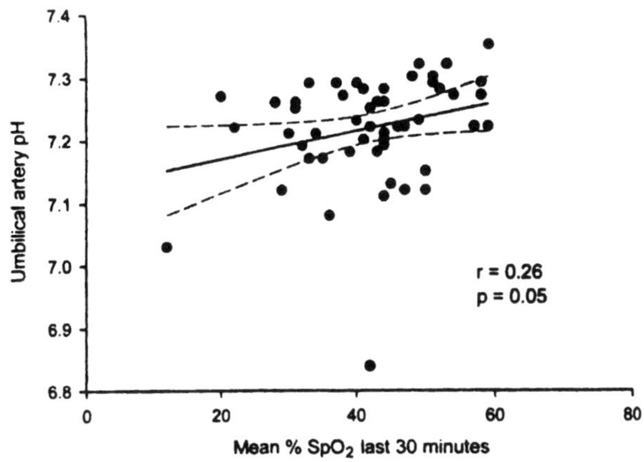

Figure 8. Relationship between umbilical artery pH at birth and mean percent fetal saturation (SpO_2) for the last 30 min of monitoring. (From reference 71, reproduced with permission.)

ment sites available (scalp or face). Therefore a special reflectance probe with light source and detector adjacent to one another had to be developed (Figure 2). Having a source and detector sitting on the same surface area close together may cause a potential error due to optical shunting (62,64,65).

Motion artifacts are a major problem of fetal pulse oximetry and challenge the development of fetal probes (62,66). Uterine contractions, maternal movements, or fetal movements can significantly affect the probe geometry (increase or decrease

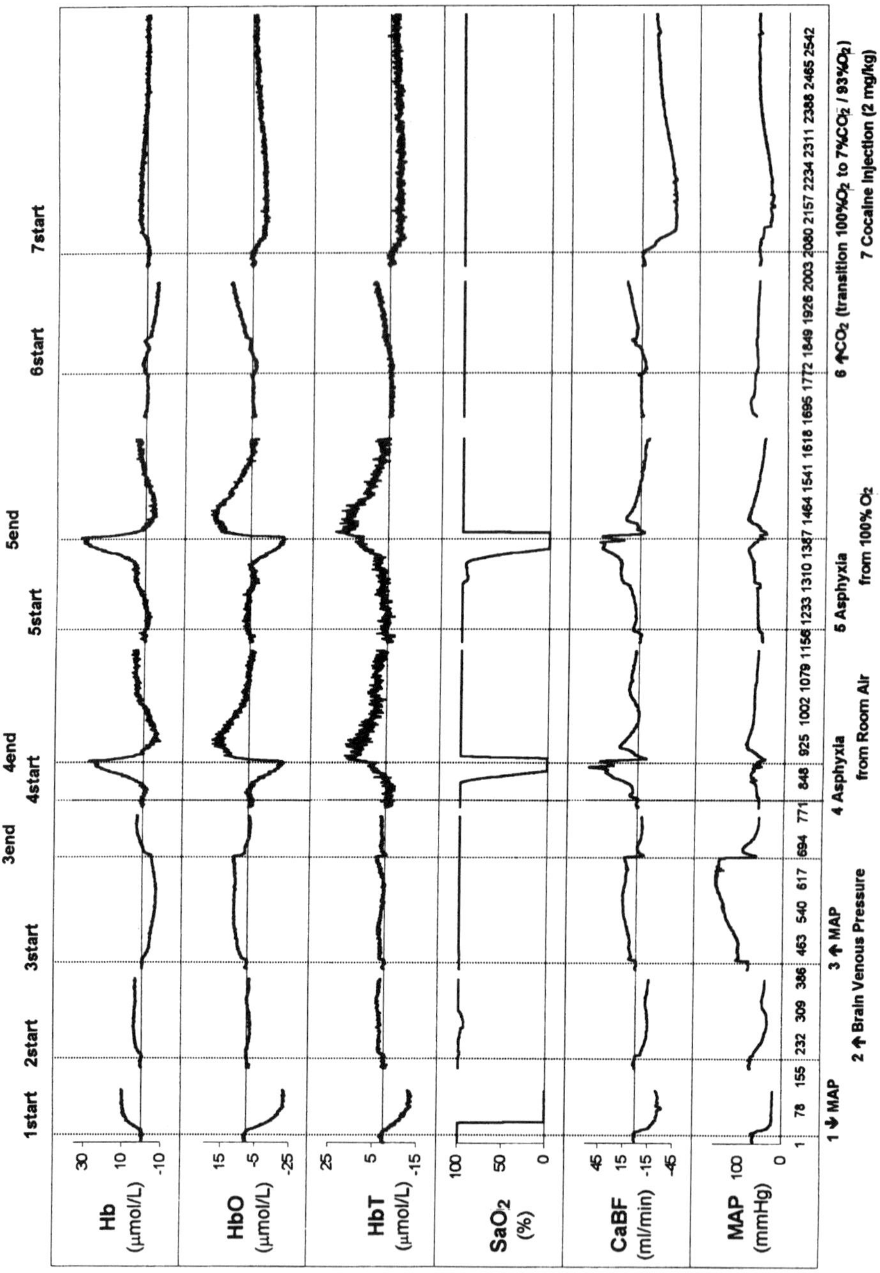

Figure 9. Continuous-wave optical spectroscopy readily detects changes in cerebral hemodynamics and oxygenation induced by variations in cerebral perfusion pressure and oxygenation in the newborn piglets (a total of 17 1- or 2-week-old piglets weighing 3.85 ± 0.84 kg, anesthetized and ventilated). Changes in cerebral and systemic hemodynamics and oxygenation during: (1) hemorrhage; (2) venous congestion; (3) hypertension; (4) asphyxia from room air; (5) asphyxia

the distance between the source and detector), inducing false-positive changes in hemoglobin concentration.

An inadequate sensor-to-skin contact, due to either (a) motion induced by contractions or maternal or fetal movements, (b) fetal skin folding, or (c) the presence of thick hair, caput succedaneum, vernix, or meconium, can cause probe lifting or detachment, optical shunting, and corruption of oxygen saturation measurements (27,62). In a study of 105 women, using a "double-clip design" probe, Gardosi and Symonds (62) could not obtain adequate readings in 44 cases (42%). The major sources of artifacts, they reported, were related to probe apposition and signal processing, and those cases were excluded. With the improved probe design, 134 (77%) out of 174 women had an adequate reading. However, frequently observed transient variations of fetal oxygen saturation have been "cured" by averaging the data over a 30-min period (64,70). This enables an average value for fetal oxygen saturation to be determined, but decreases the temporal resolution of pulse oximetry which is essential for clinical decision-making, as well as introducing the possibility of using motion artifacts as good data. To overcome the sensor-to-skin contact problems, several new probe designs have been applied: optical scalp electrodes (76), probes with balloon (62), and sensor tips (64) designed to move the optical components towards the fetal face. The latest Nellcor fetal probe includes a "sensor lifted feature" with three conductive contacts that serve to determine whether the source and detector are actually contacting tissue (64).

Finally, the bottom-line question regarding fetal pulse oximetry is, what is the relevance of peripheral (scalp or face) arterial oxygen saturation to cerebral oxygenation? The assumption that adequate peripheral saturation means adequate brain oxygenation might not be true. Indeed, using cerebral optical spectroscopy, it has been demonstrated in neonatal piglets that circumstances exist where cerebral hypoxia may develop in the presence of appropriate peripheral arterial and venous oxygen saturation (Figure 9) (35,36). To overcome this serious limitation of the fetal application of pulse oximetry, coupling of the two modalities (i.e., pulse oximetry and cerebral optical spectroscopy) in one application should be considered for the future (57).

FUTURE OF PERINATAL OPTICAL SPECTROSCOPY

Monitoring of cerebral hemodynamics and oxygenation should not be limited to the fetus only; it needs to be extended into the neonatal period when most of the brain injuries occur (6,13). The ultimate version of a fetal/neonatal optical monitor will allow

←

continued

from 100% O_2; (6) hypercarbia—transition from 100% O_2 to 7% CO_2 / 93% O_2; (7) cocaine injection (2 mg/kg). The *y* axes present optical Δ changes in optical variables [i.e., deoxyhemoglobin (Hb), oxyhemoglobin (HbO), and total Hb concentration (HbT)] as well as conventional variables [i.e., arterial oxygen saturation by pulse oximetry (SaO_2) (Nellcor, Hayward, CA), carotid blood flow by transit time Doppler technique (CaBF, change from baseline), and mean arterial pressure (MAP)]. The *x* axis presents time, where each data point equals 2 sec. Note the changes in cerebral hemodynamics and oxygenation (Hb, HbO, and HbT) despite normal peripheral oxygenation measured by pulse oximetry during venous congestion (2), hypertension (3), hypercarbia (6), and cocaine injection (7). (From reference 35 and 36, reproduced with permission.)

us to (1) continuously monitor fetal and neonatal cerebral hemodynamics and oxygenation, (2) assess the competence of cerebrovascular autoregulation important in the pathogenesis of brain hemorrhage, particularly in premature babies, (3) identify and monitor fetuses and neonates with incompetent cerebrovascular autoregulation that are at risk for brain injury, (4) detect ischemic or hemorrhagic injury itself, and (5) provide reassurance that labor and postpartum course are normal. The development of this type of instrumentation is even more urgent now, because new potentially neuroprotective agents are available for clinical testing; monitoring of their efficacy and side effects on fetal and neonatal cerebral perfusion and oxygenation will be important. The new era in fetal and neonatal management would be greatly advanced using the variety of modalities of optical spectroscopy which will allow continuous, noninvasive, and real-time monitoring and imaging of fetal and neonatal cerebral and peripheral hemodynamics, as well as the detection and clinical course of "hypoxic-hemodynamic" brain injury.

REFERENCES

1. Benaron DA, Stevenson DK. Tissue optics. *Science* 1997;276:2002–2003.
2. Nelson KB. Antecedents of cerebral palsy: multivariate analysis of risk. *N Engl J Med* 1986;315:81.
3. Volpe JJ. Intraventricular hemorrhage and brain injury in the premature infant. Neuropathology and pathogenesis. *Clin Perinatol* 1989;16:361–386.
4. Torfs CP, Oechsli FW, Cummins S. Prenatal and perinatal factors in the etiology of cerebral palsy (see comments). *J Pediatr* 1990;116:615–619.
5. Lou HC. Hypoxic-hemodynamic pathogenesis of brain lesions in the newborn. *Brain Dev* 1994;16(6):423–431.
6. Low JA, Intrapartum fetal asphyxia, definition, diagnosis and classification. *Am J Obstet Gynecol* 1997;176:957–959.
7. Horbar JD, Adler SM, et al. Variability in 28-day outcome for very low birth weight infants: an analysis of 11 neonatal intensive care units. *Pediatrics* 1988;82:554–559.
8. Calame A, Claeys V, Arazola L, Ducret S, Jaunin L. Neurodevelopmental outcome and school performance of very-low-birth-weight infants at 8 years of age. *Eur J Pediatr* 1986;145:461–466.
9. Kurth CD, Benaron D, Chance B. Near-infrared monitoring of cerebral circulation. *J Clin Monit* 1993;9:163–170.
10. Wahr JA, Samra S, Delpy DT. Near-infrared spectroscopy: theory and applications. *J Cardiothorac Vasc Anesth* 1996;3:406–418.
11. Hirtz DG. Report of the National Institute of Neurological Disorders and Stroke workshop on near infrared spectroscopy. *Pediatrics* 1993;91:414–417.
12. Volpe JJ. Hypoxic-ischemic encephalopathy: intrauterine assosment. In Volpe JJ (ed). *Neurology of the newborn,* V. Philadelphia: WB Saunders, 1995:266.
13. Low JA, Simpson LL, Temporal relationship of neuropathologic conditions caused by perinatal asphyxia. *Am J Obstet Gynecol* 1989;160:608.

14. Nelson KB. Can magnesium sulfate reduce the risk of cerebral palsy in very-low-birth-weight infants? *Pediatrics* 1995;95:263.

15. NIH. *Consensus Development Conference on the effects of corticosteroids for fetal maturation on perinatal outcomes.* Consensus Development Conference statement, Bethesda, MD, 1994.

16. Parilla BV, Cohen LS, Clark E. Lack of effect of antenatal indomethacin on fetal cerebral blood flow. *Am J Obstet Gynecol* 1997;176:1166–1171.

17. Cunningham FG, Gant NF, Leveno KJ, Gilstrap LC, Hankins GDV, Clark SL. Diseases and injuries of the fetus and newborn (fetal abnormalities: inheritied and acquired disorders). In Cunningham FG, Gant NF, Leveno KJ, Gilstrap LC, Hankins GDV, Clark SL (eds). *Williams obstetrics,* Stamford, CT: Appleton & Lange, 1997:974.

18. Hammacher K, Bokelman J, Werners PH. Foetal heart frequency and perinatal condition of the foetus and newborn. *Gynaecologia* 1968;166:349.

19. Devoe LD, Sherline DM. The nonstress test as a diagnostic test: a critical reapraisal. *Am J Obstet Gynecol* 1986;152:1047.

20. Manning FA, Harman CR, Nicolaides K, Menticologlou S, Morrison I. Fetal biophysical profile score, 6. Correlation with antepartum umbilical venous fetal pH. *Am J Obstet Gynecol* 1993;169:755.

21. Nelson KB, Ting TY, Grether JK. Uncertain value of electronic fetal monitoring in predicting cerebral palsy. *N Engl J Med* 1996;334(613–618).

22. Ellison PH, et al. Electronic fetal heart monitoring, auscultation, and neonatal outcome. *Am J Obstet Gynecol* 1991;164:1281–1289.

23. Clark SL. Intrapartum fetal surveillance: the role of fetal scalp blood sampling. *Am J Obstet Gynecol* 1985;153:717–720.

24. Small ML, Platt LD, Dirks D, Hochberg H. Continuous tissue pH monitoring in the term fetus. *Am J Obstet Gynecol* 1989;161:323–329.

25. Aarnoudse JG, Gordon H, Oesburg B, Zijlstra WG. Fetal subcutaneous scalp PO_2 and abnormal hear rate during labor. *Am J Obstet Gynecol* 1985;153:565–566.

26. Bergmans MGM, Weber T, Nickelsen C, Schmidt S, van den Berg PP. Fetal transcutaneous PCO_2 measuremens during labor. *Eur J Obstet Gynecol* 1993;51:1–7.

27. Dildy GA, Loucks CA. Intrapartum fetal pulse oximetry: past, present, and future. *Am J Obstet Gynecol* 1996;175:1–9.

28. Benaron DA, Spilman S, Van Houten JP, Stevenson DK. Tomographic time-of-flight optical imaging device. *Adv Exp Med Biol* 1994;361:609–617.

29. Chance B, He L, Weng J, Sevick, E. Highly sensitive object location in tissue models with linear in-phase and anti-phase multi-element optical arrays in one and two dimensions. *Proc Natl Acad Sci USA* 1993;90:3423–3427.

30. Jobsis FF. Noninvasive infrared monitoring of cerebral and myocardial sufficiency and circulatory parameters. *Science* 1977;198:1264–1267.

31. Cope M. System for long-term measurement of cerebral blood flow and tissue oxygenation on newborn infants by infra-red transillumination. *Med Biol Eng Comput* 1988;26:289–294.

32. Wray S, Delpu DT. Characteristics of the near infrared absorption spectra of cytochrome aa3 and hemoglobin for the noninvasive monitoring of cerebral oxygenation. *Biochim Biophys Acta* 1988;933:184–192.

33. Peebles DM, Wyatt JS, Cope M, Delpy DT, Reynolds EOR. Changes in human fetal cerebral hemoglobin concentration and oxygenation during labor measured by near-infrared spectroscopy. *Am J Obstet Gynecol* 1992;166:1369–1373.
34. Peebles DM, Edwards AD, Wyatt JS, Reynolds EOR, Cope M, Delpy DT. Relation between frequency of uterine contractions and human fetal cerebral oxygen saturation studied during labour by near-infrared spectroscopy. *Br J Obstet Gynaecol* 1994;101:44–48.
35. Stankovic MR, Fujii A, Boas D, Stubblefield PG. Monitoring of cerebral hemodynamics and oxygenation by optical spectroscopy following acute cocaine exposure in the newborn piglet. ACOG District I Junior Fellow Annual Fall Meeting, Williamstown MA, 1997.
36. Stankovic MR, Fujii A, Maulik D, Boas D, Kirby D, Stubblefield PG. Optical monitoring of cerebral hemodynamics and oxygenation in the neonatal piglet. *J Matern Fetal Invest* 1998;8:71–78.
37. Brazy JE. Cerebral oxygen monitoring with near infrared spectroscopy: Clinical application to neonates. *J Clin Monit* 1991;7:325–334.
38. Saling E. Fetal pulse oximetry during labor: issues and recommendations for clinical use. *J Perinat Med* 1996;24:467–478.
39. Brazy JE, Mitnick MH, et al. Noninvasive monitoring of cerebral oxygenation in preterm infants: preliminary observations. *Pediatrics* 1985;75:217–225.
40. Brown R, Royston D. A comparison of two systems for assessing cerebral venous oxyhemoglobin saturation during cardiopulmonary bypass in humans. *Anaesthesia* 1993;48:691–700.
41. Delpy DT, van der Zee P, et al. Estimation of optical pathlength through tissue from direct time of flight measurement. *Phys Med Biol* 1988;33:1433–1442.
42. Benaron DA, Ariagno RA, Stevenson DK. Noninvasive methods for estimating in vivo oxigenation. *Clin Pediatr* 1992;31:258–273.
43. Benaron DA, Stevenson DK. 2D and 3D images of thick tissue using time constrained times of flight and absorbance spectrometry. *Proc SPIE* 1992;1641:35–45.
44. Chance B, Zhuang Z, Chu UA, Alter C, Lipton L. Cognition activated low frequency modulation of light absorption in human brain. *Proc Natl Acad Sci USA* 1993;90:2660–2774.
45. Chance B. Comparison of time-resolved and unresolved measurements of deoxyhemoglobin in brain. *Proc Natl Acad Sci USA* 1988;85:4971–4975.
46. Brazy JE. Changes in cerebral blood volume and cytochrome AA3 during hypertensive peaks in preterm infants. *J Pediatr* 1986;108:983–987.
47. Brazy JE. Effects of crying on cerebral blood volume and cytochrome aa3. *J Pediatr* 1988;112:457–461.
48. Germon TJ, Manara AR, Nelson RJ. Near-infrared spectroscopy in adults: effects of extracranial ischemia and intracranial hypoxia on estimation of cerebral oxygenation. *Br J Anaesth* 1994;73:503–506.
49. Pollard V, DeMelo E, Deyo DJ, Uchida T, Widman R. The influence of carbon dioxide and body position on near-infrared spectroscopic assessment of cerebral hemoglobin oxygen saturation. *Anesth Analg* 1996;82:278–287.
50. Aldrich CJ, Spencer JAD, Wyatt JS, Peebles DM, Delpy DT, Reynolds EOR. Fetal cerebral oxygenation measured by near-infrared spectroscopy shortly before birth and acid–base status at birth. *Obstet Gynecol* 1994;84:861–866.
51. Aldrich CJ, Spencer JAD, Reynolds EOR, Delpy DT. The effect of maternal oxygen administration on human fetal cerebral oxygenation measured during labour by near infrared spectroscopy. *Br J Obstet Gynaecol* 1994;101:509–513.

52. Aldrich CJ, Spencer JAD, Wyatt JS, Peebles DM, Delpy DT, Reynolds EOR. Late fetal heart rate decelerations and changes in cerebral oxygenation during the first stage of labour. *Br J Obstet Gynaecol* 1995;102:9–13.

53. Aldrich CJ, Spencer JAD, Wyatt JS, Peebles DM, Delpy DT, Reynolds EOR. The effect of maternal posture on fetal cerebral oxygenation during labour. *Br J Obstet Gynaecol* 1995;102:14–19.

54. Aldrich CJ, Spencer JAD, Delpy DT, Reynolds EOR, Wyatt JS. Fetal heart rate changes and cerebral oxygenation measured by near infrared spectroscopy during the first stage of labour. *Obstet Gynecol Reprod Biol* 1996;64:189–195.

55. Wickramasinghe YABD, Houston R, Spenser SA, Rolfe P, Thorniley MS, Oeseburg B, Colier W. Effect of fetal hemoglobin on determination of neonatal oxygenation by near-infrared spectroscopy. *Pediatr Res* 1993;34:15–17.

56. Schmidt S, Eilers H, Helledie N, Krebs D. Laser spectrophotometry in the fetus. *J Perinat Med* 1989;17:57–62.

57. Seelbach-Gobel B. Correlation between NIR spectroscopy and pulse oximetry in the fetus. *J Perinat Med* 1996;24:69–75.

58. Hamilton RJ, Wickramasinghe ABD, Rolfe P. Intrapartum fetal cerebral near infrared spectroscopy: apparent change in oxygenation demonstrated in a nonviable fetus. *Br J Obstet Gynaecol* 1995;102:1004–1007.

59. Chance B, et al. Transabdominal fetal optical spectroscopy. NINDS and NICHD Workshop on Near Infrared Spectroscopy in Infants and Children, National Institutes of Health, Bethesda, MD, 1997.

60. Severinghaus JW. History of blood gas analysis. VI. Oximetry. *J Clin Monit* 1986;2: 270–288.

61. Severinghaus JW. History of blood gas analysis. VII. Pulse oximetry. *J Clin Monit* 1987;3: 135–138.

62. Gardosi JO, Symonds EM. Adaptation of pulse oximetry for fetal monitoring during labour. *Lancet* 1991;337:1265–1267.

63. Johnson N, Bannister J, Lilford RJ. Measurement of fetal peripheral perfusion with a pulse oximeter [Letter]). *Lancet* 1989;1:898.

64. Carbonne B, Goffinet F, et al. Multicenter study on the clinical value of fetal pulse oximetry. *Am J Obstet Gynecol* 1997;177:593–598.

65. Dildy GA, Loucks CA. Preliminary experience with intrapartum fetal pulse oximetry in humans. *Obstet Gynecol* 1993;81:630–635.

66. East CE, Dunster KR, Khoo SK. Human fetal intrapartum oxygen saturation monitoring: agreement between readings from two sensors on the same fetus. *Am J Obstet Gynecol* 1996;174:1594–1598.

67. Carbonne B, Segard L, Sebban E, Cabrol D, Papiernik E. Fetal pulse oximetry: correlation between changes in oxygen saturation and neonatal outcome. *Eur J Obstet Gynecol Reprod Biol* 1994;57:73–77.

68. Langer B, Haddad J, Pain L, Schlaeder G. Fetal pulse oximetry during labor of 62 patients. *Fetal Diagn Ther* 1996;11:37–45.

69. Dildy GA, Katz M, Clark SL, Jongsma HW, Nijhuis JG, et al. Intrapartum fetal pulse oximetry: fetal oxygen saturation trends during labor and relation to delivery outcome. *Am J Obstet Gynecol* 1994;171:179–184.

70. Seelbach-Gobel B, Kuhnert M, Heupel M. Fetal reflectance pulse oximetry sub partu: experiences, prognostic significance, and consequences and goals. *Z geburtshilfe Perinatol* 1994;198:67–71.

71. Alshimmiri M, Gagnon R, Natale R, Richardson BS. Prediction of umbilical artery base excess by intrapartum fetal oxygen saturation monitoring. *Am J Obstet Gynecol* 1997;177:775–779.

72. Mannheimer PD, Fein ME, Nielrlich SL. Wavelength selection for low-saturation pulse oximetry. *IEEE Trans Biomed Eng* 1997;44(3):148–156.

73. Bozzeti P, Cetin I, et. al. Respiratory gasses, acid–base balance and lactate concentrations of the midterm human fetus. *Biol Neonate* 1987;51:188.

74. Soothill P, Rodeck CH, et al. Effects of gestational age on fetal and intervillous blood gas and acid–base values in human pregnancy. *Fetal Therapy* 1986;1:168.

75. Battaglia FC. *An introduction to fetal physiology.* New York: Academic Press, 1986.

76. Buchamann J, Knitza R. Fetal oxygen saturation measurement by transmission pulse oximetry [Letter]). *Lancet* 1992;1:615.

INDEX